MEDICAL MYCOLOGY
AND
HUMAN MYCOSES

EVERETT SMITH BENEKE, PH.D.
PROFESSOR EMERITUS
MICHIGAN STATE UNIVERSITY

ALVIN LEE ROGERS, PH.D.
PROFESSOR EMERITUS
MICHIGAN STATE UNIVERSITY

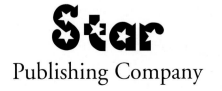

Publishing Company

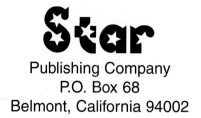

Star

Publishing Company
P.O. Box 68
Belmont, California 94002

Printed in Korea

0 9 8 7 6 5 4 3 2 1

Contents

Acknowledgments vii
Preface ix

Chapter One
CHARACTERISTICS OF FUNGI 1

Reproduction 1
Classification 3
Selected References 4

Chapter Two
COMMON CONTAMINANT FUNGI 5

Laboratory Procedures for Study of Contaminant Fungi 5
Laboratory Exercise for Study of Airborne and Soilborne Fungi 7
Representative Common Saprophytic Fungi 7

Rhizopus spp.	8	*Verticillium* spp.	17
Mucor spp	8	*Alternaria* spp.	17
Syncephalastrum spp.	9	*Aureobasidium* spp.	18
Acremonium spp.	10	*Cladosporium* spp.	18
Aspergillus spp.	10	*Curvularia* spp.	19
Botrytis spp.	11	*Drechslera* spp.	20
Fusarium spp.	12	*Epicoccum* spp.	20
Geotricum spp.	12	*Nigrospora* spp.	21
Gliocladium spp.	13	*Ulocladium* spp.	21
Paecilomyces spp.	14	*Rhodotorula* spp.	22
Penicillium spp.	14	*Saccharomyces* spp.	22
Scopulariopsis spp.	15	*Phoma* spp.	23
Sepdonium spp.	16	*Chaetomium* spp.	23
Tricoderma spp.	16	*Streptomyces* spp.	24

Chapter Three
LABORATORY PROCEDURES 27

Equipment 27
Selection and Preparation of Specimens . . . 27
Mailing of Specimens 29
Cultivation of Fungi 29
Examination of Cultures 32
Mounting Media, Stains, and
Staining Methods 32
Media 36
Serologic Techniques 45
Exoantigens 45
DNA Probe 45

In Vitro Antifungal Susceptibility Tests 46
Animal Inoculations 47
Maintenance of Stock Cultures of Fungi . . . 48

Chapter Four
SUPERFICIAL MYCOSES 51

Otomycosis 51
Piedra 52
Petyriasis Versicolor 54
Trichomycosis Axillaris 56
Tinea Nigra 56

Chapter Five
DERMATOPHYTOSES 59

Classification 59
Mycologic Classification of Dermatophytes . 59
Dermatophytoses 60
Perfect or Teleomorph States 66
Suggestions for Laboratory Study
  of Dermatophytes 68
Laboratory Diagnosis 70
Microsporum spp. 73
Epidermophyton spp. 82
Trichophyton spp. 84
Dermatomycoses 96

Chapter Six
SUBCUTANEOUS MYCOSES 99

Mycetoma 99
Clinical Specimens 100
Chromoblastomycosis 106
Sporotrichosis 110
Lobomycosis 114
Rhinosporidiosis 114
Phaeohyphomycosis 116

Chapter Seven
TRUE SYSTEMIC MYCOSES 127

Introduction To Systemic Mycoses 127
True Pathogenic Fungi 128
Blastomycosis 128
Paracoccidioidomycosis 133
Lobomycosis 135
Coccidioidomycosis 136
Histoplasmosis 141
African Histoplasmosis 145

Chapter Eight
OPPORTUNISTIC INFECTIONS—YEASTS 149

Yeasts of Medical Importance 149
Candidasis 151
Torulopsosis 160
Cryptococcosis 161
Miscellaneous Yeast Infections 167
    Malessizia 167
    Trichosporonosis 167
    Rhodotorula 168
    Saccharomyces 168
    Prototbecosis (hyaline algae) 168
    Other Yeasts 169

Chapter Nine
OPPORTUNISTIC INFECTIONS—MYCELIAL FUNGI 171

Aspergillosis 171
Hyalohyphomycosis 178
    Acremonium 179
    Beauveria 179
    Fusarium 180
    Paecilomyces 184
    Penicillium 184
    Scopulariopsis 185
    Miscellaneous Hyaline Hyphonycetes 186
    Amxiopsis 186
    Arthrographsis 186
    Chaetoconidium (Oidiodendron) 186
    Chrysosporium 186
    Coniothyrum 186
    Microascus 186
    Myriodontium 186
    Neurospora 186
    Phialenenium 186
    Scytalidium 186
    Thermomyces 186
    Trichoderma 186
Pseudallescheriasis 187
Zygomycosis 189
    Rhizopus 191
    Cunninghamella 192
    Saksenaea 192
    Absidia 193
    Apophysomyces 193
    Cokeromyces 193
    Mortierella 194
    Mucor 194
    Rhizomucor 195
    Syncephalastrum 195
    Basidiobolus 195
    Conidiobolus 196

Miscellaneous Fungal Infections
Adiaspiromycosis 198
Basidiomycosis 199
Geotrichosis 200
Keratomycocis 201
Penicilliosis 203
Pythiosis insidiosi 204

Chapter Ten
ACTINOMYCETES 207

Actinomyocis 207
Nocardiosis 214
Agents of Actinomycotic Mycetoma 217
Dermatophilosis 220

Sources of Media, Cultures, Equipment, Visual Aids, and kits.
Fungal Cultures   223
Immunodiagnostics, Kits, and Serological Tests   223
Media (prepared and dried)   223
DNA Probe Systems   224
Supplies for the Laboratory   224
Visual Aids   224
Color Slides   225
Glossary   227
Index   231

Acknowledgments

The authors are most grateful to Mr. William Dallinger, Production Manager, The Upjohn Co., 7000 Portage Road, Kalamazoo, MI 49001 for transfer of all the color plates in the 8th Edition of *Human Mycoses,* a Scope Publication by Beneke, Rogers, and Rippon to the Star Publishing Company for use in the new Edition: *Medical Mycology and Human Mycoses.* We also would like to express our appreciation to June Hillelson, D.O. for reading portions of the manuscript and to thank Ellen Pzepka, Medical Technology Program, Michigan State University, for computer services. We have used many color illustrations from the 4th Edition of the *Medical Mycology Manual with Human Mycoses Monograph* and the 8th Edition of *Human Mycoses* in addition numerous new color illustrations.

For illustrations in *Medical Mycology and Human Mycoses* we wish to acknowledge our appreciation to the following colleagues for permission to use the illustrations listed below:

Dennis E. Babel, Ph.D., Assistant Professor, Medical Mycology, Michigan State University, East Lansing, MI: Figures 46, 47, 51, 60, 65, 66, 67, 73, 75.

Beneke, E. S. Ph.D., and A. L. Rogers, Ph.D.: Figures 1, 2, 3, 4, 5a, 5b, 6a, 6b, 7a, 7b, 8a, 8b, 9a, 9b, 10a, 10b, 11a, 11b, 12a, 12b, 13a, 13b, 14a, 14b, 15a, 16a, 16b, 17a, 17b, 18a, 18b, 19a, 19b, 20a, 20b, 21a, 21b, 22a, 22b, 23a, 23b, 24a, 24b, 25a, 26b, 27a, 27b, 28a, 28b, 29a, 29b, 30a, 30b, 31a, 31b, 32a, 32b, 34, 35, 36, 37, 38, 39, 40, 41a, 41b, 55, 58, 76, 77, 78, 79, 80, 81, 82, 83, 84, 85, 86, 87, 88, 89a 89b, 93, 94, 95, 96, 97, 99, 100, 101, 102, 103, 104, 105, 106, 107, 108, 109, 110, 111, 112, 113, 114a, 114b, 115, 116, 117, 118, 122, 123, 124, 125, 126b, 127, 128, 129, 130, 131, 132, 133, 134, 135, 136, 137, 138, 139, 140, 141, 142, 143, 145, 146, 147, 148, 162, 165, 166, 168, 171, 172a, 172b, 176, 178, 183, 185, 187, 188, 193, 196, 199, 210, 212, 213, 214, 215, 216, 231, 232, 233a, 233b, 234a, 234b, 235, 236, 237, 239,240, 241, 242, 243, 247, 250, 251, 259, 260, 261, 262, 263, 264, 265, 267, 268, 269, 270, 271, 272, 273, 274.

C. Booth, Ph.D., International Mycological.Institute, Ferry Lane, Kew, Surrey TW9 3AF, United Kingdom: Figures 224, 226b, 228.

Patrick Bourke, St. Clair County Community College, Port Huron, MI: Figures 5c, 6c, 7c, 8c, 9c, 11c, 12c, 13c, 14c, 15c, 16c, 18c, 20c, 21c, 22c, 24c, 26c, 28c, 32c.

G. W. Bulmer, Ph.D., Department of Laboratory Medicine, University of Santo Tomas School of Medicine & Surgery, Manila, Philippines: Figures 144, 164, 218.

Frank Dazzo, Professor, Department of Microbiology, Michigan State University for taking of the following photographs: Figures 224, 226b, 227.

Deng, Z., et al. China. Figures 283A & B *(Penicillium marneffei.* A. SEM showing conidiophores produced in a colony grown at 25C. B. Early stages of conversion from mycelial to yeast form. From Deng, Z., et al. 1988. Infection caused by *Penicillium marneffei* in China and Southeast Asia: review of 18 published cases and report of four more Chinese cases. Rev. Infect. Dis. 10:640-652.

Richard Edelman, Ph.D., Department of Anatomy & Cell Biology, Marshall University, Huntington, WV for the scanning electron micrographs: Figures 1b, 7d, 8d, 9d, 11d, 12, 13d, 15d, 16d, 21d, 22d, 24d, 26d, 28d.

Hans Einstein, M.D., Clinical Professor of Medicine, UCLA School of Medicine, Los Angeles, CA: Figure 175.

Michael F. Furcolow, M.D., and Norman Goodman, Ph.D., Department of Community Medicine, University of Kentucky, Lexington, KY: Figures 181, 201, 208, 258.

Donald Greer, Ph.D., Department of Dermatology, Louisiana State University Medical Center, New Orleans, LA.: Figure 170.

Jacques Hochglaube, M.D., 1090 Abbott Road, East Lansing, MI: Figures 68 and 69.

Mary E. Hopper, Cornell Medical School, New York, NY:
Figures 42, 43, 44, 48, 50, 52, 53, 54, 56, 57, 59, 61, 64, 70, 71, 72.

Duane Hospenthal, M.D., Ph.D., Walter Reed Army Medical Center, Washington, DC: Figure 206.

Instructional Media Center, Michigan State University, E. Lansing, MI: Figure 86.

Michael Kolotila, Ph.D., Northern Essex Community College, Haverhill, MA for photography:
Figures 30a, 92, 115, 120, 121, 133a, 133b, 195, 197.

National Centers for Disease Control, Atlanta, GA: Figure 38.

Michael G. Rinaldi, Ph.D., Chief, Clinical Microbiology Laboratories, Audie L. Murphy Memorial Veterans' Hospital, San Antonio, TX for the color photographs:
Figures 254, 256.

John W. Rippon, Ph.D., Professor of Medicine, The University of Chicago, Chicago, IL:
Figures 33, 98, 149, 163, 169, 173, 174, 177, 180, 182, 184, 200, 202, 203, 209, 259, 264. New photographs for Figures 221, 222.

Thomas Turner, Cytologist BPA, New Jersey College of Medicine and Dentistry, New Brunswick, NJ:
Figure 130.

W. A. Shipton, D.V.M., James Cook University, Townsville, Queensland, Australia for the photograph:
Figure 255.

A. P. Ulbrich, D.O., Professor of Dermatology, Michigan State University, E. Lansing, MI:
Figures 45, 70, 72, 74, 189, 190, 191, 192.

Harold Van Velsor, M.D., Wilmington, N. Carolina:
Figures 62, 63.

Janes Veselenak, Ph.D., Sangamon State University, Springfield, IL:
Figures 119, 126a, 150, 207.

The illustrations listed below were used with the permission of the authors and the publishers in the following medical mycology books:

Kwon-Chung, KJ, Bennett, J.E. 1992. Medical Mycology. Williams & Wilkins (Lea & Febiger), Malvern, PA.

Table 20 (Fig. 20.13. Differential characteristics of the families of Mucorales that include pathogenic species); Figures 152 (Fig. 23.34. *Curvularia* spp. A. *C. lunata,* X850); 153 (Fig. 23.35. *Dactylaria gallopava.* A and B. Conidiogenous cells and conidia, X1430 and X1800); 154 (Fig. 23.23. *Exophiala dermatitidis.* D. Branched conidial structures and conidial balls, X850, and E. Conidiogenous cells on the sides and tips of hyphae, X680); 155 (Fig. 23.21. *Exophiala jeanselmei.* C. Majority of cells are yeast-like with annellides); 156 (Fig. 23.21. D. Conidial balls on side of hyphae,X1360); 157 (Fig. 23.21. E. A branched conidiophore, X1360, and F. Annellidic conidiogenous cell with conidia, X1062); 158 (Fig. 23.26. *Exserohilum rostratum.* A. Clavate, young conidia showing no dark septa at the end cells, X585); 159 (Fig. 23.26. *E. rostratum.* B. A long cylindrical conidium shows dark septa at the end cells, X585); 160 (Fig. 23.29. *Phialophora parasitica.* B. Finely roughened branched phialide with phialoconidium at the tip, X650: and C. Percurrently proliferating phialides, X650); 161 (Fig. 23.28. *Phialophora richardsiae.* C. and D. Phialides and two types of phialoconidia. Phialides with saucer-shaped collarette produce thick-walled globose conidia (dark arrow). Phialides with collarette produce elongated, sausage-shaped conidia, X1275); 217 (Fig. 11.22. Key to the tentative identification of *Aspergillus* spp. isolated from clinical specimens. From Rhodes, J. C., and Kwon-Chung, K. J. *In Medical Mycology.* Edited by Evans, E.G.V, et al. I.R.L. Press, New York, NY.). 229 (Fig. 24.9. *Scedosporium prolificans.* B and C. Conidiogenous cells showing inflated bottoms and tapering tips with annellation and terminal conidia, X759; and D. Sympodial conidia, X850); 230 (Fig. 24.4. Histopathologic features of sinusitis caused by *Pseudoallescheria boydii.* A. Hyphae with intercalary swellings GMS,X800); 245 (Fig 246 (Fig. 27.1. C. Two attached adiaspores surrounded by multinucleated giant cells caused by *Emmonsia crescens,* X160); 253 (Fig. 27.15. *Penicillium marneffei.* A. SEM showing conidiophores produced in a colony grown at 25 C. B. Early stages of conversion from mycelial to yeast form. From Deng. Z., et al: Infection caused by *Penicillium marneffei* in China and Southeast Asia. Rev. Infect. Dis. 10., 10:640. 1988).

Rippon, J.W. 1988. *Medical Mycology. The Pathogenic Fungi and the Pathogenic Actinomycetes.* Third Edition. W.B. Saunders Co, Philadelphia, PA.: Figures 151 (Fig 110-16. *Bipolaris Drechslera, and Exserohilum.* Complete plate, page 318; 179 (Fig 17-22. Coccidioidomycosis. Variation in morphology, texture, and color of isolants of *Coccidioides immitis;* 211 (Fig 23-22. Conidiophores of uniseriate and biseriate aspergilli); 238 (Fig 23-22. *Apophysomyces elegans.* B. Mature sporangium of *A. elegans* with sporangiospores and a clearly depicted apophysis); 244 (Fig 25-24. A. Zygospores of *Basidiobolus ranarum;* 245 (Fig 25-24. B. Conidia of *Conidiobolus coronatus* with basal papilla); 247 (Fig 26-3. D. Clamp connections on a hypha; 248 (Fig 26-3. F. Culture of *Schizophyllum commune.* Table ll (Modified from McGinnis, M.R., M. C. Rinaldi, and R. E. Winn. 1986. J. Clin. Microbiol. 106. Table: Chief characteristics of *Bipolaris, Drechslera, and Exserohillum*); Table 12 (Table 14-1 The Systemic Mycoses).

Rogers, A. L. and Kennedy, M. J. Table 17 (Table 2: Characteristics of a representative species of some *Aspergillus* groups grown on Czapek-Dox agar. From: *Manual of Clinical Microbiology.* Fifth Ed. American Society of Microbiology. Washington, D. C. Chapter 63, page 662. Part of Table used).

In the last few years very significant changes have occurred in the field of medical mycology. Organisms not previously causative agents of human infections have now emerged as opportunistic pathogens in greatly increase numbers. These fungi have become serious pathogens in debilitated and immunocompromised hosts as a result of steroid and chemotherapy treatments, organ transplants, hyperalimentation, AIDS, and other macrodisruptive procedures and immune diseases. Many of thee opportunistic fungi are grouped into two new disease types, phaeohyphomycosis and hyaloyhyphomycosis. The two groups are discussed in separate chapters as these organisms are among commonly encountered mycotic infections in patients. These fungi are most remarkable for their ability to adapt to many environmental conditions, thus their invasion in debilitated patients is not surprising.

MEDICAL MYCOLOGY AND HUMAN MYCOSES has a large number of color photographs in related areas throughout the ten chapters. This will aid the laboratory personnel in the recognition of the disease systems appearance of the colony, fungal characteristics in tissue, and microscopic characteristics of the fungi in culture. Additional information includes: (1) new culture media, (2) DNA probes for some of the systemic mycoses, (3) serology, (4) extensive tables and flowcharts to facilitate preliminary determination of fungal specimens in the laboratory, (5) sources of media, cultures, equipment, and instructional aids.

The last chapter incorporates information on pathogenic actinomycetes (actinomycosis and nocardiosis). Although actinomycetes are bacteria, they continue to be sent to mycologists for isolation and identification probably because they are filamentous, some with branching and the production of bacillary, coccoid or conidial-like reproductive forms.

This medical mycology manual is especially useful in the clinical laboratory and for teaching medical mycology courses. It is a valuable reference for medical and veterinary students, practicing clinicians, medical technologists, and clinical microbiologists.

Everett S. Beneke, Ph.D., HCLD
Alvin L. Rogers, Ph.D., HCLD

Chapter 1

CHARACTERISTICS OF FUNGI

To be acquainted with some of the many thousands of fungi in the world, one needs to know the systematic arrangement of these organisms. Identification of fungi is made easier if one is familiar with basic terminology, the major classification system, and a few representative organisms. Acquaintance with some of the contaminant and pathogenic fungi also leads to better understanding of the behavior of fungi that become pathogenic in humans or other animals.

Fungi are eukaryotic, distinctly different from bacteria. The main parameters of difference are: (1) size, (2) wall composition and structure, (3) arrangement of nuclear material, (4) presence or absence of mitochondria and endoplasmic reticulum, and (5) response to antibiotics. Many fungi have tubular somatic or vegetative structures. These branching tubes or threads contain numerous nuclei distributed throughout and are known as **hyphae** (a single thread is a **hypha**). Hyphae that have cross-walls or septa with openings or perforations are called **septate hyphae.** Hyphae without regularly occurring septa are designated aseptate (or coenocytic). A large, intertwined mass of hyphae is known as **mycelium.** The terms "hyphae" and "mycelium" may be used interchangeably. An example of an organism with aseptate hyphae is *Rhizopus* spp. Many organisms have septate hyphae, viz., *Penicillium* spp.

The commonly used term "molds" refers to the filamentous fungi; those that are usually single-celled with buds or cell division are commonly known as yeasts. Yeasts vary in type from single cell forms to filamentous forms. Yeasts or yeastlike fungi may grow by elongation of cells in sequence to resemble hyphae except for the loose terminal attachments of one cell wall to the other. This situation is called **pseudohyphae.** Many of the fungal pathogens are **dimorphic,** with a yeast and a mycelial form. The yeast or yeast-like form will develop on special media at 37°C or in human or animal tissues, while the mycelial form will develop at room temperature, or 24° to 28°C.

A glossary is at the end of this manual (page 227).

REPRODUCTION

Two types of reproduction occur in the fungi: asexual (imperfect, or anamorph) and sexual (perfect, or teleomorph).

Asexual Reproduction (Imperfect, or anamorph)

Asexual spores arise by differentiation of spore-bearing hyphae without nuclear fusion. The following spore types are most common:

1. **Sporangiospores** form inside a terminal sac or **sporangium** attached to a stalk (**sporangiophore**) (Figures 5b and 6b, pages 8–9) on aseptate hyphae. Some genera have a columella, which is an extended stalk or sterile evagination inside the sporangium. An example of sporangial production is *Rhizopus oryzae*.

2. **Conidia** (singular, conidium) are specialized, non-motile spores that do not develop by cytoplasmic cleavage or free-cell `formation. The specialized branches or stalks that give rise to conidia are **conidiophores,** while the cells from which or within which conidia are directly produced are referred to as **conidiogenous** or **sporogenous** cells. Small conidia are termed **microconidia,** while large, many-celled conidia are called **macroconidia.**

The two major modes of conidiogenesis are thallic and blastic (Kendrick and Carmichael, 1973). In thallic conidiogenesis, an entire preexisting hyphal cell develops into a conidium called a thallic conidium, an example is **arthroconidium (arthrospore).** Blastic conidiogenesis involves only a part of a preexisting cell. The blastic conidia differentiate from fertile hyphae either by a "blowing out" or by de novo growth of part of the hyphal elements. When all cell wall layers of conidiogenous cells are involved in cell wall formation of conidia, the conidia are referred to as **holothallic** or **holoblastic.** If the outer layer of the conidiogenous cells does not become part of the cell wall of the conidia, the conidia are said to be **enterothallic** or

enteroblastic. Names for the types of conidia are derived from the methods of conidial development. The conidial types are as follows (modified after Barron, 1968):

Phialoconidia: Conidia produced by **phialides (sterigmata),** which are vase-shaped conidiogenous cells. Examples: *Penicillium* spp., (Figures 15b and 15c, page 15), *Phialophora* spp. (Figures 142, page 108)

Annelloconidia: Conidia formed from **annellides,** which are usually vase-shaped conidiogenous cells with the apex of the neck of each cell lengthening as each new conidium develops. A ring or annulus is left as each conidium secedes. Example: *Scopulariopsis* spp. (Figures 16b and 16c, page 15).

Blastoconidia: Conidia produced by budding from the conidiogenous cells of pre-existing conidia as in *Cladosporium* spp. (Figures 22b and 22c, page 19).

Poroconidia: Conidia produced through pores in the conidiogenous cells. Example: *Alternaria* spp. (Figures 20b and 20c page 18). The conidiogenous cell may continue to lengthen by sympodial development, giving a "bent knee," or a geniculate appearance to the conidiophore. Example: *Drechslera* spp. (Figures 24b and 24c, page 20).

Chlamydoconidia: Any filamentous fungus may develop thick-walled, round or irregular, resting cells (spores) that are capable of reproducing the fungus. These asexual spores are called chlamydoconidia and may be referred to as thallic conidia. The spores may be terminal or intercalary within the hyphae. Examples: *Microsporum audouinii, Candida albicans.* Chlamydoconidia are very common in older hyphae.

Arthroconidia: Conidia formed from separation of entire preexisting hyphal cells. Example: *Geotrichum* spp. (Figures 12b and 12c, page 13).

Blastoconidia (buds): Spores produced by budding and separation from the parent cell. Examples: *Rhodotorula* spp. (Figures 28b and 28c, page 22) and *Candida* spp.

Sexual Reproduction (Perfect, or teleomorph)

This process involves nuclear fusion and meiosis. It occurs at some point in the life history of many fungi. The process differs in different fungi.

The sexual stage is not ordinarily observed in the clinical laboratory; special culture conditions are usually necessary for development of sexual spores. Sexual spores that may develop in the pathogenic fungi characteristically are of three types: zygospores, ascospores, and basidiospores, and fit into three groups: zygomycetes (Zygomycota), ascomycetes (Ascomycota), and basidiomycetes (Basidiomycota).

Zygospores: Organisms such as species of *Rhizopus* or *Mucor* may develop thick-walled spherical zygospores from two swollen hyphal tip cells (gametangia). This is characteristic of the class Zygomycetes (Figure 1).

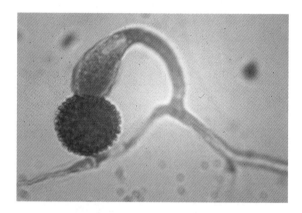

Figure 1a. Zygospore of a zygomycete

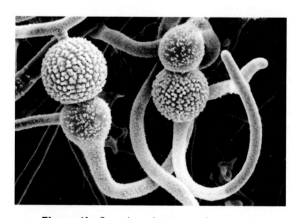

Figure 1b. Scanning microscope of a zygospore

Ascospores: Some pathogens, such as *Blastomyces dermatitidis* or species of *Arthroderma* (teleomorph form of imperfect species in the genus, *Microsporum* spp)., as well as many nonpathogens produce a spherical fruiting body (**cleistothecium,** or **gymnothecium**) with a wall (**peridium**) of woven hyphae, containing many sacs, or **asci,** each of which contain ascospores. This is characteristic of the class Ascomycetes (Figure 2). Asci may also be formed without the spherical fruiting body (**cleistothecium**) in yeasts (example: *Saccharomyces* spp.).

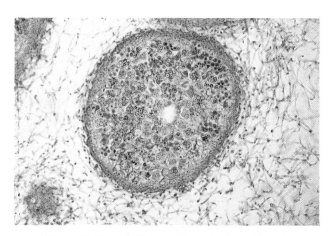

Figure 2. *Eupenicillium* sp. Cleistothecium with asci

Basidiospores: One pathogenic yeast, *Cryptococcus neoformans,* has a sexual state, **Filobasidiella,** in which basidiospores develop on the tips of club-shaped structures, the **basidia** (Figure 3). In this genus, four chains of basidiospores are produced from the tip of the **basidium.** Basidiospores characterize the class Basidiomycetes. The shapes of the basidia and the number of basidiospores vary.

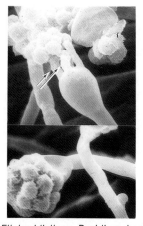

Figure 3. *Filobasidiella* sp. Basidium, basidiospores

CLASSIFICATION

The same categories or groupings applied to other organisms to classify and separate them are also applied to fungi. The categories include kingdom, phylum, subphylum, class, subclass, order family, genus, and species. Although classification systems differ, there are phyla that contain most fungi pathogenic to humans and other animals.

Zygomycota: This group of fungi usually lack cross-walls, and the organisms reproduce asexually by means of sporangia with spores (sporangiospores), sporangioles, or conidia. Sexual reproduction results in formation of a thick-walled resting spore, such as a **zygospore.** Only a few

pathogens are in this group. Examples: *Rhizopus* spp. and *Mucor* spp.

Ascomycota: The fungi in the Ascomycota have cross-walls or septa in the mycelium. The yeasts in this group are commonly cellular in form. Organisms reproduce asexually by means of budding cells, cell division, arthroconidia, chlamydoconidia, and conidiophores bearing conidia. The typical sexual reproductive structure is the **ascus,** varied in shape, with usually 8 ascospores. In some cases a fruiting body (cleistothecium) may surround the asci. Most pathogenic fungi with a known perfect state belong to this phylum. Example: *Arthroderma* spp. for the perfect state of the dermatophytes.

Basidiomycota: These fungi have septate hyphae with uninucleate or binucleate cells. The binucleate mycelium that arises from sexual reproduction usually forms clamp connections or bulges on the side of the cells where the nuclei divide in the formation of new cells. The typical sexual reproductive structure is the **basidium,** a club-shaped structure usually bearing four basidiospores on the surface. Basidiomycetes are of little importance in causing human or animal diseases. Example: *Filobasidiella* spp., the sexual state of *Cryptococcus neoformans.* Mushroom poisoning is of importance in medical practice.

Deuteromycota (Fungi Imperfecti): This is an artificial grouping of fungi that reproduce by asexual means only. Many apparently would be ascomycetes and some would be basidiomycetes if the sexual stage was found to occur. Many of the pathogenic fungi in humans and other animals belong to this phylum.

The categories used in classification of fungi are shown below, with the perfect state of *Blastomyces dermatitidis, Ajellomyces dermatitidis,* used for an illustration.

Kingdom: Fungi
    Phylum: Ascomycota
        Class: Plectomycetes
            Order: Onygenales
                Family: Gymnoascaceae
                    Genus: *Ajellomyces*
                        Species: *dermatitidis*

For the reader to develop a better background concerning fungi, it is suggested that reference be made to a textbook on mycology, such as *Introductory Mycology* by Alexopoulos and Mims. A number of other reference books or textbooks also may be helpful in the study of fungi.

Selected References

General Mycology

Ainsworth GC, Sussman AS (eds). 1965, 1966, 1968, 1973. *The Fungi.* Vols. I, III, IVA, and IVB. Academic Press, New York

Alexopoulos CJ, Mims CW. 1979. *Introductory Mycology.* 3rd ed. John Wiley and Sons, Inc., New York

Arx JA. von. 1981. *The Genera of Fungi Sporulating in Pure Culture.* 3rd Edition. J. Cramer, Vaduz. Germany

Barnett HL, Hunter BB. 1987. *Illustrated Genera of Imperfect Fungi.* 4th ed. MacMillan Publishing Co., New York

Barron GL. 1968. *The Genera of Hyphomycetes from Soil.* Williams and Wilkins Co., Baltimore

Cole GT, Samson RA. 1979. *Patterns of Development in Conidial Fungi.* Pitman, London.

Ellis MB. 1971. *Dematiaceous Hyphomycetes.* Commonwealth Mycological Institute, Kew, Surrey, England

Gilman JC. 1957. *A Manual of Soil Fungi.* 2nd ed. Iowa State University Press, Ames, Iowa

Hanlin R, Ulloa M. 1988. *Atlas of Introductory Mycology.* 2nd ed., Winston-Salem, NC, Hunter Textbook.

Hanlin R. 1990. *Illustrated Genera of Ascomycetes.* APS Press, The American Phytopathological Society. St. Paul, Minnesota

Hawksworth DL, Sutton BC, Ainsworth GC. 1983. Ainsworth & Bisby's *Dictionary of the Fungi.* 7th ed. Kew, England, Commonwealth Mycological Institute.

Kendrick WB, Carmichael JW. 1973. *Hyphomycetes. In* Ainsworth GC, Sparrow FK, Sussman AS (eds). *The Fungi.* Vol. IVA. Academic Press, New York, pp 323-509.

Kendrick WB. 1985. *The Fifth Kingdom.* Ontario, Canada. Mycological Publications

Moore-Landecker E. 1990. *Fundamentals of the Fungi.* 3rd ed. Prentice Hall. Englewood Cliffs, New Jersey

Webster J. 1980. *Introduction to Fungi.* 2nd ed. Cambridge University Press. Cambridge, New York

Medical Mycology

Baker RD (ed). 1971. *Human Infection with Fungi, Actinomycetes and Algae.* Springer Verlag, New York

Beneke ES, Rogers AL, Rippon JW. 1984. *Human Mycoses.* 8th ed. The Upjohn Co., Kalamazoo, Michigan

Conant NF, Smith DT, Baker RD, et al. 1971. *Manual of Clinical Mycology.* 3rd ed. W. B. Saunders Co., Philadelphia

Delacretaz J, Grigoriu D, Ducel G. 1976. *Color Atlas of Medical Mycology.* Hans Huber, Berne, Switzerland

Evans EGV, Richardson MD. 1989. *Medical Mycology: A Practical Approach.* I.R.L. Press, Oxford

Kane J. (ed). 1996. *Laboratory Handbook of Dermatophytes.* Star Publishing Co, Belmont, CA

Koneman EW, Roberts GD, 1985. *Practical Laboratory Mycology.* 2nd ed. Williams and Wilkins Co Baltimore

Kwon-Chung KJ, Bennett JE, 1992. *Medical Mycology.* Lea & Febiger, Baltimore, MD

Lacaz CS. 1984. *Micologia Medica.* 7th ed. Sarvier, Editora de Livros Medicos, Ltda, Sao Paulo

Maresca, B, Kobayashi, BS, eds. 1994. Molecular Biology Pathogenic Fungi, A Laboratory Manual. Telos Press, New York.

McGinnis MR. 1980. *Laboratory Handbook of Medical Mycology.* Academic Press. New York

Odds. 1988. *Candida and Candidosis.* 1988. W. B. Saunders. Orlando, Florida

Rippon JW. 1988. *Medical Mycology. The Pathogenic Fungi and the Pathogenic Actinomycetes.* W.B. Saunders Co., Philadelphia

Sabouraud R. 1910. *Les Teignes.* Masson and Cie, Paris

Seeliger HPR, Heymer T. 1981. Diagnostik Pathogener Pilze des Menschen und seiner Umwelt. Georg Thieme Verlag. Stuttgart; New York

Smith JMB. 1989. *Opportunistic Mycoses of Man and Other Animals.* CAB International, United Kingdom

Zapater RC. 1973. Atlas de Diagnostico Micológico. 3rd ed. El Ateneo, Barcelona

Scientific Periodicals, Abstracts, and Memoranda

Mycologia. Lancaster Press, Lancaster, PA

Mycopathologia. Dr. W. Junk, PO Box 13713. The Hague, Netherlands

Mykosen, Organ für Experimentelle and Klinische Mykologie. Berliner Medizinische Verlasanstalt, BerlinLichterfeld-West

Review of Medical and Veterinary Mycology. 1943 to date. Commonwealth Mycological Institute, Kew, Surrey, England (Abstracts in medical mycology)

Journal of Medical and Veterinary Mycology (Sabouraudia). Journal of the International Society for Human and Animal Mycology. Blackwell Scientific Publications. London; Boston

In addition to these references, numerous articles may be found in the various medical journals and in certain journals of biological science.

Chapter 2

COMMON CONTAMINANT FUNGI

One good way for the microbiologist or laboratory technician to become acquainted with the characteristics of growth, the colonies, and the appearance of the somatic (or vegetative) and reproductive structures of fungi is to study the common contaminant fungi, beginning with the more readily identifiable genera. The atmosphere usually contains many spores of the fungi that cause contamination of cultures. Many of these saprophytic fungi are present in soil, decaying vegetation, or as a contaminant on clinical specimens. Sometimes it is difficult to determine whether the fungus isolated was or was not involved in the clinical specimen. This is especially true with the increasing number of opportunistic fungal infections, discussed in later chapters. Some of these fungi may become pathogenic or cause allergies. Some contaminants may be confused with pathogenic fungi. Both contaminant and pathogenic fungi may be isolated from skin lesions, sputum, or other clinical specimens from patients.

Saprophytic fungi may behave as pathogens and invade the tissues of patients whose normal immunologic defenses are impaired by prolonged use of antibacterial, antineoplastic, or immunosuppressive drugs. Invasion may occur in patients with lowered resistance suffering from cancer, uncontrolled diabetes, organ transplants, AIDS, or other diseases. An "opportunistic" saprophyte should be (1) demonstrated microscopically in the clinical material, (2) cultured repeatedly from several clinical specimens, and (3) if possible confirmed by serologic tests using serum from the patient.

The initial study of mycology should be devoted to an introduction to the major classification systems and terminology related to fungi, with specific examples being used to illustrate the different classes in case students or clinical laboratory personnel lack previous background in mycology.

LABORATORY PROCEDURES FOR STUDY OF CONTAMINANT FUNGI

In the laboratory study of the common contaminant fungi, the following procedures are useful:

1. Aseptic technique: Use at all times.

2. Petri dish culture: Place a small amount of hyphae or spores or both on the center of the agar medium in a petri dish, using a stiff 22-gauge nichrome wire in an inoculating needle holder, and observe the rate of growth, color changes, and sporulation. Sabouraud glucose agar and many other types of media will support growth of contaminant fungi. Observe the development of the colony over several weeks, noting rate of growth, texture, pigmentation on the surface and reverse side, and folds or ridges on the surface. These morphologic changes are important aids in recognition of certain genera and species of contaminants and pathogens.

3. Fungus on test tube surface: The arrangement of the asexual reproductive structures of fungal cultures that have developed against the glass surface of test tubes may be observed directly under the 10X objective of the microscope. It is necessary to know the arrangement of the conidia on the conidiophores. A slide mount disturbs the arrangements of these structures.

4. Direct mounts: Using aseptic technique, remove a small portion of the colony from near the center. Place material in a drop of lactophenol with or without cotton blue or trypan blue mounting medium. The cotton blue dye is desirable for light-colored or colorless fungi. If material is dense, tease it apart with two sterile needles and add a coverglass. Examine under low (10X) magnification of the microscope, then higher magnification for smaller organisms.

5. Cellophane tape-coverglass mounts: This method (see Endo, 1966) will keep more of the reproductive structures of the fungus intact than the direct mount method. Use only on saprophytes and dermatophytes.

5

a. Place a 12-millimeter (mm) piece of Scotch double-sided tape on the surface of the fungus colony by means of a forceps. Apply pressure gently and remove.

b. Press the sticky side without the fungus on a coverglass. Press gently to remove bubbles.

c. Place the coverglass over a drop of lactophenol cotton blue or other suitable mounting medium. Alcohol or surfactants added to the mounting medium help reduce bubbles.

NOTE: If human or animal pathogens are not involved, the tape may be placed on the coverglass at the beginning of the procedure.

6. Riddell slide culture: Growing the fungus on a slide culture will result in beautiful preparations with the sporulation characteristics of the organism remaining undisturbed. For a quick observation of spore and hyphal characteristics, a direct mount or a cellophane tape mount should be made rather than a slide culture.

Fungi to be studied in detail should be grown in a van Tieghem cell or on a slide culture. A good method for obtaining permanently stained slides has been published by Riddell (1950). This procedure works for most of the filamentous fungi. Briefly the method is as follows:.

a. Pour about 15 milliliters (ml) of melted 2% agar medium into a sterile petri dish.

b. After the medium has solidified, mark it rapidly into 1-centimeter (cm) squares using a flamed dissecting needle or knife and a flamed glass rod.

c. Place a bent glass rod after flaming into a sterile petri dish containing about 7 to 8 ml of sterile water (10% sterilized glycerin may be added). Using aseptic technique, place a slide that has been passed through a flame several times on top of the bent glass rod.

d. Lift out an agar square and place it on the flamed slide.

e. Inoculate the four sides of the agar block with spores or mycelial fragments of the fungus to be grown.

f. Place a flamed coverglass centrally upon the agar block (see Figure 4).

g. Check the culture periodically for growth and sporulation. After sporulation has occurred, two permanently stained slides may be obtained from the slide culture by proceeding as follows:

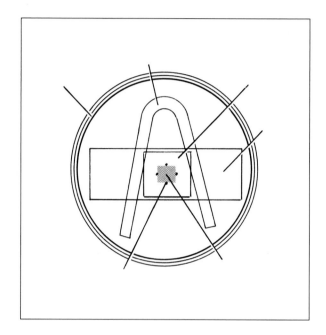

h. Remove the coverglass from the agar block. To hold conidia on coverglass, pass the coverglass 10 cm above flame, two or three times (apply a drop of 95% alcohol to the center of the coverglass to wet the fungus for better penetration of the mounting medium in case of *Penicillium* or *Aspergillus*).

i. Place a drop of lactophenol cotton blue or trypan blue on a clean slide and lower the coverglass (h) gently.

j. Similarly, using the slide with the fungus growing on it, proceed as in steps h and i, with a clean coverglass.

k. If the correct amount of mounting medium has been used, the slides may be sealed immediately with fingernail polish. The corners of the coverglass may be sealed first to hold it in position on the slide, and more lacquer may be applied after the corners are secured. If there is excess mounting medium around the edges, it is necessary to let the slides dry overnight and then to absorb the excess medium with blotting paper before sealing. These slides should keep indefinitely if well sealed. Substitutes for nail polish may be used for sealing the slides. When a slide does dry out, the nail polish may be removed from one side of the coverglass, a drop of mounting medium added, and, after the dry area under the coverglass is filled, the slide is resealed.

7. Microscopic examination: Examine the slide mounts under the microscope and note the characteristic spore structures, sporangiophore or conidiophore structure if present, and mycelial characteristics for the particular fungus being studied.

LABORATORY EXERCISE FOR STUDY OF AIRBORNE AND SOILBORNE FUNGI

Airborne Fungi

Each member of the class should select one of the following locations to expose a petri dish containing Sabouraud glucose agar (or another medium) for different periods of time:

    a.   Atmosphere in building

    b.   Atmosphere outside building

    c.   Atmosphere in basement

    d.   Atmosphere in barn or chicken house

    e.   Atmosphere in crowd-filled room

Soilborne Organisms

After using a dilution plate technique or sprinkling particles on four or five spots on the Sabouraud glucose agar, compare types of fungi that grow from soil samples with those in the plates that contain airborne fungi. Use the following sources for samples:

    a.   Soil with high organic content

    b.   Soil with low organic content

    c.   House dust

    d.   Manure from chicken house or cow or horse stable

Results

With the aid of reference books and knowns that have been studied in class, identify the genus of as many organisms as possible. Keep a record of the number of genera and the number of colonies that occur. Compare the class results on airborne fungi with the fungi that are most frequently reported in the atmosphere at various times in the year, as follows:

Alternaria spp.	*Streptomyces* spp.
Cladosporium spp.	*Rhizopus* spp.
Penicillium spp.	*Phoma* spp.
Aspergillus spp.	*Trichoderma* spp.
Monilia spp.	*Chaetomium* spp.
Botrytis spp.	Unknowns
Mucor spp.	Miscellaneous

Alternaria and *Cladosporium* have been reported as the fungi most frequently isolated from the atmosphere throughout the year. For further details on occurrence of atmospheric spores, see *Allergy in Practice* by Feinberg or other publications.

REPRESENTATIVE COMMON SAPROPHYTIC FUNGI

Some of the more common contaminant fungi are described on the following pages. These saprophytic fungi, often found in clinical materials as laboratory contaminants, may become pathogenic under special conditions, and some genera resemble the pathogenic fungi. Since a large number of genera and species may be in the phylum Deuteromycota (Fungi Imperfecti), identification to genus is sufficient for the beginner, as more training and experience is required to determine species in most cases. Learning to recognize some of the common genera of the normally saprophytic fungi will help the laboratory worker when many of these organisms become opportunistic pathogens. An increasing number of the dematiaceous hyphomycetes which have dark pigments in the cell walls are causative agents of phaeohyphomycosis (Chapter 6). In addition a rapidly increasing number of the hyaline (colorless) Hyphomycetes are causative agents of hyalohyphomycosis (Chapter 9).

The fungi included in this section are separated into three groups based on distinctive characteristics. The chief distinguishing characteristics help separate the following three groups:

1. **Zygomycetous fungi:** These fungi have broad, nonseptate (coenocytic) mycelium, asexual reproduction usually by sporangiospores, and sexual reproduction by zygospores.

2. **Hyaline Hyphomycetes:** This group of fungi has septate mycelium without evidence of melanin pigment in the cell walls either in tissue or in culture, and asexual reproduction is by conidia with no sexual reproduction.

3. **Dematiaceous Hyphomycetes:** These fungi have evidence of melanin (dark brown to black pigments) in their cell walls in culture and usually in tissue sections, and asexual reproduction is by conidia with no sexual reproduction.

Zygomycetes (Phycomycetes)

Species from the genera *Rhizopus, Cunninghamella,* and *Saksenae* are the most likely to be isolated from clinical cases of Zygomycosis. Other generally less frequently isolated genera include: *Absidia* spp., *Apophysomyces* spp., *Cokeromyces* spp., *Mucor* spp., *Rhizomucor* spp., and *Syncephalastrum* spp.

1. *Rhizopus* spp.

Colonies: Very fast growing, quickly filling the culture plate with a dense, cottony, aerial mycelium, at first white, later becoming gray (Figure 5a).

Microscopic: Mycelium aseptate, with many stolons (hyphal branches) connecting groups of unbranched sporangiophores. At the point of connection, a cluster of rhizoids (rootlike structures) are attached to the substrate. The sporangiophores terminate with a dark brown or black, spherical sporangium containing a columella. Spores oval, bluish, or brown (Figures 5b and 5c). Zygospores formed with compatible strains.

Usually *R. oryzae* is the most prevalent etiologic agent of zygomycosis. *R. microsporus* is the second most likely cause of zygomycosis, mainly from cutaneous cases and rarely from subcutaneous abscesses or rhinocerebral infections.

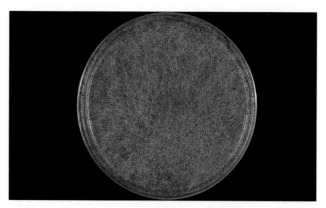

Figure 5a. *Rhizopus* sp., Colony

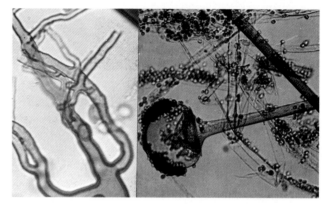

Figure 5b. *Rhizopus* sp., Microscopic of sporangiophore

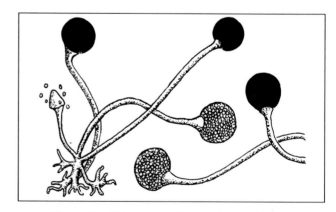

Figure 5c. *Rhizopus* sp., Diagram of sporangiophore

2. *Mucor* spp.

Colonies: Very fast growing, quickly filling a petri plate with cottony, aerial mycelium, at first white, later becoming dark gray, brown, or yellow (Figure 6a).

Microscopic: Mycelium aseptate, forming many upright, single or branched sporangiophores. The tip of the sporangiophore bears a globose sporangium with the wall readily breaking off, leaving a collarlike base around the central columella. Spherical to elliptical spores are formed between the sporangial wall and the columella (Figures 6b and 6c). No rhizoids at the base of the sporangiophores. Some species are pathogenic.

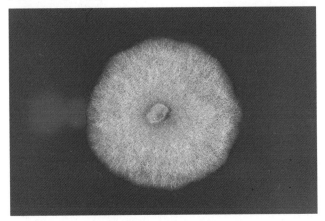

Figure 6a. *Mucor* sp. Colony

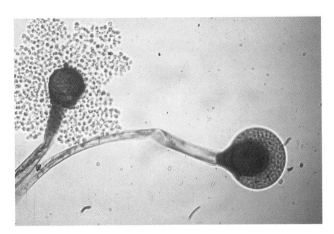

Figure 6b. *Mucor* sp. Microscopic of sporangiophore

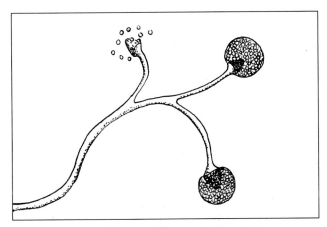

Figure 6c. *Mucor* sp. Diagram of sporangiophore

Species of *Mucor* have causative agents in a case of rhinocerebral zygomycosis, an erythematous skin lesion, and a gastric zygomycosis case.

3. *Syncephalastrum* spp.

Colonies: Very fast growing, quickly covering the surface of the agar medium with dense, cottony, aerial mycelium which is at first white, then dark gray (Figure 7a).

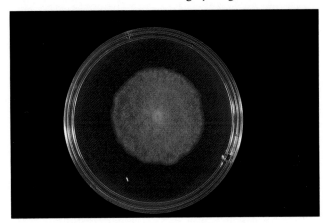

Figure 7a. *Syncephalastrum* sp. Colony

Microscopic: Mycelium aseptate, forming short sporangiophores sympodially, and terminated by an enlarged globose vesicle with many tubular sporangia (merosporangia) containing chains of spores radiating from it. Two to many single-celled spores are in a sporangium (Figures 7b, 7c and 7d).

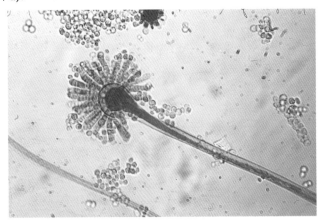

Figure 7b. *Syncephalastrum* sp. Microscopic of merosporangia

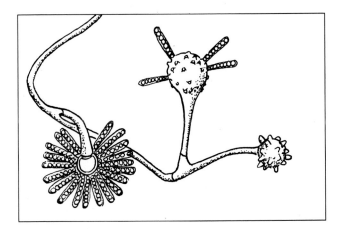

Figure 7c. *Syncephalastrum* sp. Diagram of merosporangia

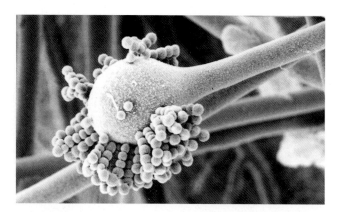

Figure 7d. *Syncephalastrum* sp. SEM merosporangia

Deuteromycota (Fungi Imperfecti)

Many fungi with septate hyphae apparently lack a sexual state and are commonly called "imperfect fungi." Fungi that produce conidia on hyaline (colorless) conidiophores or directly on hyaline hyphae are in the Class Hyphomycetes, family Moniliaceae (hyphae and conidia hyaline). Organisms with one or both of the hyphae and conidia dark in color are in the family Dematiaceae. These dark-brown, green, or black pigmented fungi are commonly known as dematiaceous fungi.

Class Hyphomycetes

Family Moniliaceae—hyaline or brightly colored hyphae

4. Acremonium (Cephalosporium) spp.

Colonies: Fast growing, at first compact and moist, becoming overgrown with loose, cottony, aerial hyphae, white, gray, or rose in color (Figure 8a).

Microscopic: Septate hyphae, phialides erect, unbranched, with a cluster of conidia (phialoconidia) at the tip. Conidia elliptical, one-celled, occasionally several-celled, held together by a mucoid substance (Figures 8b, 8c, and 8d).

Occasionally a causative agent of mycetoma. In cases of hyalohyphomycosis, infections have involved invasive pulmonary and paranasal sinus cases, as well as cutaneous and subcutaneous tissues, cornea, and other body locations including cellulitis, bursitis, nephritis, endocarditis, peritonitis, and fungemia.

5. Aspergillus spp.

Colonies: Slow to rapid growing, white at first, then shades of blue-green, yellow-green, black, tan, or white. Surface velvety to cottony (Figure 9a).

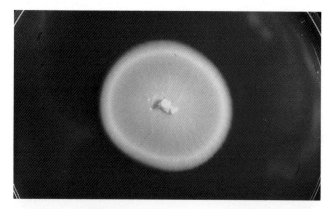

Figure 8a. *Acremonium* sp. Colony

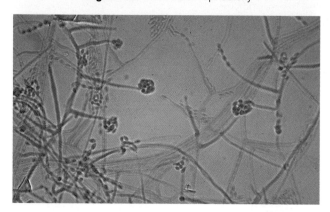

Figure 8b. *Acremonium* sp. Conidiophores and conidia

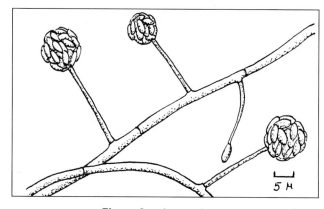

Figure 8c. *Acremonium* sp.
Diagram of conidiophore and conidia

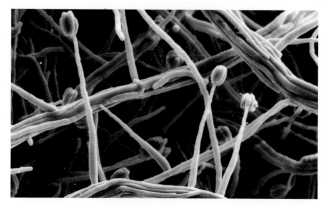

Figure 8d. *Acremonium* sp.
SEM of conidiophore and conidia

Microscopic: Mycelium septate, conidiophores long with vesicle-like tips, surface containing many flask-shaped phialides and chains of conidia (phialoconidia) which are one-celled, spherical to elliptical, smooth or rough-walled (Figures 9b, 9c, and 9d). Some species develop cleistothecia with asci and ascospores. *A. fumigatus, A. flavus, A. terreus,* and *A. niger* are the most likely species encountered in pathologic material.

See aspergillosis (page 171) for more information on types of infections.

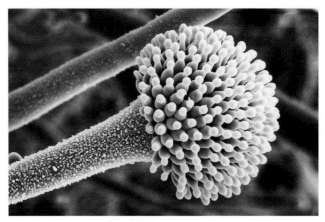

Figure 9d. *Aspergillus* sp.
SEM of conidiophore and conidia

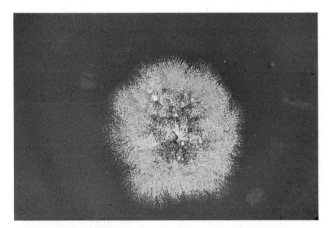

Figure 9a. *Aspergillus* sp. Colony

6. *Botrytis* spp.

Colonies: Moderately fast growing, white to gray colonies with a fluffy surface (Figure 10a).

Microscopic: Mycelium septate, conidiophores simple or with many branches. The branches are thin or thick, and narrowing toward the tips, ending in swollen truncate or oval conidiogenous cells which bear numerous conidia, or ending in a narrow point with one conidium (Figures 10b). Rarely involved in cases of hyalohyphomycosis.

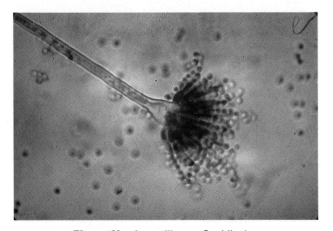

Figure 9b. *Aspergillus* sp. Conidiophore

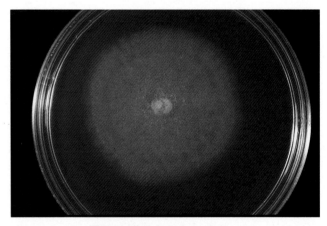

Figure 10a. *Botrytis* sp. Colony

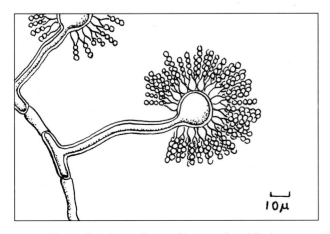

Figure 9c. *Aspergillus* sp. Diagram of conidiophore

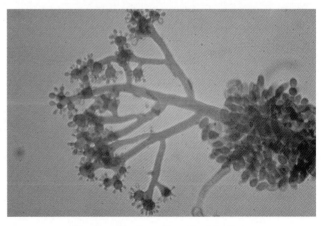

Figure 10b. *Botrytis* sp. Conidiophore

7. *Fusarium* spp.

Colonies: Fast growing, at first white, cottony or woolly, frequently becoming pink, purple, or yellow in the hyphae or in the substrate (Figure 11a).

Microscopic: Mycelium septate, phialides borne singly or in packed groups (sporodochia). Conidiophores short, branched irregularly, or in whorls. Conidia (phialoconidia) of two types: macroconidia sickle-shaped, curved with pointed ends, many-celled; microconidia one-celled, oval or elongated; some conidia two- or three-celled, elongated and curved (Figures 11b, 11c and 11d).

Most of the human cases involve trauma, burns, organ transplants, bone marrow transplants, facial granuloma, fungemia, bone marrow, and general dissemination. At times the organisms are involved in keratinomycosis and isolated from skin lesions of burn patients.

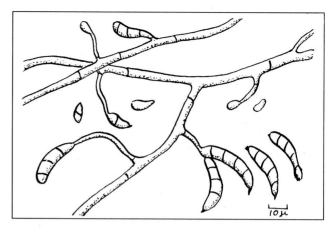

Figure 11c. *Fusarium* sp.
Diagram of conidia

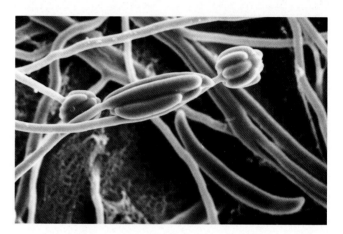

Figure 11d. *Fusarium* sp. SEM of conidia

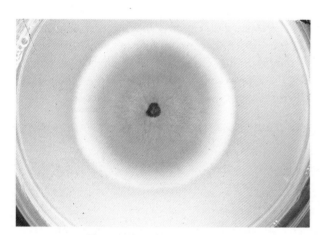

Figure 11a. *Fusarium* sp. Colony

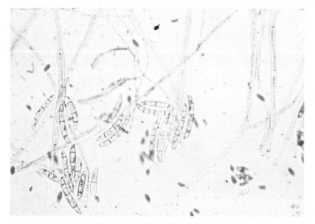

Figure. 11b. *Fusarium* sp.
Macroconidia and microcondida

8. *Geotrichum* spp.

Colonies: Fast growing, producing cottony, aerial mycelium, white or becoming cream, tan, or greenish. Some species smoother and more granular on the surface on certain media (Figure 12a).

Microscopic: Septate hyphae, breaking up to form one-celled, thin-walled rectangular cells, arthroconidia (Figures 12b, and 12c). Nonpathogenic strains are commonly found in cottage cheese, in rot of tomatoes, and in soil.

Geotrichum spp. has been reported numerous times from human specimens but most of the time there was no association with any specific disease. The fungus is considered opportunistic.

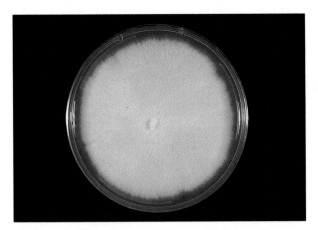

Figure 12a. *Geotrichum* sp. Colony

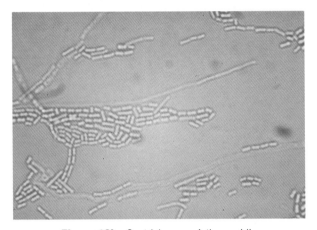

Figure 12b. *Geotrichum* sp. Arthroconidia

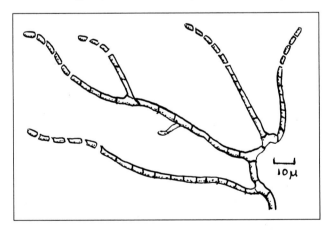

Figure 12c. *Geotrichum* sp. Diagram of arthroconidia

9. *Gliocladium* spp.

Colonies: Fast growing, at first white, spreading over surface of plate and becoming green, rose, or cream or remaining white (Figure 13a).

Microscopic: Septate hyphae with conidiophores like *Penicillium*, branched with flask-shaped phialides at tips. Conidia (phialoconidia) one-celled, spherical, hyaline or brightly colored in mass, forming clusters or balls held together by a mucilaginous material (Figures 13b, 13c, and 13d). No conidial chains formed, an important distinction from *Penicillium*.

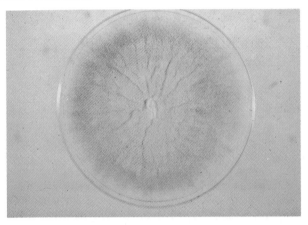

Figure 13a. *Gliocladium* sp. Colony

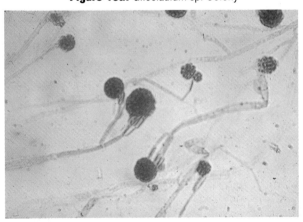

Figure 13b. *Gliocladium* sp. Coniophore and conidia

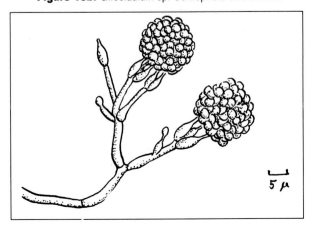

Figure 13c. *Gliocladium* sp. Diagram of conidiaphore and conidia

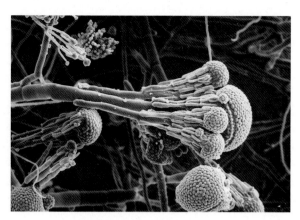

Figure 13d. *Gliocladium* sp.
SEM of conidiophore and conidia

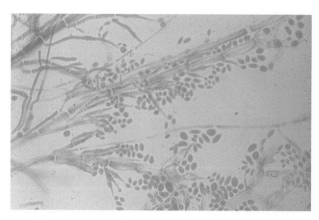

Figure 14b. *Paecilomyces* sp. Conidiophore and conidia

10. *Paecilomyces* spp.

Colonies: Rather rapid growing, thin, spreading, powdery to velvety, becoming yellowish-brown, tan, gray-green, violet, or white, depending upon species (Figure 14a).

Microscopic: Mycelium septate, with single phialides arising along hyphae with characteristic long, tapering, conidia-bearing tubes. Also "penicillus" or *Penicillium* like conidiophores with phialides having elongated tips. Conidia (phialoconidia) in chains, and elliptical (Figures 14b and 14c).

Majority of cases have occurred in immunocompetent patients. Infections have occurred as fatal endocarditis, complications in prosthetic heart valves, in a cerebrospinal fluid shunt, and causes of endophthalmitis.

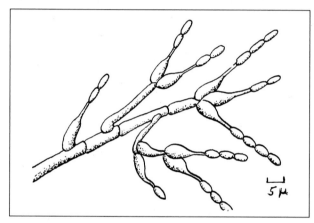

Figure. 14c. *Paecilomyces* sp.
Diagram of conidiophore and conidia

11. *Penicillium* spp.

Colonies: Fast growing, at first white, becoming shades of green, blue-green, or other colors after conidia mature. Surface velvety to powdery due to abundance of conidia (Figure 15a).

Microscopic: Brush-like conidiophores or "penicillus" developed from septate hyphae. Chains of conidia, one-celled, globose to elliptical, smooth or rough, cut off from flask-shaped phialides (Figures 15b, 15c and 15d). Species separated on the basis of variations in branches (metulae) of the conidiophores, conidia, and colonial characteristics.

The only known primary pathogen of humans is *P. marneffei,* a thermal dimorphic species (see *penicilliosis marneffei,* page 203).

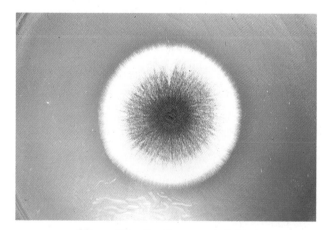

Figure 14a. *Paecilomyces* sp. Colony

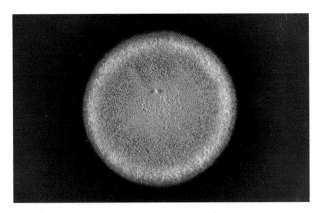

Figure 15a. *Penicillium* sp. Colony

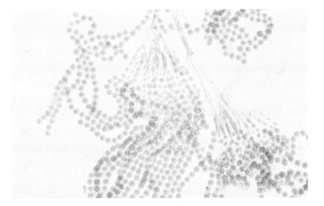

Figure 15b. *Penicillium* sp. Conidiophore and conidia

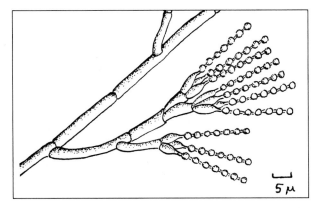

Figure 15c. *Penicillium* sp.
Diagram of conidiophore and conidia

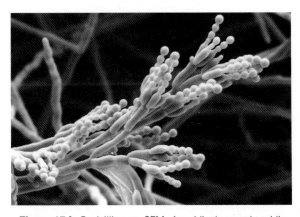

Figure 15d. *Penicillium* sp. SEM of conidiophore and conidia

12. *Scopulariopsis* spp.

Colonies: Moderately slow growing, white at first, thin, becoming brown and powdery from heavy sporulation. Color and appearance somewhat like those of *Microsporum gypseum* (Figure 16a).

Microscopic: Mycelium septate, with single, unbranched conidiophores or branched "penicillus"—like conidiophores. Annellides produce chains of lemon-shaped conidia (annelloconidia) with a pointed tip and truncate base (Figures 16b, 16c and 16d). Conidia usually echinulate.

Occasionally in nail infections, in deep-seated granulomatous lesions, and in subcutaneous infections.

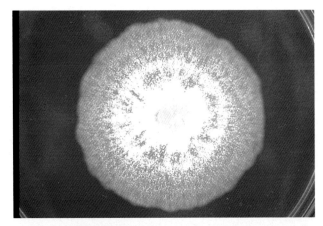

Figure 16a. *Scopulariopsis* sp. Colony

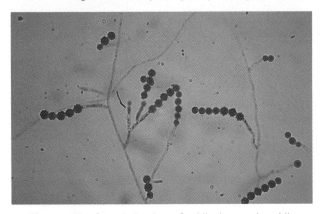

Figure 16b. *Scopulariopsis* sp. Conidiophore and conidia

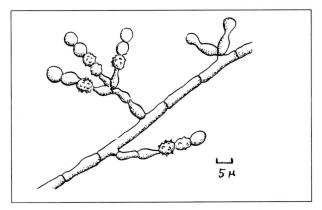

Figure 16c. *Scopulariopsis* sp. Diagram of conidiophore and conidia

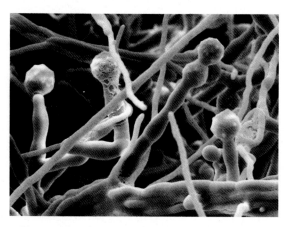

Figure 16d. *Scopulariopsis* sp. SEM of conidiophore

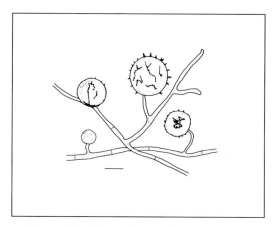

Figure 17c. *Sepedonium* sp. Diagram of conidia

13. *Sepedonium* spp.

Colonies: Hyphae widespread, growing rapidly, forming a thick white turf, sometimes becoming yellow (Figure 17a).

Microscopic: Septate hyphae form conidiophores, indistinguishable from the hyphae, simple or branched, producing spiny to warty macroconidia (Figures 17b and 17c). This fungus resembles *Histoplasma capsulatum* at 25°C.

14. *Trichoderma* spp.

Colonies: Fast growing, woolly or cottony, thin, white at first, becoming green or yellow-green or remaining white due to dense mats of conidia on surface (Figure 18a).

Microscopic: Septate hyphae, with short, branched conidiophores, with ultimate flask-shaped phialides, opposite or in whorls. Single-celled conidia (phialoconidia) formed in rounded clusters at tips of conidiophores, colorless to green (Figures 18b and 18c).

Reported in cases of septicemia following contaminated intravenous dextrose infusions, in a case of peritonitis, and in a pulmonary fungus ball.

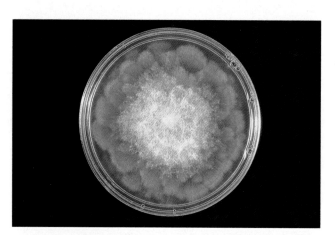

Figure 17a. *Sepedonium* sp. Colony

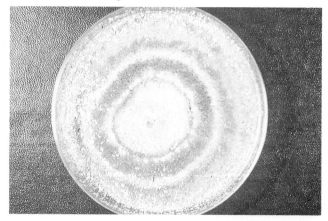

Figure 18a. *Trichoderma* sp. Colony

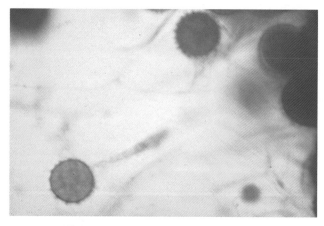

Figure 17b. *Sepedonium* sp. Macroconidia

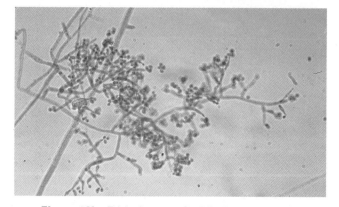

Figure 18b. *Trichoderma* sp. Conidiophores and conidia

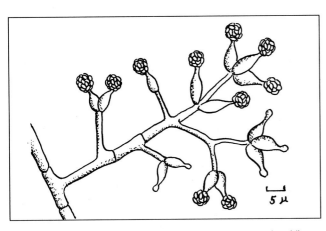

Figure 18c. *Trichoderma* sp. Diagram of conidiophores and conidia

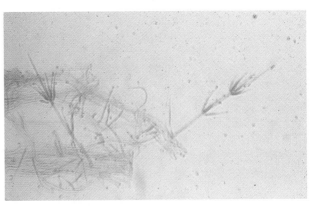

Figure 19b. *Verticillium* sp. Conidiophores

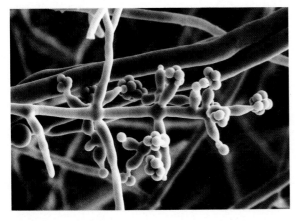

Figure 18d. *Trichoderma* sp. SEM of conidiophores and conidia

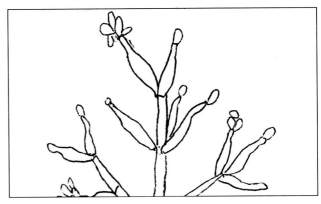

Figure 19c. *Verticillium* sp. Diagram of conidiophore

15. *Verticillium* spp.

Colony: Fast growing, floccose, white at first, then becomes powdery, later the color may change to green, blue-green, yellow, red or rose as the conidia mature (Figure 19a).

Microscopic: Septate hyphae develop simple or branched verticils, and hyaline or pigmented. The phialides with tapering tips are borne in whorls on the branches of the conidiophores. The conidia are ovoid or cylindrical, produced in balls, and are hyaline to green, or red to pink in color (Figures 19b and 19c).

A saprophytic fungus, plant diseases.

Class Deuteromycota

Family Dematiaceae: Hyphae and/or conidia with melanin pigments (brown to black). This group is commonly known as dematiaceous fungi. The genera are separated on the basis of number of cells and septations, or type of spore development.

16. *Alternaria* spp.

Colonies: Fast growing, dense, grayish at first, becoming greenish-gray, brown, or black with gray edges. Surface overgrown with loose gray-to-white aerial hyphae. Reverse side of colony black (Figure 20a).

Microscopic: Mycelium dark, septate. Multicellular conidia (poroconidia) produced at end of conidiophores (hyphal branches) in chains, dark brown, with transverse and longitudinal septa (muriform), variable in shape (Figures 20b and 20c), with youngest conidia produced at tip of chain. *Alternaria* resembles *Stemphyllium,* if conidia not in chains. *Alternaria* is of importance in allergies.

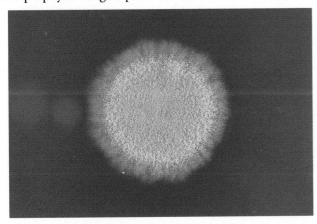

Figure 19a. *Verticillium* sp. Colony

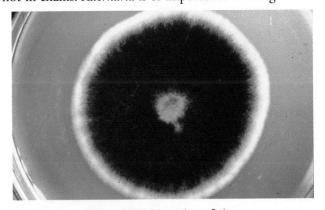

Figure 20a. *Alternaria* sp. Colony

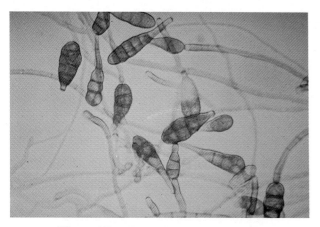

Figure 20b. *Alternaria* sp. Muriform conidia

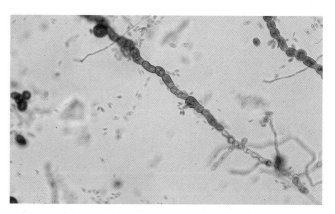

Figure 21b. *Aureobasidium* sp. Light and dark hyphae and conidia

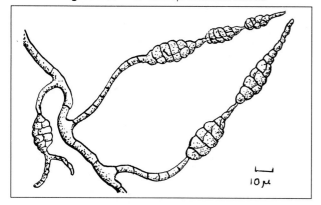

Figure 20c. *Alternaria* sp. Diagram of conidial chains

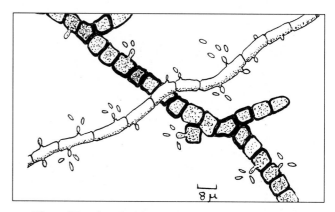

Figure 21c. *Aureobasidium* sp. Diagram of hyphae and conidia

Infections involve bone, cutaneous tissue, paranasal sinuses, urinary tract and patients with immunosuppressive conditions.

17. *Aureobasidium (Pullularia) pullulans*

Colonies: Young colonies at first white or pinkish and yeastlike, later becoming wrinkled, black, leathery, and shiny when masses of conidia are formed (Figure 21a).

Microscopic: Young mycelium thin-walled, producing many elliptical conidia (blastoconidia) by budding. Older hyphae are dark, thick-walled, with a short tube developed after germination to bud off elliptical conidia (Figures 21b, 21c and 21d). The conidial mass makes up the shiny surface of the colony.

This fungus has been involved in cases of visceral infections, in blood in acute myeloid leukemia, and in a splenic abscess.

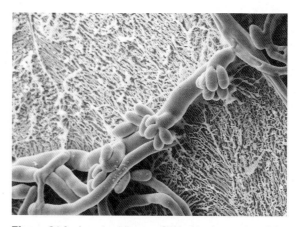

Figure 21d. *Aureobasidium* sp. SEM of hyphae and conidia

18. *Cladosporium*

Colonies: Moderately slow growing dark gray-green, reverse side brownish-gray or black. Surface powdery to velvety, becoming heaped and folded in some species (Figure 22a).

Microscopic: Hyphae septate, brown to olive in color; conidiophores dark, varied in length, forming branches with repeated forking, termination in chains of conidia (blastoconidia). Conidia one-celled (occasionally two-celled, ovate to cylindrical with pointed ends, in some cases lemon-shaped, smooth to rough-walled (Figures 22b, 22c and 22d).

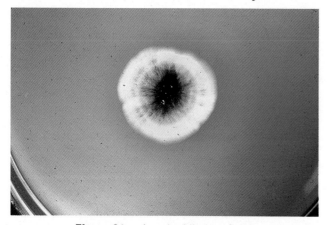

Figure 21a. *Aureobasidium* sp. Colony

Species of *Cladosporium* are etiologic agents of subcutaneous phaeohyphomycosis as well as cutaneous, eye and nail infections.

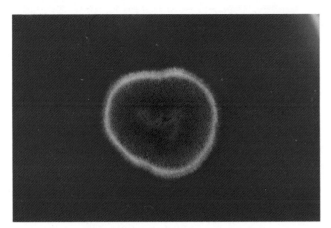

Figure 22a. *Cladosporium* sp. Colony

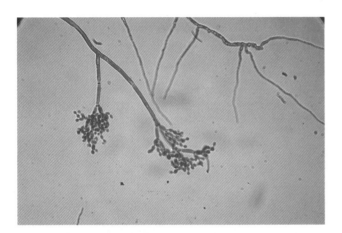

Figure 22b. *Cladosporium* sp.
Conidiophore and conidia

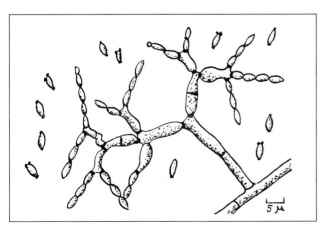

Figure 22c. *Cladosporium* sp.
Diagram of conidiophore and conidia

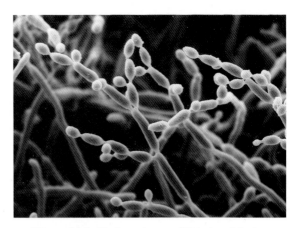

Figure 22d. *Cladosporium* sp. SEM of conidiophore

19. *Curvularia*

Colonies: Fast growing, dark gray, brown or nearly black, with the reverse side black (Figure 23a).

Microscopic: The conidiophores are simple, brown, bearing conidia at the apex or on new sympodial growth. The conidia are transversely septate and cylindrical or slightly curved with one of the central cells larger and darker (Figure 23b).

Curvularia has been the causative agent of paranasal sinusitis in immunosuppressed patients, and the cause of a lung lesion.

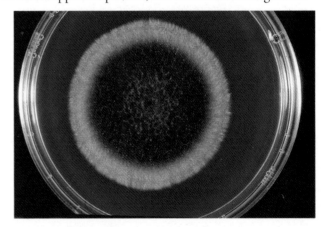

Figure 23a. *Curvularia* sp. Colony

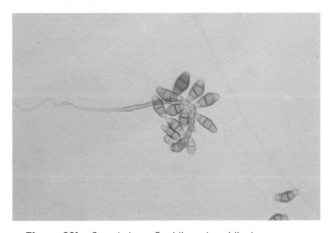

Figure 23b. *Curvalaria* sp. Conidia and conidiophore

20. *Drechslera* spp.

Colonies: Fast growing, grayish-brown, becoming darker or black in center, velvety to woolly surface (Figure 24a).

Microscopic: Hyphae septate, dark, with long or short, simple or branched, septate conidiophores that are twisted or bent at the tip. Conidia (poroconidia) cylindrical to elliptical, dark, with usually more than three cells, loosely attached to the twisted or bent tip of conidiophore (Figures 24b, 24c, and 24d) brown, indeterminate, extended by sympodial growth. *Drechslera* resembles *Helminthosporium* in appearance but differs by sympodial development of the conidiophores.

Drechslera biseptata has been isolated from a brain biopsy.

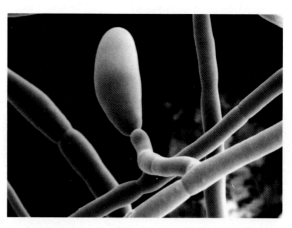

Figure 24d. *Drechslera* sp. SEM of conidiophore

21. *Epicoccum*

Colonies: Fast growing, floccose, yellow to orange with a deep purple-red diffusible pigment on the reverse side in some species. Colony becomes dark with conidial formation (Figure 25a).

Microscopic: The conidiophores are short, dark, and aggregated together (sporodochia), with conidiogenous cells producing dark multiseptate conidia with both longitudinally and transverse netlike septation (Figure 25b).

A laboratory contaminant.

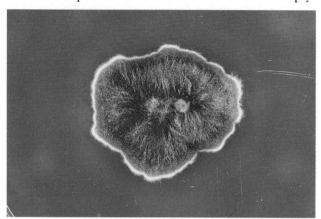

Figure 24a. *Drechslera* sp. Colony

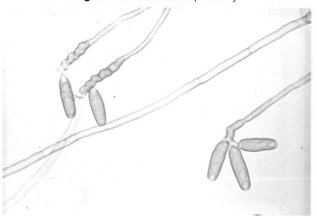

Figure 24b. *Drechslera* sp. Conidiophore and conidia

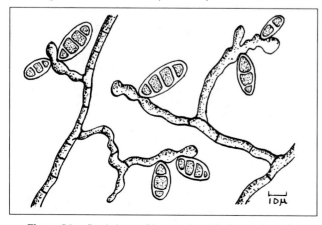

Figure 24c. *Drechslera* sp. Diagram of conidiophore and conidia

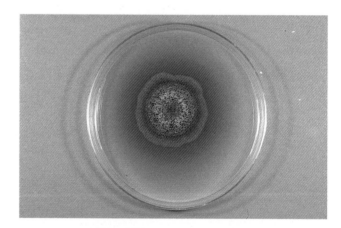

Figure 25a. *Epicoccum* sp. Colony

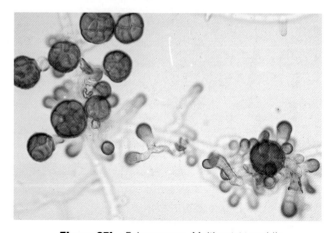

Figure 25b. *Epicoccum* sp. Multiseptate conidia

22. *Nigrospora* spp.

Colonies: Fast growing, forming a compact, cottony or woolly, white aerial mycelium that becomes gray after sporulation. The reverse side of the colony is black (Figure 26a).

Microscopic: Hyphae septate, with short, simple or branched, inflated conidiophores bearing jet-black, large subspherical conidia (blastoconidia). The vesicle or inflated tip of the conidiophore is hyaline (Figures 26b, 26c and 26d).

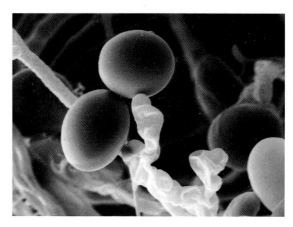

Figure 26d. *Nigrospora* sp. SEM of conidia

Nigrospora has been isolated from scrapings of an ulcerated lesion on the nose of a patient.

23. *Ulocladium* spp.

Colonies: Fast growing, dark brown, with a black reverse side (Figure 27a).

Microscopic: Conidiophores are simple with dark terminal swellings, producing conidia from sympodial growth. Conidia formed from pores (poroconidia), dark brown, muriform, ovoid to broadly elliptical, and born singly at the apex of new sympodial growing points of the conidiophores (Figure 27b).

Usually a laboratory saprophyte. It has been reported in a case of phaeohyphomycosis.

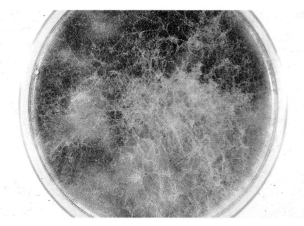

Figure 26a. *Nigrospora* sp. Colony

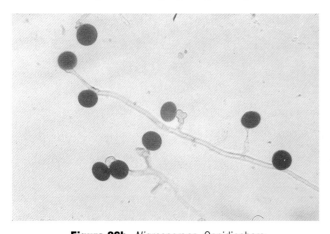

Figure 26b. *Nigrospora* sp. Conidiophore

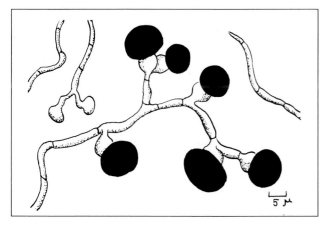

Figure 26c. *Nigrospora* sp. Diagram of conidia and conidiophore

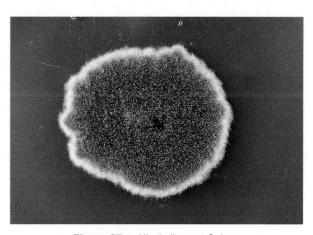

Figure 27a. *Ulocladium* sp. Colony

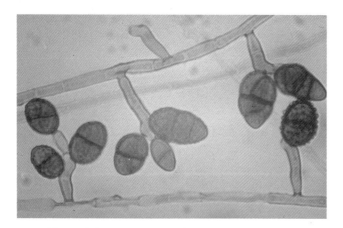

Figure 27b. *Ulocladium* sp. Conidiophore and conidia

Phylum Deuteromycota

Class Blastomycetes: yeast fungi

24. *Rhodotorula* spp.

Colonies: Yeast-like, developing rapidly at 37°C on most mycologic agar media, pasty or mucoid, glistening, coral-red, pink, or salmon in color (Figure 28a). Occasionally some strains may form a rudimentary pseudomycelial formation.

Microscopic: Yeast cells vary in shape from short ovoid (2.5 to 6.5 μm) to elongate cells up to 14 μm long (Figures 28b, 28c, and 28d). Reproduction is by multilateral budding. Microscopically *Rhodotorula* is similar in appearance to *Saccharomyces.*

Species of *Rhodotorula* may invade and multiply rapidly in organs of patients with chronic debilitating diseases in the terminal stages. Infection is rather rare with reports including fungemia, endocarditis, peritonitis, meningitis, and ventriculitis.

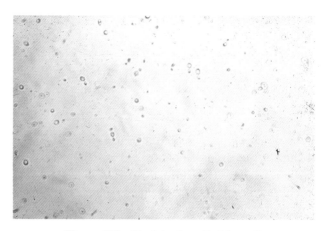

Figure 28b. *Rhodotorula* sp. Budding cells

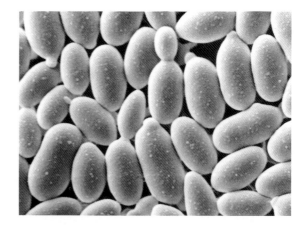

Figure 28c. *Rhodotorula* sp. Diagram of budding yeast cells

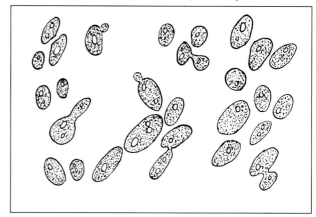

Figure 28d. *Rhodotorula* sp. SEM of budding cells

25. *Saccharomyces* spp.

Colonies: On malt extract agar the colony at 25°C is butyrous, cream color, slightly raised and smooth. *S. cerevisiae* is known as baker's or brewer's yeast (Figure 29a).

Microscopic: The cells are globose or subglobose (5 to 10 by 5.0 to 12 μm), or ellipsoidal to cylindrical, up to 21 μm long (Figure 29b). Asci may form with 1 to 4 ascospores on certain media.

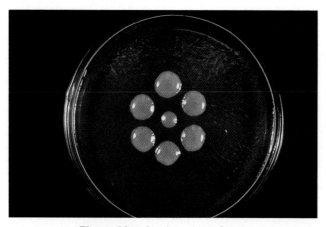

Figure 28a. *Rhodotorula* sp. Colony

This yeast has been reported in cases of fungemia, invasive infections of the prosthetic heart valves, indwelling catheters, and in cases of peritonitis.

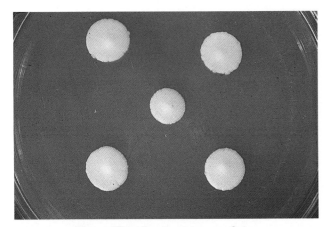

Figure 29a. *Saccharomyces* sp. Colony

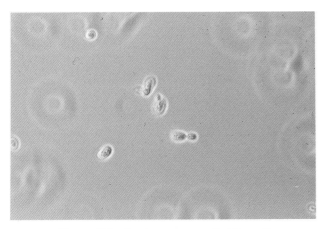

Figure 29b. *Saccharomyces* sp. Budding cells

Phylum Deuteromycota

Class Coelomycetes

26. *Phoma* spp.

Colonies: On Sabouraud glucose agar the colony is slow-growing, dark gray-olive (Figure 30a). The fruiting body is a pycnidium, a tough, leathery to membranous structure that is globose to lens-shaped, with an ostiole, an opening.

Microscopic: Conidia are produced in abundance on threadlike conidiophores inside the pycnidium. At maturity the hyaline, one-celled, elliptical to rod shaped (2.5 by 5 µm) conidia ooze out of the pycnidium through the ostiole (Figure 30b).

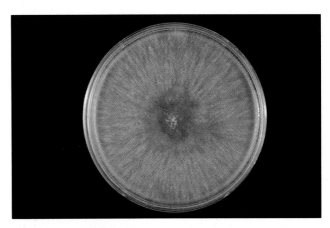

Figure 30a. *Phoma* sp. Colony

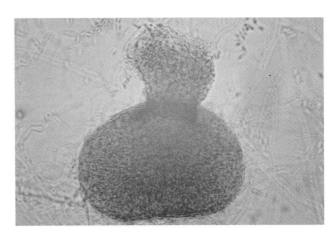

Figure 30b. *Phoma* sp. Pycnidium and conidia

Case reports include isolation of the fungus from a cystic abscess near the Achilles tendon of a renal transplant patient, a pustular lesion on a leg, on the foot and a perioral lesion in the mouth of an individual. The tissue had moniliform cells or septate hyphae with or without yeast cells.

Phylum Ascomycota

Class Plectomycetes

27. *Chaetomium* spp.

Colony: The fungus is fast growing, gray with darker areas containing matured perithecia (Figure 31a).

Microscopic: These fruiting bodies (perithecia) are flask-shaped, or pyriform with many straight or curly dark hairs on the outside and with ostioles (openings at apex) for release of ascospores. The pyriform asci have an evanescent wall (disintegrates). The ascus contains 8 dark, lemon-shaped ascospores (Figure 31b).

Three species have been implicated in phaeohyphomycosis, including a case of subcutaneous abscess, a cerebral infection in a renal transplant patient, and in a cutaneous lesion.

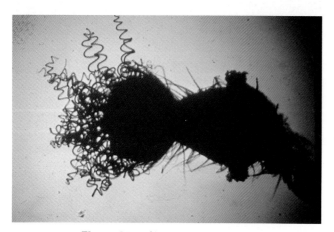

Figure 31a. *Chaetomium* sp. Colony

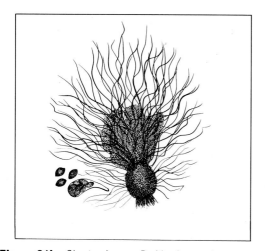

Figure 31b. *Chaetomium* sp. Perithecium and ascospores

Phylum Schizomycota

Class Actinomycetales

28. *Streptomyces* spp.

Colonies: Slow growing, small (less than 12 mm in 14 days), dry, leathery, wrinkled, with a chalky surface, white in some species, colored in others, adherent to agar surface. Frequently with a musty odor and discoloration in the medium (Figure 32a).

Microscopic: Thin mounts or slide cultures show slender branched hyphae 1 μm wide with straight or coiled conidiophores breaking up into chains of conidia (Figures 32b

and 32c). Aerial conidia and less extensive fragmentation of hyphae help distinguish this fungus from *Nocardia*.

This genus is important in the fermentation industry including antibiotics and other chemicals.

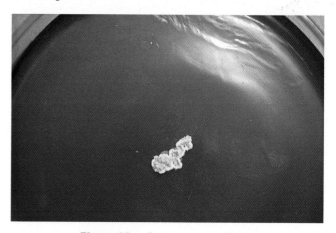

Figure 32a. *Streptomyces* sp. Colony

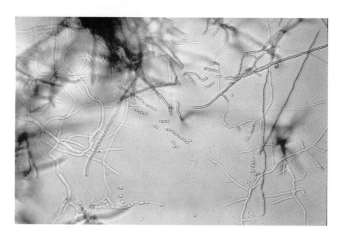

Figure 32b. *Streptomyces* sp. Hyphae and conidiophore

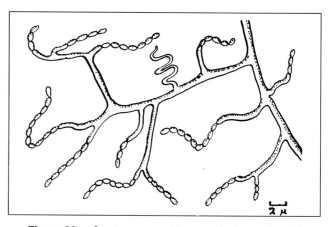

Figure 32c. *Streptomyces* sp. Diagram of hyphae and conidia

Selected References for Study of Contaminant Fungi:

Arx JA von. 1981. *The Genera of Fungi Sporulating in Pure Culture.* 3rd ed. J. Cramer, Vaduz, Germany

Barnett HL, Hunter BB. 1987. *Illustrated Genera of Imperfect Fungi.* 4th ed. Macmillan Publishing Co, New York

Barron GL. 1968. *The Genera of Hyphomycetes from Soil.* Williams and Wilkins Co., Baltimore

Carmichael JW, Kendrick WB, Conners IL, Sigler L. 1980. *Genera of Hyphomycetes.* University of Alberta Press, Edmonton

Domsch, et al. 1980. *Compendium of Soil Fungi,* Vols. 1 and 2. Academic Press. New York

Ellis MB. 1971. *Dematiaceous Hyphomycetes.* Commonwealth Mycological Institute, Kew, Surrey, England

Endo RM. 1966. A cellophane tape-cover glass technique for preparing microscopic slide mounts of fungi. Mycologia 48:655

Gilman JC. 1957. *A Manual of Soil Fungi.* 2nd ed. Iowa State University Press, Ames, Iowa

Hamlin R. 1990. *Illustrated Genera of Ascomycetes.* APS Press. The American Phytopathological Society. St. Paul, Minnesota

Kendrick WB, Carmichael JW. 1973. *Hyphomycetes.* In Ainsworth GC, Sparrow FK, Sussman AS. (eds). *The Fungi.* Vol. IVA. Academic Press, New York, pp 323-509.

Kreger-van Rij NJW. 1984. *The Yeasts, a Taxonomic Study.* Elsevier Science Publishers B.V. Amsterdam, The Netherlands

Raper KB, Fennel DF. 1965. *The Genus Aspergillus.* Williams and Wilkins Co., Baltimore

Raper KB, Thom C. 1949. *Manual of the Penicillia.* Williams and Wilkins Co., Baltimore

Riddell RW. 1950. Permanent stained mycological preparations obtained by slide culture. Mycologia 42:265

Samson RA, Pitt JI. 1989. *Modern Concepts in Penicillium and Aspergillus Classification.* Plenum Press, New York and London

Chapter 3

LABORATORY PROCEDURES

The most rapid method to determine whether a fungus is present in clinical specimens is the direct examination of part of the specimen on a microscope slide. Negative results do not rule out the possibility that a fungus is present. Additional procedures that may be needed to establish the diagnosis are culture, use of Wood's light, stained smears, or histologic sections; roentgenologic examination; immunologic, serologic tests, and DNA Probes. Animal inoculation is not needed in routine clinical laboratory procedures.

EQUIPMENT

Sterilized equipment should be used at all times to avoid contamination by nonpathogenic fungi and by bacteria. The following equipment may be useful in the collection of specimens.

Bard-Parker scalpel	Syringe
Epilating forceps	Nail clippers
Scissors	Sterile cotton swabs
Vacutainer tube	Sterile test tubes
Coverglasses	Petri dishes
Clean slides for smears	Collection bottles
70% alcohol	Media, reagents
Sterile brush	Safety hood

Regulations in the Clinical Laboratory

There are numerous regulations that must be followed in the operation of a clinical laboratory. Under the Clinical Laboratory Improvement Amendments of 1988 (CLIA '88) there are a number of regulations concerning the operation of the bacteriology and mycology laboratories that *must* be followed including the safety of personnel, safety in the laboratory, handling of specimens, hazardous chemicals, quality control, equipment maintenance, proficiency testing, etc. More information is available from the Health Care Financing Administration in Washington, D. C. The OSHA regulations concerning biologic and chemical hazards and safety in the laboratory are available from a number of sources (See Selected References).

Under CLIA '88 there are two types of laboratories for mycology: level 1, moderately complex laboratory for isolation with limitations on identification, and level 2, highly complex laboratory for isolation and identification of all fungi, and need for interpretative skills. The fungi include yeasts, dimorphic fungi, dermatophytes, filamentous fungi and aerobic actinomycetes.

SELECTION AND PREPARATION OF SPECIMENS

The selection of material is important because it is difficult to know prior to microscopic examination whether the fungus is in the sample selected. Collection of sufficient material for both direct examination and culture is necessary. The specimens collected may include: skin, nails, hair, scrapings from ulcers, pus, cerebrospinal or other body fluids, urine, sputum, blood, bone marrow, stools, bronchial washings, and biopsies (Table 1). Prompt delivery of specimens to the laboratory is necessary to avoid overgrowth with bacteria or rapidly growing saprophytic fungi.

Superficial Mycoses

The fungi causing superficial mycoses are *Malassezia furfur* (pityriasis versicolor), *Trichosporon beigelii* (white piedra), *Piedraia hortai* (black piedra), and *Exophiala werneckii* (tinea nigra).

For skin scrapings of pityriasis versicolor, the affected area should be washed with 70% alcohol to remove dirt or medication and scraped with a sterile scalpel. Place the scales in a small sterile container or a petri dish for laboratory examination. Special media is needed for isolation of *M. furfur.*

The same procedures are applicable for the affected areas of tinea nigra.

In piedra cases, the hair of the scalp or beard should be cut or clipped from the areas of infection and placed in a sterile container for laboratory examination.

Cutaneous Mycoses

Infected areas of skin, nails, and hair should be removed and examined directly under the microscope and cultured for the presence of organisms.

Skin scrapings: The area of infection should be washed with 70% alcohol to remove surface contaminants. Scrapings should be taken from active border areas of the lesion and placed in a sterile container for laboratory study. Direct examination in 10% to 20% potassium hydroxide (KOH) solution or potassium hydroxide-calcofluor white are the most rapid methods. The latter requires an epifluorescence microscope. Other media or stains, including KOH-glycerin, KOH-ink, and periodic acid-Schiff stain, may be used. Cultures should be made for species identification.

In lesions that might contain *Candida albicans,* smears should be made on slides for staining and scrapings placed on mycological media for culture, as materials from lesions dry out rapidly if kept too long.

Nail scrapings: Scrapings or clippings of nails, especially near the bed of the nail, should be collected in a sterile container for examination. The same procedure is used as for skin, except that the nail requires a longer period of time to clear in KOH even with gentle heating.

Hair: The basal portion of the hair or hair stubs should be plucked out with tweezers, as the fungus usually is found in this part. The edges of the patches are likely to contain the best material. Wood's light (ultraviolet light rays of 3,660 angstrom units) under darkened conditions is a useful aid for collecting infected hairs in scalp ringworm caused by most species of *Microsporum.* The infected hairs usually fluoresce with a bright yellowish-green color. Most species of *Trichophyton* and *M. gypseum* in hair infections do not fluoresce. The hair may be placed in sterile paper containers, petri dishes, directly on slides, or on agar medium and examined later in the laboratory.

Subcutaneous Mycoses

The diseases in this group include mycetoma, chromoblastomycosis, sporotrichosis, phaeohyphomycosis, lobomycosis, and rhinosporidiosis. The specimens best collected for this group include crusts and pus from open abscesses; exudate from lesions; aspirated fluids from unopened sinus tracts or abscesses, by syringe; and tissue from biopsy. The organism *Rhinosporidium seeberi,* causing rhinosporidiosis, has not been cultured at present; thus scrapings or biopsy material should be examined directly or fixed for histologic examination.

Systemic Mycoses

The agents of the deep or systemic mycoses may be identified in the laboratory from examination of pus or exudate, spinal fluid, sputum, bone marrow and blood, or material from abscesses, biopsies, autopsies or direct examination, or cultures. Animal inoculations may be made from material collected or from cultures for development of the dimorphic form. This is useful for demonstrating the yeast form or spherules for verification of the fungus or for students to examine.

Pus or exudate: Specimens should be placed in sterile containers or as a drop on a slide with a coverglass placed over the material and pressed down to make a thin smear. A drop of 10% to 20% KOH solution may be added before adding the coverglass, if clearing is necessary. Budding cells, large cells (spherules) with endospores, or hyphae may be seen. The specimens in the sterile containers should be cultured on appropriate media.

Cerebrospinal fluid: The fluid should be collected in a sterile container, centrifuged, and a portion of the sediment checked directly. Some of the sediment should be checked in India ink for oval or budding cells and capsule formation. Sediment should be stained by Gram's method as well as by the acid-fast method in case actinomycetelike hyphae are evident. Cultures should be made.

Sputum: The sputum specimen should be obtained early in the morning before anything has been eaten or drunk. After a mouth wash has been used, the sputum should be brought up from the lungs and placed into a sterile, glass, screw-capped container. The specimen should not be kept long in the laboratory before examination. The same procedure for examination as that for pus should be followed. Gram's method should be used to check for hyphae of actinomycetes, yeast cells of *Candida,* and arthroconidia of *Geotrichum.* If there is blood in the sputum, a blood stain should be made and checked for *Histoplasma capsulatum.* An acid-fast stain will help indicate if *Nocardia* is present.

If cryptococcosis is suspected, an India ink mount should be made. Cultures should be made either directly from the material taken from the patient or from the material in the sterile container.

Bone marrow: The initial needle aspiration or core biopsy specimen is used for making a bone marrow smear. Additional bone marrow and blood are removed and placed into a sterile container with 0.5 ml of 1:1,000 heparin (for 3 to 4 ml of bone marrow) for culture on brain-heart infusion blood agar.

Blood: Fungemia and septicemia is expected to increase in debilitated immunocompromised patients. In the past blood cultures have been unreliable for detection of opportunistic fungal infections or fungal sepsis. The most reliable factor for isolation of fungi from blood is the volume of the blood sampled, conditions of incubation and the culture medium. A higher rate of fungal recovery is from culture of 10 ml or more of blood. Two to three different blood samples shoud be cultured. The blood should be diluted 1:10 to 1:20 in the culture bottle of 45 to 90 ml. A biphasic blood culture medium containing brain heart infusion broth/agar is better than other blood culture media (Roberts and Washington, 1975) for isolation of fungi (Septi-Chek, Roche Laboratories). All blood cultures should be vented and incubated at 30° C for 30 days. then checked for fungal growth on days 1,2,7, and weekly. The biphasic blood culture medium will allow the detection of yeast growth as small colonies on the agar surface. The non-biphasic blood cultures may be checked for growth by subculturing a portion of the blood culture onto Sabouraud glucose agar.The lysis-centrifugation system is better for isolation of filamentous fungi than other systems (Isolator, DuPont deNemours). There is a decreased time for detection of fungal growth on the radiometric and non-radiometric detection systems (Johnston Laboratories).

Tissue biopsies: Tissue samples should be placed on sterile moistened gauze for smears, direct examination, culture, and histologic sections.

NOTE: In handling of pathogenic fungi, routine precautions should be taken, including washing of hands, use of aseptic technique, disinfecting of any contaminated surfaces with good fungicides, and sterilizing or burning of all cultures or contaminated materials ready to be discarded.

MAILING OF SPECIMENS

Skin, nail, and hair placed in envelopes or bottles and placed in the designated biohazard containers in accordance with postal regulations. These specimens will usually arrive in viable condition.

Other specimens, such as sputum, urine, and exudates from lesions, are usually of no value after shipment by mail, because saprophytic fungi and bacteria multiply rapidly, reducing the chance of isolating the pathogenic fungus. If the specimens must be mailed, contaminating microorganisms may be controlled by the addition of 20 units of penicillin and 40 units of streptomycin or of 0.05 milligrams (mg) of chloramphenicol for each ml. Postal regulations

need to be followed for mailing of certain pathogens. For specific details on mailing and labeling of specimens, the individual should consult the State Health Department or another agency.

Selected References

Ajello L. 1951. Collecting specimens for the laboratory demonstration and isolation of fungi. JAMA 146:1581

Bille J, Edson, RS, Roberts GD. 1984. Clinical evaluation of the lysis-centrifugation blood culture system for the detection of fungemia and comparison with a conventional biphasic broth blood culture system. J. Clin. Microbiol. 19:126.

Caplan LM, Merz WG. 1978. Evaluation of two commercially prepared biphasic media for recovery of fungi from blood. J Clin Microbiol 8:469

Hageage GJ, Harrington BJ. 1984. Use of calcofluor white in clinical mycology. Lab. Med. 1984. 15:190.

Haley LD, Callaway BS. 1978. *Laboratory Methods in Medical Mycology.* HEW Publication, CDC #78-8361. US Government Printing Office, Washington, DC (Stock #01 7-023-00 1 24-8)

Ilstrup DM, Washington JA II. 1983. The importance of volume of blood cultured in the detection of bacteremia and fungemia. Diagn. Microbiol. Infect. Dis. 1:107

McCarthy LR, Senne JE. 1980. Evaluation of acridine orange stain for detection of microorganisms in blood cultures. J. Clin. Microbiol. 1980. 11:281

Merz WG, Roberts GD. 1991. Detection and Recovery of Fungi from Clinical Specimen. Chapter 58:588 in 5th edition of *Manual of Clinical Microbiology* by Balows A, et al.

Prevost E, Bannister E. 1981. Detection of yeast septicemia by biphasic and radiometric methods. J. Clin. Microbiol. 13:655

Roberts GD, Washington, JA II. 1975. Detection of fungi in blood cultures. J. Clin. Microbiol. 1:309

Thompson AN. 1955. Mycological teaching material. Am. J. Med. Tech. 21:57

CULTIVATION OF FUNGI

The techniques used for cultivation of fungi are somewhat similar to those used by the medical bacteriologist. There are important differences to consider when handling fungi. A stiff nichrome wire needle (22-gauge) should be used for transferring cultures. A pair of dissecting needles is useful for teasing masses of mycelium apart on slides before mounting the material for better observation.

It is best to use test tubes or prescription bottles for culture of clinical specimens and for the study of cultures. Petri dishes are not recommended, as these containers afford less protection from the more virulent organisms, and dry out more rapidly.

Sabouraud glucose agar with chloramphenicol and cycloheximide (Commercially available as Mycosel, BBL, Cockeysville, Md, Mycobiotic Agar, Difco, Detroit, MI) is useful for isolation of many clinical specimens, especially the dermatophytes. Dermatophyte Test Medium, (Charles Pfizer, Diagnostic Div., New York) is useful for presumptive tests of skin, nail, or hair material. Sabouraud glucose agar with antibiotics, blood agar, and other special media are useful for isolation of fungi causing systemic mycoses. Saprophytic fungi as opportunistic organisms can be isolated on a number of mycological media with antibiotics. (See Table 1).

Table 1. Type of Specimen and Suggested Media for Isolation of Fungi Causing Mycoses

DISEASE	CULTURE MEDIUM	TYPE OF SPECIMEN
Superficial Mycoses		
Pityriasis versicolor	Not necessary	Skin scrapings
Tinea nigra	Sabouraud agar + antibiotics*	Skin scrapings
Piedra	Sabouraud agar	Cut hair
Cutaneous Mycoses		
Tinea capitis	Sabouraud agar + antibiotics* Dermatophyte Test Medium (presumptive; use other media for identification)	Epilated hair
Tinea corporis, etc.		Skin scrapings
Tinea unguium (onychomycosis)	Sabouraud agar + chloramphenicol	Nail scrapings
Candidiasis		Skin and nail scrapings, mucocutaneous scrapings, vaginal scrapings
Subcutaneous Mycoses		
Chromoblastomycosis	Sabouraud agar + antibiotics*	Scrapings, crust, exudate from lesion
Mycetoma (maduromycosis)	Sabouraud agar Brain-heart infusion agar Brain-heart infusion blood agar	Pus from draining sinuses Aspirated fluids Biopsy material
Phaeohyphomycosis (also systemis)	Sabouraud Agar + chloramiphenicol	Sputum, bronchial washings and scrapings, body fluids, pus, corneal scrapings
Sporotrichosis (also systemic)	Sabouraud agar + antibiotics*	Pus from ulcerating lesions, aspirated fluid, lung washings
Rhinosporidiosis	None	Biopsy of nasal or ocular polyps, skin scrapings
Systemic Mycoses		
Yeastlike fungi		
Candidiasis	Sabouraud agar + chloramphenicol Brain heart infusion biphasic Blood culture medium	Sputum, bronchial washings, biopsy Cerebrospinal fluid, urine, stools, blood

Table 1 *(cont.)* Type of Specimen and Suggested Media for Isolation of Fungi Causing Mycoses

DISEASE	CULTURE MEDIUM	TYPE OF SPECIMEN
Yeastlike fungi (continued)		
Cryptococcosis	Sabouraud agar + chloramphenicol Bird (niger) seed	Cerebrospinal fluid, sputum Pus from abscesses, sinus tracts, scrapings from skin lesions, urine, blood, bone marrow
Geotrichosis	Sabouraud agar + chloramphenicol	Sputum, bronchial washings. stools
Dimorphic fungi		
Blastomycosis (North American)	Sabouraud agar + antibiotics[*] Brain heart infusion agar Yeast extract phosphate medium	Scrapings from edges of lesions Pus from abscesses, sinus tracts Urine, sputum, bronchial washings
Paracoccidioidomycosis	Same as Blastomycosis	Scrapings from edges of lesions Scrapings from mucous membranes Biopsied lymph nodes Sputum, bronchial washings
Coccidioidomycosis	Sabouraud agar + antibiotics[*] Yeast extract phosphate medium	Sputum, bronchial washings Cerebrospinal fluid, urine, scrapings from lesions, pus from abscesses, sinuses
Histoplasmosis	Yeast extract phosphate medium Blood agar Emmons' modified Sabouraud agar plus blood	Blood, bone marrow Sputum, bronchial washings Cerebrospinal fluid, pus from sinus tracts or ulcers, skin scrapings from lesions
Miscellaneous Mycoses		
Aspergillosis	Sabouraud agar + chloramphenicol	Sputum, bronchial washings
Zygomycosis (mucormycosis)	Sabouraud agar + chloramphenicol	Sputum, bronchial washings, biopsy material
Hylohyphomycosis	Sabouraud agar + chloramphenicol	Sputum, bronchial washings, nail scrapings, biopsy, blood, body fluids, pus, corneal scrapings
Otomycosis (External otitis)	Sabouraud agar + chloramphenicol	Epithelial scales and detritus
Actinomycetes		
Actinomycosis	Brain-heart-infusion blood agar (all anaerobic, 37°C)	Pus from draining sinuses, aspirated fluid, sputum, spinal fluid, bronchial washings
Nocardiosis	Sabouraud agar, brain-heart-infusion blood agar (incubate at room temperature and 37°C) Paraffin bait technique	Same as above

[*] Addition of chloramphenicol and cycloneximide to the medium. Commercially available culture media, such as Mycosel (BBL, Bioquest, Cockeysville, MD) and Mycobiotic Agar (Difco Laboratories, Inc. Detroit, MI), contain these two antibiotics.

Clinical material or a small portion from a known stock culture should be cut into the surface of the medium on the slant, using aseptic technique at all times. The cultures should be incubated for two weeks or more at 24° to 28°C and observed for colony formation. A portion of the colony should be mounted on a slide for microscopic examination of spore development in order to learn the morphologic characteristics of the fungus. Cultures should be kept for four to six weeks.

Before and after working with pathogenic fungi, the area should be wiped down with a fungicide, such as 2% Amphyl or other similar antiseptics, or a wet paper towel may be kept below the area where the cultures are being handled. A biologic safety hood should be used for most fungi causing systemic fungal diseases, especially *Histoplasma capsulatum, Blastomyces dermititidis, Paracoccidioides brasiliensis,* and *Coccidioides immitis.*

Examination of Cultures

When fungi are cultured on different media in slants, the characteristics of the fungus may be observed under the low-power objective of the microscope by looking along the edges of the medium and colony.

Direct examination: Portions of colonies should be removed from the culture and placed on a slide with lactophenol cotton blue, teased apart, and covered with a coverglass for observation under the microscope. If spores or other structures allow identification of the fungus, no further procedures are necessary. However, many organisms must be grown on special media, subjected to special physiologic tests, or cultured on a slide culture for genus and species determination.

Slide culture: To avoid disturbing the arrangement of the fungus structures, one can use a slide culture technique, with permanently stained mounts being made from the slide and coverglass. The following slide culture technique may be of use for class or laboratory study of fungi. This method should not be used for fungi causing the deep mycoses.

Riddell slide culture method: This involves growing the fungus on the sides of an agar block between a glass slide and a coverglass in a moist chamber. For more details see the description of this procedure on page 6 of this manual (Riddell, 1950).

Cellophane tape-coverglass mounts: This method keeps more of the fungus structures intact than does the direct mount method. See description of this procedure on page 5 of this manual.

Slanted coverglasses placed in the culture medium. The 18mm coverglasses can be slanted into the agar medium near a fungus colony for 3 to 5 days to let the fungus grow up on the sides of the slanted coverglasses. The slanted coverglass can be removed and double mounted with a 22mm coverglass on top of the 18 mm coverglass.

Mounting Media, Stains, and Staining Methods

These media may be used for temporary mounts and in some cases for more permanent slide mounts. Nail polish or other material may be used to seal the slides.

Potassium hydroxide (KOH): 10% to 20% solution. Use of KOH is one of the most rapid methods for direct examination of infected material. Gently heating the slide increases the rate of clearing, and the fungus elements should be readily observed. These specimens have been made permanent (Taschdjian, 1954) by drawing off the alkaline mixture, neutralizing in 10% acetic acid, dehydrating in absolute alcohol, clearing in xylol, and mounting.

Potassium hydroxide (KOH)-Calcofluor white: Calcofluor white (CFW) combined with KOH will enhance the appearance of fungal elements in the specimens for microscopic examination. The CFW nonspecifically binds to the chitin and cellulose in the cell wall of the fungus and fluoresces a bright green-blue. Use an epifluorescence microscopic with a mercury vapor lamp along with a UV excitation filter to get maximum absorbance of CFW.

Preparation: 15% KOH solution
                       KOH ....15 ml
                       Glycerol...............................20 ml
                       Distilled water ....80 ml

Dissolve KOH in glycerol and water, then store at 25°C.

0.1% (wt/vol) CFW solution
Use a commercial solution of Cellufluor (Polysciences, Washington, PA) or fluorescent brightener (Sigma Chemical Co., St. Louis, MO).

Mix, gently heat, filter if precipitate occurs, store at 25°C in dark.

Procedure:

Place specimen on a glass microscope slide.
Mix and add coverglass. Gently heat to speed clearance.
Examine for fluorescence microscopically.

KOH and fountain pen ink: A mixture of 9 parts KOH (10%) and 1 part blue-black ink is useful for examination of scrapings containing such fungi as *Malassezia furfur* and *Candida albicans*. KOH and glycerin: Pus and sputum can be maintained for a long period of time by placing in an aqueous solution containing 5% KOH and 25% glycerin.

Lactophenol cotton blue (Aman's medium): This is an excellent medium for mounting most fungi:

Lactic acid	20 g
Phenol crystals	20 g
Glycerin	40 g
Water	20 ml
Cotton blue (Poirier blue)	0.05 g

Cotton blue, a potential carcinogen, has been used extensively in the past. A suggested substitute is trypan blue (Borelli and Salas, 1975).

India ink: A drop of India ink is placed on a glass slide with a drop of cerebrospinal fluid or a loopful of the *Cryptococcus neoformans* culture and the two are stirred together. A coverglass is added quickly and the slide examined for capsules, which are readily demonstrated by this method. If the India ink is too dark, it may be diluted by 50% with water or saline. Sterilize the slide after cautious examination.

Other mounting media: A number of other media for mounting fungi are described in the literature.

Direct staining on vinyl plastic tape (Keddie et al, 1961): Scotch brand tapes #681 and #473 are recommended for use in stripping and staining for fungal infection of the horny epidermis. Place tape with material, adhesive side up, on a slide and stain one minute with Hucker crystal violet, Loeffler methylene blue, or Giemsa solution. Rinse with alcohol for a moment, dry, and mount in permanent or temporary mounting media.

Periodic acid-Schiff stain: This stain is excellent for differentiating fungi in skin scrapings and tissue sections.

Skin scrapings: Spread thin scrapings on a slide coated with Mayer's albumen or coat the lesion with the fixative, scrape surface scales off, and immediately press them on the surface of a clean slide. Heat gently and check to see if scrapings are fast on the slide before proceeding.

Procedure:

Use 3 or 4 drops of periodic acid-Schiff stain to cover, or immerse the fixed scrapings:

1. Immerse one minute in 95% alcohol.

2. Immerse five minutes in 5% periodic acid.

3. Immerse two minutes in basic fuchsin solution.

4. Rinse in tap water.

5. Immerse ten minutes in zinc (or sodium) hydrosulfite solution.

6. Rinse in tap water.

7. Counterstain with either saturated aqueous solution of picric acid for two minutes or light green stain for five seconds.

8. Rinse for a short time in tap water.

9. Dry well and observe under immersion oil; gently blot excess oil off slide before storage, or

10. After step 8, dehydrate about ten seconds in 95% alcohol and one minute in 100% alcohol, rinse twice in xylol for about one minute each time, and mount in permount or other mounting media.

Reagents:

Basic fuchsin solution:

Basic fuchsin	0.1g
95% alcohol	5.0 g
Water	95.0 ml

Zinc (sodium) hydrosulfite solution:

Zinc (sodium) hydrosulfite	1.0g
Tartaric acid	0.5 g
Water	100.0 ml

Saturated aqueous solution of picric acid (do not let dry out).

Light green stain:

Light green	1.0 g
Glacial acetic acid	0.25 ml
80% alcohol	100.0 ml

The fungi stain a bright red or purplish-red after periodic acid hydrolysis to release aldehydes that can combine with

Schiff reagent. The carbohydrates in the cell walls take the red stain as a result of the reaction.

Tissue sections: Tissues should be fixed, dehydrated, embedded in paraffin, and sectioned by the routine method:

Procedure:

1. Place in xylol to deparaffinize.

2. Rinse in 100% alcohol.

3. Wash in distilled water.

4. Immerse ten minutes in 1% periodic acid.

5. Rinse in tap water five to ten minutes.

6. Immerse two minutes in basic fuchsin solution.

7. Rinse in tap water 30 seconds.

8. Immerse 30 minutes (or possibly up to two or three hours for some material) in zinc (or sodium) hydrosulfite solution.

9. Rinse in tap water three to five minutes.

10. Immerse two minutes in light green stain.

11. Rinse for a short time in tap water.

12. Dehydrate about ten seconds in 95% alcohol and one minute in 100% alcohol, rinse twice in xylol for about one minute each time, and mount in permount or other mounting media.

NOTE: Hematoxylin and eosin (H and E) stained slides may be restained by removal of the coverglass with xylol and rehydration. The slide is then placed in 1% periodic acid for ten minutes and the rest of the procedure is continued. This technique is useful when the H and E stain does not differentiate the fungus from the tissue sufficiently well.

Gram's method (Hucker modification): All fungi are Gram-positive when stained by the Gram method.

Procedure:

1. Fix the smear.
2. Place crystal violet on slide for one minute.

3. Wash with water.

4. Apply Gram's iodine solution for one minute.

5. Wash with water.

6. Decolorize in 95% alcohol (or equal parts of alcohol and acetone).

7. Counterstain with safranine for ten seconds.

8. Wash and dry.

Reagents:

1. Ammonium oxalate-crystal violet solution:

   Crystal violet (85% dye content) ....4.0 g
   Ethyl alcohol (95%) ....20.0 ml

Dissolve crystal violet in alcohol; dilute solution 1:10 with distilled water.

   Ammonium oxalate ....0.8 g
   Water ....80.0 ml

Dissolve ammonium oxalate in water. Mix 1 part of crystal violet solution with 4 parts of ammonium oxalate solution.

2. Gram's iodine solution:

   Iodine ....1.0 g
   Potassium iodide...2.0 g

Dissolve in 5 ml of distilled water, then make up to 250 ml with water. Add 60 ml of a 5% solution of sodium bicarbonate.

3. Counterstain:

   Safranine (2.5% solution in 95% alcohol)...10.0 ml
   Water...100.0 ml

Acid-fast stain (Kinyoun's modification): This stain is especially useful as an aid in differentiation of *Nocardia* spp. The hyphae of *N. asteroides* and *N. brasiliensis* appear partially acid-fast or acid-fast. Acid-fast organisms stain red.

Procedure:

1. Make smear and either heat-fix slide or use a slide warmer at 65° to 75°C for at least two hours.

2. Apply Kinyoun carbol fuchsin over smear. Stain at room temperature for five minutes.

3. Rinse off stain with distilled water. Decolorize with acid alcohol for three to ten seconds or until no red appears or use 1% aqueous H_2SO_4 for destaining.

4. Rinse in distilled water.

5. Counterstain three to four minutes with methylene blue or other counterstain.

6. Rinse with water, dry in air or with gentle heat, and examine under oil.

Reagents:

Kinyoun carbol fuchsin:

```
Basic fuchsin.................................4.0 g
Ethyl alcohol (95%) .....................20.0 ml
(Add alcohol slowly while shaking to dissolve)
Phenol (liquified or melted crystals) ...........8.0 g
Water (distilled)...............................100.0 ml
```

Acid alcohol:

```
Hydrochloric acid, concentrated................3.0 ml
Ethyl alcohol, 95%.................................97.0 ml
```

Methylene blue:

```
Methylene blue chloride ...........................0.3 g
Distilled water.......................................100.0 ml
```

Giemsa stain: This stain and some others—Gridley, periodic acid-Schiff, Gomori methenamine-silver nitrate—are useful to locate *Histoplasma capsulatum* in the reticuloendothelial cells.

Procedure:.

1. Fix the smear with 100% methyl alcohol for about three to five minutes.

2. Add mixed staining solution on slide for about 15 minutes.

3. Wash well in tap water.

4. Dry by blotting with bibulous paper.

Reagents:

Stain solution (stock):

```
Giemsa powder..........................................600.0 mg
Methyl alcohol (acetone-free) ......................50.0 ml
Glycerin (neutral, freshly opened supply) ....50.0 ml
```

Grind the powder in a mortar and weigh. Then place it in the mortar again with a portion of the glycerin and regrind. Pour the upper one-third into a chemically clean flask, add more glycerin, and regrind. Add stopper to flask and place in water bath at 55°C for two hours. Shake (lightly) every half hour. Use part of the alcohol to wash out the mortar. Remove the mixture from the bath at the end of the two hours, cool, and add alcohol washings from mortar. After stain has ripened for about two weeks it is ready for use. The undissolved portion can be filtered or may settle out. The solution can be placed in a dropper bottle.

Buffer solution (pH 7.2):

```
Na2HPO4 (anhydrous) ...........................6.77 g
KH2PO4.........................................2.59 g
Distilled water to.................................1,000 ml
```

Staining solution:

```
Stain solution (stock) ...............................2.0 ml
Buffer solution .........................................6.0 ml
(Mix well before using)
```

Acridine orange stain: See reference for procedure under (Chick, 1961).

Other staining methods: Additional staining techniques, including Gomori methenamine-silver nitrate technique, Gridley histologic stain, and others, are described in various references and textbooks.

Selected References

Borelli D, Salas J. 1975. El empleo del azul tripan en sustitución del azul algodón en micologia. Rev. Latinoamer. Microbiol. 17:185 Chick EW. 1961. Acridine orange fiuorescent stain for fungi. Arch. Dermatol. 3:305

Cohen MM. 1954. A simple procedure for staining tinea versicolor with fountain pen ink. Appl. Microbiol. 17:486

Cunningham JL. 1972. A miracle mounting fluid for permanent whole-mounts of microfungi. Mycologia 64:906

Gordon A. 1951. Rapid permanent staining and mounting of skin scraping and hair. Arch. Dermatol. Syph. 63:343

Gridley MF. 1953. A stain for fungi in tissue sections. Am. J. Clin. Pathol. 23:303

Kaplan W, Kaufman L. 1961. The application of fluorescent antibody techniques to medical mycology—a review. Sabouraudia 1: 137

Keddie F, Orr A, Liebes D. 1961. Direct staining on vinyl plastic tape, demonstration of the cutaneous flora of the epidermis by the strip method. Sabouraudia 1:108

Kligman AM, Mescon H. 1950. The periodic acid-Schiff stain for demonstration of fungi in animal tissues. J. Bacteriol. 60:415

Littman ML. 1949. Improved slide culture technique for study and identification of pathogenic fungi. Am. J. Clin. Pathol. 19:278

McGinnis ML. 1974. Preparation of temporary or permanent mounts of microfungi with undisturbed conidia. Mycologia 66:169

Padhye AA. 1969. Cellophane mounts of ascigerous states of dermatophytes and other keratinophilic fungi. Mycologia 60:1242.

Riddell RW. 1950. Permanent stained mycological preparations obtained by slide culture. Mycologia 42:265

Sharvill D. 1952. The periodic acid-Schiff stain in the diagnosis of dermatomycosis. Br. J. Dermatol. 64:329

Swartz JH, Medrek TF. 1969. Rapid contrast stain as a diagnostic aid for fungus infections. Arch. Dermatol. 99:494

Taschdjian CL. 1954. Simplified technique for growing fungi in slide culture. Mycologia 46:681

MEDIA

Materials from suspected cases of mycotic infection should be cultured, even though direct examination of the material fails to reveal the presence of a fungus. Routinely, cultures should be made on appropriate media (see Table 1) and incubated at 24° to 30°C (37°C if the infection is thought be a subcutaneous or systemic type). Skin, nail, or hair specimens from cases of dermatomycoses are usually isolated on Sabouraud glucose agar slants or plates with the addition of cycloheximide and chloramphenicol (commercial brands: Mycobiotic Agar, or Mycosel) or on Dermatophyte Test Medium at 24° to 30°C.

MEDIA FOR PRIMARY ISOLATION OF FUNGI FROM CLINICAL SPECIMENS

Media can be obtained commercially in dehydrated form. Addition of antibiotics is desirable in some cases.

Brain heart infusion agar (commercially prepared): For isolating fungi and for maintaining the yeast phase of some of the systemic fungi, with or without blood, at 37°C.

Brain heart infusion agar, biphasic vented blood culture bottles: For isolation of yeasts and other fungi from blood (Roberts et al, 1976).

Formula:

    Brain-heart infusion....................................37 g
    Agar..17 g
    Distilled water..1,000 ml

Procedure:

Boil the medium to liquify the agar, pour 50 ml into a bottle and cap with a rubber stopper. Sterilize and slant. After 24 hours prepare a solution of brain heart broth and add 60 ml of the sterile medium through a sterile hypodermic needle into the rubber stopper.

Commercial sources of media for recovery of fungi from blood include: biphasic blood culture systems (Septi-Chek, Roche Laboratories), radiometric detection systems (Bactec 460, Johnston Laboratories), nonradiometric detection systems (Bactec NR 660, Johnston Laboratories), and lysis centrifugation (Isolator, DuPont deNemours).

Brain heart infusion agar with cycloheximide (Actidione) and chloramphenicol (Chloromycetin.) For primary isolation of *Histoplasma capsulatum* and *Blastomyces dermatitidis* at room temperature (24°–30°C). At 37°C the yeast phases of dimorphic fungi should be grown without cycloheximide in the medium.

Formula:

    Brain-heart infusion...................................37.0 g
    Cycloheximide...0.5 g
    Chloramphenicol.......................................0.05 g
    Agar...20.0 g
    Distilled water..1,000 ml

50 ml of sheep blood may be added aseptically when the medium is cooled to 50°C before dispensing.

Dermatophyte Test Medium: (Taplin et al, 1969): Color indicator medium for presumptive identification of dermatophytes. Most dermatophytes produce a red color in the medium while most saprophytic fungi, yeasts, and bacteria do not modify the yellow color. Subculture needs to be made on Sabouraud agar or other medium for identification.

Formula:

Phytone ....10.0 g
Glucose...10.0 g
Agar..20.0 g
Phenol red solution ....40.0 ml
HCl, 0.8 M 6.0ml
Cycloheximide......................................0.5 g
Gentamicin sulfate ....100 ug/ml
Chlortetracycline HCl........................100 ug/ml

Preparation:

Ingredients must be obtained from sources indicated. Substitution of other brands changes the specificity and effectiveness of the medium:

1. Add the phytone, dextrose, and agar to 1,000 ml of distilled water and boil to dissolve the agar.

2. Add 40 ml of phenol red solution while stirring. (Phenol red solution: 0.5 g of Bacto-phenol red dissolved in 15 ml of 0.1 N NaOH made up to 100 ml with glass-distilled water.)

3. Adjust pH of medium by adding 6 ml of 0.8 M HCl while stirring.

4. Dissolve 0.5 g of cycloheximide in 2 ml of acetone and add to hot medium while stirring.

5. Dissolve gentamicin sulfate in 2 ml of glass-distilled water and add to medium while stirring.

6. Autoclave at 12 lb pressure for ten minutes and cool to approximately 47°C.

7. Dissolve chlortetracycline in 25 ml of sterile glass-distilled water in sterile flask. Add to medium while stirring.

8. Dispense 8-ml amounts in sterile 1-oz screw-cap bottles, slant, and cool. The final pH is about 5.5 and the medium should be yellow in color.

9. For maximum shelf life, store in refrigerator.

Procedure:

Microscopic features must be checked for positive identification, although a nonmycologist can now recognize most dermatophytes by the red color change in the colony. If there is bacterial or soil contamination on the skin or nails, the surface must be cleaned first or the medium loses its value as too many contaminants increase the number of false positives. Organisms contributing to false-positive results may be some of the saprophytic fungi, yeasts, and bacteria. Cultures should be incubated at 22° to 30°C with the caps loose for up to 14 days before the color is evaluated for change from yellow to red for the dermatophytes.

Niger (thistle) seed agar (Staib's Medium): Colonies of *Cryptococcus neoformans* produce a brown pigment between 24° and 37°C. Other species of *Cryptococcus* and species of *Candida* grow on this medium without pigment production.

Formula:

Glucose...10.0 g
Creatinine...0.78 g
Chloramphenicol...................................0.05 g
Diphenyl (dissolved in 10 ml of
    95% ethanol)....................................0.10 g
Guizotia abyssinica (thistle) seeds ....70.0 g
Agar..20.0 g
Distilled water.......................................1,000 ml

Procedure:

Grind the seeds in a blender after adding 350 ml of water. Autoclave and filter. Bring the volume to 1,000 ml. Add the other constituents except diphenyl. Autoclave and cool to 45°C, then add the 10 ml of diphenyl before pouring plates.

Sabouraud-cycloheximide-chloramphenicol agar[*]: Useful for isolation of pathogenic fungi from clinical materials heavily contaminated with bacteria and saprophytic fungi. Some of the organisms inhibited or partially inhibited by cycloheximide are: *Cryptococcus neoformans, Trichosporon beigelii, Pseudallescheria boydii, Aspergillus fumigatus, Candida krusei, C. tropicalis, C. parapsilosis, Nocardia asteroides,* and many of the agents of phaeohyphomycosis and hyplohyphomyosis.

Formula:

Sabouraud glucose agar, plus 5 g of agar if firmer agar is needed (2% agar content per liter (l) 20.0 g).

Cycloheximide (Actidione) ....0.5 g
Chloramphenicol (Chloromycetin)............0.05 g
Distilled water......................................1,000 ml

[*]Commercial products are: Mycobiotic Agar (Difco, Detroit, MI) and Mycosel Agar (BBL, Cockeysville, MD).

Procedure:

Add the 65 g of dehydrated Sabouraud glucose agar to 1,000 ml of distilled water and heat to boiling. Add and mix 0.05 g of chloramphenicol that has been suspended and heated quickly in 10 ml of 95% alcohol. Add the cycloheximide in a 10-ml acetone solution to the medium and mix well, tube, and autoclave for ten minutes.

Sabouraud glucose agar: For primary isolation and maintenance of cultures. Commercially available. This medium with chloramphenicol or other antibiotics is useful for isolation of opportunistic filamentous fungi in immunosuppressed patients.

Formula:

```
Glucose...................................................40 g
Neopeptone...........................................10 g
Agar.......................................................15 g
Water ............................................1,000 ml
```

Procedure: Adjust pH to 5.6.

The addition of 10 mg of thiamine per liter enhances the growth of some of the dermatophytes, especially *Trichophyton verrucosum*. If the dehydrated product is used or the medium is used for slide cultures, 2% agar should be used to insure a firm dry surface.

Emmons' modification of Sabouraud glucose agar: A lower carbohydrate concentration is more conducive to growth and sporulation. Commercially available.

Formula:

```
Glucose...................................................20 g
Neopeptone...........................................10 g
Agar.......................................................20 g
Distilled water..................................1,000 ml
```

Procedure: Adjust pH to 6.8–7.0 and autoclave.

Sabouraud-Brain-Heart-Infusion (Sabhi) Agar: Sabhi agar is mainly used for the isolation of some of the systemic pathogens including *Histoplasma capsulatum* and *Blastomyces dermatitidis*. The medium is commercially available.

Formula:

```
Calf brain (infusion from) ...........100 g
Beef heart (infusion from) ...........125 g
```

```
Proteose peptone ...........................................5 g
Glucose...........................................................21 g
NaCl...............................................................2.5 g
Na₂HPO₄ .....................................................1.25 g
Agar..............................................................14 g
Distilled water.........................................1,000 ml
```

Procedure:

Mix the ingredients, heat to boiling, and dispense into tubes or bottles and autoclave for 15 min. at 121°C. Aseptically add sterile antibiotics to the medium at 50°C.

Yeast Extract Phosphate Medium: Useful for isolation and sporulation of *Histoplasma capsulatum*, *Blastomyces dermatitidis*, and *Coccidioides immitis*.

Formula (Formerly Smith's systemic fungal medium):

```
Yeast extract ...............................................1 g
Phosphate buffer .........................................2 ml
Agar.............................................................20 g
Distilled water.........................................1,000 ml
```

Procedure:

The medium when in solution has 50 ug/ml of chloramphenicol and 0.5 mg/ml of cycloheximide added. The stock solution of phosphate is made by dissolving 40.0 g of Na₂HPO₄ in 300 ml of distilled water and adding 60.0 g of KH₂PO₄. The pH is about 6.0. Raise the volume to 400 ml and store at 4°C until needed. Autoclave the medium with the 2 ml of phosphate buffer, cool to 45°C, and add streptomycin, 20 ug/ml. To culture specimens, one drop of concentrated NH₄OH (0.05 ml) is added to the surface of the agar and allowed to diffuse.

Special Media for Specific Uses:

Acetate Agar: Useful for sporulation of yeasts.

Formula:

```
Potassium acetate.........................................10 g
Bacto-yeast extract .......................................1 g
Glucose .........................................................0.5
Agar.............................................................20 g
Distilled water.........................................1,000 ml
```

Heat to melt the agar and sterilize for 15 minutes at 121°C.

Alphacel-yeast extract agar (Kwon-Chung, 1973): Used for cleistothecial formation in *Histoplasma capsulatum* and *H. capsulatum* var *duboisii*.

Formula:

> Alphacel......................................20.0 g
> $MgSO_4$......................................1.0 g
> KH_2PO_4....................................1.5 g
> $NaNO_3$......................................1.0 g
> Yeast extract..............................0.5 g
> Agar..20.0 g
> Distilled water......................1,000 ml

After the medium is in solution, adjust the pH to 5.7 with NaOH and autoclave for 20 minutes.

Assimilation medium for carbohydrates: Widely used auxanographic method for identification of genera and species of the yeasts. Many methods are used in laboratories for determination of assimilation patterns, including a carbohydrate-nutrient disk method (Huppert et al, 1975), and a pour plate-disk method (Land et al, 1975). Commercially developed kits are now available for identification of genera and species of yeasts (API 20C, Analytak Products, Inc., Plainview, NY, Minitek System, BBL, Cockeysville, MD, etc).

Formula (modified after Land et al, 1975):

> Agar..20.0 g
> Yeast nitrogen base...................0.67 g
> Distilled water......................1,000 ml

Procedure:

After the medium is put into solution by heating and stirring, add 20 ml of a stock solution of bromcresol purple (1 g/L) and 4 ml of 0.1 N NaOH. The pH should be 7.0 to 7.2. The medium should be dispensed into screw-capped bottles (60 ml) and autoclaved for storage at 4°C for up to six months. The melted medium should be poured with or without a suspension of yeast cells at a temperature of 45°C into petri plates (150 mm × 15 mm). Two or 5 ml of a moderately heavy suspension of yeast cells (McFariand standard of 4–7) is added to the 60 ml of melted medium and poured, or the yeast cells may be streaked on the surface of the plates with a swab.

Carbohydrate disks (0.64 or 1.27 cm): These may be ordered commercially with or without the sugars: Examples of disks are: glucose, maltose sucrose, lactose, galactose, trehalose, inositol, melibiose, cellibiose, raffinose, dulcitol, xylose. The disks may be dispensed on the medium in the petri dish by means of a 12 place dispensor or template. The disks should be approximately 30 mm apart. The cultures should be incubated between 25°–30°C and read after 24 and 48 hours. A change in color and growth around the disk indicates utilization of the carbohydrate.

Asparagine Broth (coccidioidin, histoplasmin broth):

Formula:

> L-asparagine..............................7 g
> Ammonium chloride ....7 g
> K_2HPO_4 anhydrous...............1.31 g
> Ammonium chloride ....7 g
> Sodium citrate ....0.9 g
> $MgSO_4 \cdot 7H_2O$ ....15 g
> Ferric citrate, USP ....0.3 g
> Glucose (cerelose grade)............10 g
> Glycerin......................................25 g
> Distilled water ....1000 g

Dissolve asparagine in 300 ml of hot distilled water at 50°C. To this solution add the salts in order starting with KH_2PO_4 and mixing well for each salt. Add the remaining items . Dispense in a Fernbach culture flask after sterilization. This medium is useful for preparation of fungal antigens. The medium is inoculated with conidia, incubated on a shaker at 25°–30°C for 3 to 4 weeks, then filtered to collect the broth.

Canavanine-glycine-bromthymol blue (CGB) agar. This medium is useful for deparation of the two varieties of *Cryptococcus neoformans*.

Solution A

> Glycine.......................................10 g
> KH_2SO_4 ....1 g
> $MgSO_4$....................................1 g
> Thiamine-HCl ....1 mg
> l-canavanine sulfate (Sigma) ......30 mg
> Distilled water.........................100 ml

Adjust to pH 5.6 and filter sterilize

Solution B

> Sodium bromthymol blue............0.4 g
> Distilled water..........................100 ml

Procedure:

Mix 880 ml of distilled water, 20 ml of solution B, and 20 g of agar. Sterilized for l5 minutes. Add 100 ml of solution A, while the agar is hot. Stir and dispense aseptically in tubes and plates. *C. neoformans* var *gattii* (serotypes B and C) will turn the surface medium blue in 1 to 5 days. *C. neoformans* var. *neoformans* leaves the medium greenish-yellow.

Casein Medium. For differentiation of *Nocardia* and *Actinomadura.* For hydrolysis by fungi.

Formula:

Solution A

> Skim milk (dehydrated or instant nonfat).....10 g
> Distilled water..100 ml

Solution B

> Distilled water..100 ml
> Agar...20 g

Procedure:

Autoclave both solutions separately, cool, and mix together. Pour into petri dishes.

Chlamydospore agar: A commercially prepared medium that is good for chlamydoconidial formation.

Cornmeal agar: Can be used to stimulate chlamydoconidial production in *Candida albicans* (see Cornmeal Tween 80 agar). The addition of 1% glucose to the agar can be used to differentiate *Trichophyton rubrum* and *T. mentagrophytes,* based on pigment formation. Useful in stimulating sporulation of many fungi and for slide culture studies. Commercially available.

Formula:

> Cornmeal ....40 g
> Water ....1,000 ml
> Agar...20 g

Procedure:

Simmer cornmeal and water for one hour. Filter or decant, bring volume up to 1,000 ml and add agar, melt, and filter again if necessary. Autoclave at 121°C for 15 minutes.

Cornmeal (modified) agar: Good for sporulation of many fungi.

Formula:

> Cornmeal agar (commercial) ....17 g

> Glucose..2 g
> Sucrose ....3 g
> Yeast extract ....1 g
> Distilled water ....1,000 ml

Dissolve the ingredients with heat, tube, and autoclave.

Cornmeal Tween 80 agar: See procedure under cornmeal agar . Add 10 g of Tween 80 to the medium to enhance chlamydoconidial formation.

Cysteine blood agar: Useful for development and maintenance of the *Histoplasma capsulatum* yeast form.

Formula:

Add to blood agar base 10% rabbit or sheep blood agar, 1% glucose and 0.1% cysteine.

Czapek's agar: Especially useful in the study of the colony characteristics of *Nocardia* spp., *Penicillium* spp., and *Aspergillus* spp. Commercially available.

Formula:

> Sucrose ....30.0 g
> Sodium nitrate...3.0 g
> Dipotassium phosphate ....1.0 g
> Magnesium sulfate......................................0.5 g
> Potassium chloride......................................0.5 g
> Ferrous sulfate ....0.01 g
> Water ....1,000 ml
> Agar...15.0 g

Preparation:

Add reagents to water, boil until solids are dissolved. Dispense into tubes and autoclave for 15 minutes at 121°C.

L-Dopa medium (Modified Chaskes-Tyndall medium): Useful for identification of *Cryptococcus neoformans.* In 48 to 72 hours both varieties of *C. neoformans* produce chocolate-brown to black colonies.

Formula:

> L-asparagine...1 g
> Glucose..1 g
> KH_2PO_4..3 g
> $MgSO_4 \cdot 7H_2O$ ....0.25 g
> Thiamine HCl...1 mg
> Biotin ....5 ug
> L-dopa...100 mg
> Agar...20 g

Preparation:

Add agar to 900 ml of distilled water and autoclave for 15 minutes. To the remaining 100 ml of distilled water the remaining ingredients except thiamine HCl and adjust the pH to 5.6 then add the vitamins, filter sterilize the cooled agar (50°C). Dispense into plates or sterile tubes.

Fermentation medium for carbohydrates: For use in differentiation of *Candida* spp.

Formula:

```
Beef extract.....................................3.0 g
Peptone..........................................10.0 g
NaCl..............................................5.0 g
Distilled water.......................................1,000 ml
Bromcresol purple, stock solution .............1.0 ml
```

Procedure:

Heat to dissolve, adjust pH to 7.2, tube in 9-ml quantities, and sterilize at 120°C for 15 minutes. Inverted Durham tubes should be placed in test tubes prior to sterilization.

Bromcresol purple solution for stock:
```
Bromcresol purple ........................................1.6 g
Alcohol, 95% .........................................100.0 ml
```

Stock carbohydrate solutions:
10% aqueous solutions of dextrose, maltrose, sucrose, lactose, galactose, and trehalose sterilized by filtration.

Add 1 ml of carbohydrate to one tube containing 9 ml of sterile beef extract broth.

Germ tube: For production of germ tubes (Taschdjian, et al, 1960).

Serum:

Fresh or inactivated human serum and deep-frozen stored serum are satisfactory, as are sheep, rabbit, guinea pig, horse, and bovine sera. Heat-coagulated serum is not satisfactory.

Incolate 0.5 ml of human or sheep serum in a small tube with the organism.

Incubate at 37°C for two to three hours.
Check for germ tubes or short filamentous outgrowths without constrictions from the oval or rounded cells

of *Candida albicans.* The germ tubes are characteristic of this species. A 1% peptone broth is useful for germ tube development.

Gelatin medium: Useful for demonstation of proteolytic activity.

Formula:

```
Gelatin .......................................120 g
Distilled water.......................................1,000 ml
```

Procedure:

Suspend the gelatin in distilled water, heat to boiling. Tube the medium and autoclave for 15 minutes at 121°C. After inoculation with the fungus incubate at 25°C for 7 to 14 days. Place the tubes in a refrigerator for 1 hr before reading. If there is proteolytic activity, the gelatin will remain liquid in the refrigerator. This medium is useful for separation of pathogenic and nonpathogenic *Cladosporium* or other dematiaceous fungi. The pathogenic *Cladosporium* spp. do not liquify gelatin.

Hair-bait technique (Orr, 1969): The addition of cycloheximide with penicillin and streptomycin to sterile distilled water in the hair-bait technique increases the number of keratinophilic fungi recovered from soil samples. Use a moat with mineral oil in cans under each leg of the stand. This will keep mites from entering or leaving.

Procedure:

Soil is placed in sterile petri plates containing 3 × 9-cm filter disk to aid in maintaining moisture. The soil is moistened with sterile distilled water containing 500 µg of penicillin, 300 µg of streptomycin, and 0.5 mg of cycloheximide[1]/ml. The soil is baited with human hair or horsehair (sterilized).

Check hair periodically for about one month. Identify colonies if possible, or place hair with fungal growth on medium with cycloheximide and chloramphenicol. Later identify colonies.

Litmus milk: Medium for actinomycetes, etc.

Formula:

```
Skim milk powder ......................................100 g
Litmus...............................................750 mg
Yeast extract....................................5 g
```

Glucose..3 g
Distilled water...............................1,000 ml

Procedure:

Dissolve, adjust pH to 7.0, tube, and autoclave at 10 lb of pressure. Inoculate, then add the pyrogalol-carbonate seals on cotton plugs, incubate for four weeks at 37°C.

Nitrate assimilation test medium (rapid) for yeasts (Hopkins and Land, 1977): This swab nitrate method yields results in 15 minutes.

Formula (for 5x concentration):

KNO$_3$...2.0g
NaH$_2$PO$_4$................................1.14 g
Zephiran chloride, 17% solution...............1.2 ml
Distilled water................................200 ml

Six-inch cotton swabs are saturated in the 5x concentration with 0.1 ml (equivalent of 0.5 ml of medium). The swabs are dried in vacuum at room temperature for 24 hours, autoclaved, and put into a sealed container for extended storage.

Procedure:

The tip of the swab containing medium is coated with yeasts by sweeping it over yeast colonies several times and then swirling against the bottom of the test tube to imbed the yeast cells into the swab. After incubation for ten minutes at 45°C, the swab is inserted into a second tube containing 2 drops each of a-naphthylamine and sulfanilic acid. The swabs containing all nitrate-positive yeasts turn a bright cherry red.

Oatmeal tomato-paste agar: Useful for ascospore formation in dermatophyes (Weitzman and Silva-Hutner, 1967).

Formula:

Beech-nut baby oatmeal ....10 g
Hunt's tomato paste.....................................10 g
MgSO$_4$ · 7H$_2$O ....1 g
KH$_2$PO$_4$..1 g
NaNO$_3$..1 g
Agar...18 g
Distilled water.......................................1,000 ml

Procedure:

Adjust the pH to 5.6 with NaOH and autoclave for 20 minutes. The tomato paste may be omitted with little loss of ascospore development in dermatophytes with perfect stages.

Paraffin bait technique (Mishra and Randhawa, 1969): *Nocardia asteroides* may be isolated by appplication of the paraffin bait technique. This organism has been isolated repeatedly from soil by this method.

Carbon-free broth formula:

NaNO$_3$..2.0 g
K$_2$HPO$_4$...0.8 g
MgSO$_4$ · 7H$_2$O ....0.5 g
FeCl$_3$..10.0 mg
MnCl$_2$ · 4H$_2$O..8.0 mg
ZnSO$_4$...2.0 mg
Distilled water.......................................1,000 ml

Procedure:

Adjust pH to 7.0.

Homogenize sputa or gastric washings by shaking with glass beads. Mix 2 ml of the homogenized specimen with 5 ml of sterile carbon-free broth, put in a sterile test tube, and introduce a paraffin-coated glass rod (previously immersed for 10 to 12 hours in 95% alcohol) after the alcohol has drained off. Incubate at 37°C. Check growth after one, two, four, and six weeks.

Potato dextrose agar: Useful for spore production. Commercially available.

Formula:

Peeled, diced potatoes, infusion from ....200 g
Glucose...20 g
Agar..15 g (or 20 g)
Distilled water.......................................1,000 ml

Procedure:

Preparation as for cornmeal agar if infusion is made. The use of 2% agar insures a drier surface on the agar medium. For pigment production of *Trichophyton rubrum*. Production of red pigment on this medium is useful in separation of *Trichophyton mentagrophytes* and *T. rubrum*.

Rice grain medium: *Microsporum canis* grows well and forms conidia on this medium while *M. audouinii* grows poorly and forms no conidia.

Formula:

White rice (not enriched)	8.0 g
Distilled water	25.0 ml

Procedure:

Put rice and water into a flask and autoclave for 15 minutes and dispense into plates.

Soil extract agar: Useful for mating *Blastomyces dermatitidis.*
Formula:

Garden soil	500 g
Tap water	1,200 ml

Autoclave the water and soil for 3 hr at 121°C, and filter while hot through a Whatman No. 2 filter paper. Add water to the supernatant to make the volume of the filtrate at 1,000 ml.

Soil filtrate	1,000 ml
Glucose	2 g
Yeast extract	1 g
KH_2PO_4	0.5 g
Agar	15 g

Adjust the pH to 7.0. Dispense 8.0 ml into test tubes and autoclave for 15 minutes at 121°C.

Starch hydrolysis test medium:

Formula:

Heart infusion broth	25 g
Casitone	4 g
Yeast extract	5 g
Soluble starch	5 g
Agar	15 g
Distilled water	1,000 ml

Procedure:

Heat until ingredients are dissolved, adjust the pH to 7, and autoclave at 121°C for 15 minutes. Inoculate and incubate for 7 to 14 days. Pour Grams iodine over the plate or tube. A clear halo will form around the colony, indicating starch has been hydrolyzed.

Sucrose-yeast extract agar: This medium is useful for mating *Filobasidiella* species.

Formula:

Sucrose	20 g
Biotin	5.0 ug
Yeast extract	0.5 g
KH_2PO_4	1 g
$MgSO_4$	0.5 g
$CaCl_2$	0.1 g
NaCl	0.1 g
Agar	40 g
Distilled water	1,000 ml

Procedure:

Dissolve sucrose, biotin, yeast extract in 100 ml of distilled water and filter sterilize. Add the rest of the ingredients to 900 ml of distilled water and sterilize. Add the sucrose solution aseptically to the cooled agar base and dispense.

Thioglycollate medium: For primary isolation of *Actinomyces* species.

Formula:

Trypticase	20.0 g
NaCl	5.0 g
Dipotassium phosphate	2.0 g
Sodium thioglycollate	1.0 g
Methylene blue	0.002 g
Agar	0.5 g
Distilled water	1,000 ml

Trichophyton agars for species identification (Georg and Camp, 1957):

1. Casein agar base

Formula:

Casamino acid, vitamin free	2.5 g
Glucose	40.0 g
$MgSO_4$	0.1 g
KH_2PO_4	1.8 g

Agar...20.0 g
Distilled water up to ....1,000 ml

Procedure:

Adjust pH to 6.8. Heat to dissolve ingredients, tube or put in flasks, and sterilize.

2. Casein agar base plus inositol

Formula:

Casein agar base
i-inositol ....50.0 µg/ml of medium

3. Casein agar base plus thiamine-inositol

Formula:

Casein agar base
Thiamine hydrochloride ..,.0.2 µg/ml of medium
i-inositol ....50.0 µg/ml of medium

4. Casein agar base plus thiamine

Formula:

Casein agar base
Thiamine hydrochloride ....0.2 µg/ml of medium

5. Casein agar base plus nicotinic acid

Formula:

Casein agar base
Nicotinic acid ....2.0 µg/ml of medium

6. Ammonium nitrate agar base

Formula:

Same as that for casein agar base except substitute 1.5 g of NH_4NO_3 for casamino acid.

7. Ammonium nitrate agar base plus histidine

Formula:

Ammonium nitrate agar base
Histidine.........................30.0 µg/ml of medium

Stock solutions of vitamins: After sterilizing for ten minutes, store at 5°C.

Histidine solution......150 mg/100 ml of distilled water

Inositol solution—250 mg/100 ml of distilled water

Nicotinic acid solution—10 mg/100 ml of distilled water

Thiamine solution—10 mg/1,000 ml of distilled water at a pH of 4 to 5.

Urease test medium (Philpot, 1967): Useful for separation of *Trichophyton mentagrophytes* from *T. rubrum*. Within seven days *T. mentagrophytes* strains should hydrolyze urea and the medium becomes deep red, while action of *T. rubrum* is less rapid.

Formula (modification of Christensen's test medium):

Peptone...1 g
NaCl...5 g
KH_2PO_4 ....2 g
Glucose..5 g
Agar...20 g
Distilled water...............................1,000 ml

Procedure:

Dissolve by heat, add 5 ml of phenol red solution (0.2% in 50% alcohol). Autoclave at 115°C for 15 minutes, cool, and add 100 ml of urea (20% aqueous solution, sterilized by filtration). Tube and slant. Place a small amount of colony in the medium and incubate at 24° to 26°C. Read in seven days. A deep-red color through the medium is a positive reaction.

Urea medium: Species of *Cryptococcus* are urease positive (+); occasionally *Rhodotorula* spp. are positive. *Trichophyton mentagrophytes* also produces urease, although not one hundred perent of the time.

Procedure:

Prepare 100 ml of urea agar base and sterilize by filtering. A second medium contining 15 gm of agar in 900 ml of distilled water is heated to dissolve the agar, and sterilized before the urea agar base is added, which should be done when the second medium has cooled to about 50°C. The medium is put in tubes and slanted (Seeliger, 1955). Development of red color denotes positive urease reaction.

V-8 juice agar (neutral): Used for mating *Filobasidiella neoformans*.

Formula:

> V-8 juice......................................50 ml
> KH$_2$PO$_4$...................................0.5 g
> Agar..40 g
> Distilled water...........................1,000 ml

Adjust the pH to 7.2 and autoclave at 121°C for 30 minutes then dispense into plates.

Tyrosine or xanthine agar: For aerobic actinomycetes.

Formula

> Nutrient agar ....23 g
> Tyrosine.......................................5 g
>   or
> Xanthine..4 g
> Demineralized water......................1,000 ml

Procedure:

Dissolve the nutrient agar in 500 ml of water and add either tyrosine or xanthine and mix. Make up to 1 l and distribute crystals evenly. Adjust pH to 7.0. Autoclave for 15 minutes at 121°C. Pour into plates with crystals distributed evenly in the medium.

Serologic Techniques

Serologic techniques employing a patient's serum or cerebrospinal fluid have proved to be of great value in recent years in the diagnosis and prognosis of fungal infections. An excellent coverage on serodiagnosis of fungal disease is covered by Kaufman and Reiss (1992). Three areas are discussed: immunologic procedures, antigen detection, and identification of fungi. The tests discussed are: complement fixation (CF), counterimmunoelectrophoresis (CIE), enzyme immuno assay (EIA), immunodiffusion (ID), latex agglutination (LA), radioimmunoassay (RIA), and tube agglutination. For more detailed information on the serology of aspergillosis, blastomycosis, coccidioidomycosis, histoplasmosis, and candidosis see serology in the chapters on these diseases. Test kits are available from the following commerical sources: Greer Laboratories, Inc., Lenoir, NC; Hollister-Stier Laboratories, Spokane, Wash.; Immuno-Mycologics, Inc., Norman, OK; Meridian Diagnostics, Inc., Cincinnati, OH, M.A. Bioproducts, Walkersville, MD; and Nolan-Scott Biological Laboratories, Inc., Tucker, GA.

The complement fixation test is more difficult technically and requires more time and special training. Most state departments of health and the Center for Disease Control, Atlanta, may be contacted for assistance in these serologic techniques.

Exoantigen Test

At times clinical laboratories may have isolates of *Histoplasma capsulatum*, *Blastomyces dermatitidis*, *Coccidioides immitis*, and *Paracoccidioides brasiliensis* that fail to sporulate or are not typical. Some isolates of *H. capsulatum* are difficult to convert to the yeast form. Exoantigen testing is useful for these variants that occur in fungi. Preparation of the exoantigen is as follows:

1. A mature fungus culture is covered with 5 to 10 ml of an aqueous merthiolate solution, 1:5,000. The culture is left for 24 hours at 25°C to ensure killing.

2. Filter the solution with the exoantigen through a 0.45 um size membrane filter inside a safety hood.

3. The filtered extracts should be concentrated to 50x for *H. capsulatum* and *B. dermatitidis* and to 25x for *C. immitis* with a Minicon B-15 concentrator (Amicon Co, Lexington, MA).

4. The concentrated extract is placed into microdiffusion wells next to the control antigen well and is allowed to react with a control antiserum from commercial sources (Immunomycologic, Meridian Diagnostics, and Scott-Nolan Laboratories).

5. After 24 hrs at 25°C the ID plates are checked for the presence of precipitin bands of identity with the reference reagents.

C. immitis may be identified with the presence of the DF, TP or HL antigens while *B. dermatitidis* and *H. capsulatum* are identified by the presence of H or M bands.

DNA Probes

Four commercially available acridinium ester-labeled DNA probes directed against rRNA have been evaluated for *B. dermatitidis*, *C. immitis*, *H. capsulatum*, and *C. neoformans* in culture. The specificity and sensitivity for all four fungi were near 100%. The high sensitivities and specificities of the probes with less than one hour to perform the assay and the availability of standardized reagent kits make the acridinium ester-labeled DNA probes very useful in laboratories in need of a rapid,accurate method for identification of the fungal pathogens. The probes are useful to identify these fungal pathogens as soon as colonies appear on the primary recovery media. Commercially available

AccuProbes are available from GenProbes, San Diego, CA.

In Vitro Antifungal Susceptibility Tests

Antifungal dilution tests are important to determine the MIC and/or the lowest concentration of antifungal agents required to inhibit or kill a particular kind of fungus. Due to the wide variations in antifungal tests in different laboratories it became necessary to work on a standardization of the test for yeasts and other fungi. A Subcommittee on Antifungal Susceptibility Testing has been established. The objective of the National Committee for Clinical Laboratory Standards (NCCLS) was to study the standardization of antifungal susceptibility testing by laboratories and develop recommendations. A standardization recommendation has been made for antifungal susceptibility testing of yeasts. Announcements and publications are published by NCCLS, 771 E. Lancaster Ave, Villanova, PA, 19085.

Selected References

Bille J, Edson RS, Roberts GD. 1984. Clinical evaluation of the lysis-centrifugation blood culture system for the detection of fungemia and comparison with a conventional biphasic broth blood culture system. J. Clin. Microbiol. 19:126.

Bojalil LF, Cerbon J. 1959. Scheme for the differentiation of *Nocardia asteroides* and *Nocardia brasiliensis.* J. Bacteriol. 78:852

Borelli D, Salas J. 1975. El empleo del azul tripan en sustitución dei azul algodón en micologia. Rev. Latinoamer. Microbiol. 17:185

Campbell CC. 1945. Use of Francis' glucose cystine blood agar in the isolation and cultivation of *Sporotrichum schenckii.* J Bacteriol 50:233

Caplan LM, Merz WG. 1978. Evaluation of two commercially prepared biphasic media for recovery of fungi from blood. J. Clin. Microbiol. 8:469

Connel SL, Padgett DE. 1988. An improved technique for making permanent slide cultures of fungi. Mycopathologia 101:165

Evron R. Ganor, S. 1968. The use of sodium taurocholate medium for identifying *Candida albicans.* J. Invest. Dermatol. 51:108

Florek KK, Rogers AL. 1978. Viability of lactophenol exposed endospores and spherules of *Coccidioides immitis* (Abst). Annual Meetings, American Society of Microbiology, Las Vegas

Fromtling RA, et al. 1993. Multicenter evaluation of a broth macrodilution antifungal susceptibility tests for yeasts. Antimicrob. Agents Chemother. 37:39

Georg LK, Ajello L, Papageorge C. 1954. Use of cyclohex-

imide in the selective isolation of fungi pathogenic to man. J. Lab. Clin. Med. 44:422

Georg LK, Camp LB. 1957. Routine nutritional test for the identification for dermatophytes. J. Bacteriol. 74: 113

Gorman JW. 1967. Sabhi, a new culture medium for pathogenic fungi. Am. J. Med. Tech. 33:151

Hopkins JM, Land GA. 1977. Rapid method for determining nitrate utilization by yeasts. J. Clin. Microbiol. 5:497

Hageage GJ, Harrington BJ. 1984. Use of calcofluor white in clinical mycology. Lab. Med. 15:109

Huppert M, Harper G, Sun SH, et al. 1975. Rapid methods for identification of yeasts. J. Clin. Microbiol. 2:21

Joshi KR, Gavin JB, Bremner DA. 1973. The formation of germ tubes by *Candida albicans* in various peptone media. Sabouraudia 11:259

Kaufman L, Reiss, E. 1992. Serodiagnosis of fungal diseases. *In* Rose, NF, Friedman, H (eds). *Manual of Clinical Immunology.* Am. Soc. Microbiol. 2nd ed. Washington , DC

Kaufman L, Standard PG. 1978. Improved version of the exoantigen test for identification of *Coccidioides immitis* and *Histoplasma capsulatum* cultures. J. Clin. Microbiol. 8:42

Kwon-Chung KJ, Poacheck J, Bennett JE. 1982. Improved diagnostic medium for separation of *Cryptococcus neoformans* var *neoformans* (serotytes A and C), and *Cryptococcus neoformans* var. *Gatti* (serotypes B and C). J. Clin. Microbiol. 15:535.

Land GA, Vinton EC, Adcock GB, et al. 1975. Improved auxanographic method for yeast assimilations: A comparison with other approaches. J. Clin. Microbiol. 2:206

Lombardi, et al. 1989. Exoantigen tests for the rapid and specific identification of *Apophysomyces elegans* and *Saksenaea vasiformis.* J. Med. Vet. Mycol. 27:113.

Mishra SK, Randhawa HS. 1969. Application of paraffin bait technique to the isolation of *Nocardia asteroides* from clinicai specimens. Appl. Microbiol. 18:686

Orr GF. 1969. Keratinophilic fungi isolated from soil by a modified hair bait technique. Sabouraudia 7:129.

PER. 1992. *Guide to OSHA Requirements.* Address: PER, 818 Olive St, Suite 918, St. Louis, MO 63101

Philpot C. 1967. The differentiation of *Trichophyton mentagrophytes* from *T. rubrum* by a simple urease test. Sabouraudia 5:189.

Roberts JA, Counts JM, Creselius HG. 1970. Production in vitro of *Coccidioides immitis* spherules and endospores as a diagnostic aid. Am. Rev. Resp. Dis. 102:811

Seeliger, H. 1955. Ein neues Medium zür Pseudomycelbildung von *Candida albicans.* Zeitschr. Hygiene 141:488

Smith CD, Goodman NL. 1975. Improved culture method for the isolation of *Histoplasma capsulatum* and *Blastomyces dermatiditis* from contaminated specimens. Am. J. Clin. Pathol. 63:276

Stockman L, Clark KA, Hunt JM., Roberts GD. 1993. Evaluation of commercially available acridinium ester-labeled chemiluminescent DNA probes for culture identification of *Blastomyces dermatitidis, Coccidioides immitis, Cryptococcus neoformans,* and *Histoplasma capsulatum.* J. Clin. Microbiol. 31:845.

Sun SH, et al. 1976. Rapid in vitro conversion and identification of *Coccidioides immitis.* J. Clin. Microbiol. 3: 186.

Taplin D, Azias N, Rebell G, Blank H. 1969. Isolation and recognition of dermatophytes on a new medium (DTM). Arch Dermatol 99:203.

Taschdjian CL. 1954. Simplified technique for growing fungi in slide culture. Mycologia 46:681

Wiegand SE, Ulrich JA, Winkelmann RK. 1968. Diagnosis of superficial pathogenic fungi; use of ink blue method. Mayo. Clin. Proc. 43:795

ANIMAL INOCULATIONS

Inoculation of the laboratory animal is of value in establishing the pathogenicity of fungi as well as in observing the tissue phase characteristics of some of the pathogenic fungi. In some cases, infected material that fails to grow in culture may cause disease symptoms in the animals. Specific information on animal inoculation is given under laboratory procedures for each pathogenic fungus.

Types of Animals Used

Some commonly used laboratory animals are mice, guinea pigs, rabbits, and hamsters.

Method of Inoculation

Animals are inoculated either intracerebrally, intravenously, intraperitorneally, or intratesticularly with saline suspensions of the organism by means of a syringe and the proper size needle. Equipment should be sterilized before and after use, and care should be taken to see that all of the suspension is put into the animal. For mice, the following quantities of a saline suspension may be sufficient for injection, depending upon concentrations:

Intracerebral: About 0.25 ml in a tuberculin syringe with a 26-gauge needle. The needle is inserted posteriorly to the right of the midline of the skull, penetrating only slightly inside.

Intravenous: 0.2 ml or less, depending on concentration, with a 1 ml or smaller syringe and a 26-gauge needle. The inoculum should be injected into one of the four veins in the mouse's tail.

Intraperitoneal: About 0.5 ml in a 1-ml or larger syringe and a 24-gauge needle. The needle is inserted through the skin and peritoneum, but not deep into the abdominal cavity.

Animals should be sacrificed periodically to observe the course of the infection.

Gastric mucin

A 5% hog gastric mucin may enhance the virulence of the fungi when the suspension is inoculated I.P. into the animal.

Procedure:

1. Put 5 g of gastric mucin in 95 ml of distilled water; emulsify with a blender for five minutes.

2. Autoclave for 15 minutes at 120°C; cool

3. Adjust pH to 7.3 with NaOH (sterile).

4. Check for sterility and store in refrigerator.

5. Use equal parts of the gastric mucin and the fungus suspension and inject the mixture (1 ml) intraperitoneally into the laboratory animal.

Isolation of Pathogenic Fungi from Soil Utilizing Mice

Soil screening through laboratory animals, especially mice, has been one of the most fruitful methods for increasing knowledge concerning the natural habitats of pathogenic fungi. A number of modified procedures have been used, including variations in the ratio of the soil sample to the physiologic saline solution, variations in antibiotics used, and variations in length of time the mice are held prior to sacrifice and culture of fungi from internal organs.

Procedure for isolation (Ajello, 1960; Emmons, 1961):

1. Press the open mouth of a sterile 4 oz screw-cap bottle or large test tube against the surface of the soil and scoop up a sample.

2. Make up a soil and physiologic saline solution in the proportion of about 1:5, without antibiotics.

3. After thoroughly stirring or shaking the suspension of soil, allow the sample to settle for about one hour.

4. Remove an 8 ml portion of the supernatant and combine it with 2 ml of an antibiotic solution (2 mg streptomycin and 5 mg penicillin per ml of water).

5. Inject 1 ml suspensions intraperitoneally into a total of five mice.

6. Sacrifice the mice in one month.

7. Isolate portions of infected spleen, omentum, liver, or other organs on modified Sabouraud agar with antibiotics, or another medium. Mince the tissue with scissors, spread with inoculating needle, and incubate at 24°C for four weeks.

Cultures may be placed on a moat to prevent infecting mites from spreading to other cultures. The legs of a shelf or table can be placed in cans containing mineral oil. No mites can enter the moat.

Selected References

Ajello L. 1960 *Histoplasma capsulatum* soil studies. Mykosen 3:43

Burrell R. 1970. Improved device for the administration of fungal spores to small animals via the respiratory route. Appl. Microbiol. 20:984

Emmons CW. Isolation of *Histoplasma capsulatum* from soil in Washington, DC. Pub Health Rep. 76:591

Haley LD. 1964. *Diagnostic Medical Mycology.* Appleton-Century-Crofts, New York, Ch. 20

Huppert M, Sun SH, Gross AJ. 1972. Evaualtion of an experimental animal model for testing antifungal substances. Antimicrob. Agents. Chemother. 1:367

Strauss RE, Kligman AM. 1951. The use of gastric mucin to lower resistance of laboratory animals to systemic fungus infections. J. Infect. Dis. 88:151

Vogel RA, Conant NF. 1952. The cultivation of *Coccidioides immitis* in the embryonated hen's egg. J. Bacteriol. 64:83

MAINTENANCE OF STOCK CULTURES OF FUNGI

There are several ways to maintain culture collections. With the exception of lyophilization and cryogenic storage, all methods are easy and do not demand special equipment

Room temperature (22° to 24°C): Stock cultures are maintained in racks or baskets for up to three months before subculturing. The length of time before the medi-um dries out with consequent death of the culture varies, depending upon the type of plug, relative humidity, and the size of the test tube. A sealed or capped tube will not dry out as rapidly.

Sterile distilled water: After cultures are grown on potato dextrose agar slants for two weeks at 25°C, 6 to 7 ml of sterile distilled water is pipetted aseptically into each tube. The spores and some hyphae are disolved by the same pipette, transferred into a sterile, glass, 1 g vial, and the cap tightened. The labeled vials are stored at 25°C. Survival time varies from ten or more years.

Refrigeration (5° to 10°C or lower): Stock cultures may be maintained for up to four months before they are transferred to new slants. Capped tubes or sealed tubes usually may be kept for six months. Some of the *Trichophyton* species that do not produce microconidia readily, *Epidermophyton floccosum,* and *Microsporum audouinii* should be maintained at room temperature, as they usually die when refrigerated.

Deep Freeze (–20°C or lower): This method is satisfactory for most fungi that sporulate. After growth of the fungus on phytone yeast extract agar, as recommended by Carmichael (1962), or on other media, such as mycophil agar, for 10 to 14 days, the tubes with caps tightened are placed in the freezer at approximately –20°C. Viability should be maintained for a number of years.

Mineral oil: The stock culture is maintained by pouring sterile mineral oil (Saybolt viscosity 330 at 100° F) over the entire agar slant containing an actively growing colony. The entire agar surface must be completely covered to prevent loss of water from the medium. The culture may be viable for up to twenty years if slant is kept in an upright position at 25°C.

To make a transfer, a small portion of the fungus is removed from below the surface of the mineral oil and, after excess oil drains off, is placed in a new agar slant.

About 100 ml of mineral oil in a flask should be sterilized for 45 minutes at 120°C before use.

Lyophilization: This method is excellent to preserve certain types of fungi in a stable condition for an indefinite number of years. Many small-spored fungi, such as *Penicillium* spp., *Aspergillus* spp., some of the yeasts, *Actinomyces* spp., and other microorganisms, have been preserved for years by this method. A number of large-spored or poorly sporulating pathogenic fungi are not suitable for lyophilization. The procedure is described in Bosmans (1974), Hesseltine (1960), and Raper and Alexander (1945).

Cryogenic storage: This method is increasing in usage as small liquid nitrogen refrigerators are presently available for a reasonable price. This method is particularly useful for organisms that do not survive well when lyophilized. More information may be found in Hwang (1966) and Muggelton (1964).

Selected References

Bosmans J. 1974. Ten years lyophilization of pathogenic fungi. Mycopathologia 53: 13

Butterfield W, Jong SC, Alexander MT. 1974. Preservation of living fungi pathogenic for man and animals. Can J. Microbiol. 20: 1665

Carmichael JW. 1962. Viability of mold cultures stored at -20 C. Mycologia 54:432

Hartung de Capriles C, Mata S, Middelveen M. 1989. Preservation of fungi in water (Castellani): 20 years. Mycopathologia 106:73

Hesseltine CW, Bradle BJ, Benjamin CR. 1960. Further investigations on the preservation of molds. Mycologia 52:762

Hwang SW. 1976. Investigation of ultralow temperature for fungal cultures. III. Viability and growth rates of mycelial cultures following cryogenic storage. Mycologia 68:377

Nakase T, et al. 1989. Maintenance of yeasts on agar under mineral oil: 20 years storage.

Odds FC. 1991. Long-term laboratory preservation of pathogenic yeasts in water. J. Med. Vet. Mycology 29:413

Pasarell L, McGinnis MR. 1992. Viability of fungal cultures maintained at -70°C. J. Clin. Microbiol. 330:1000

Raper KB, Alexander DF. 1945. Preservation of molds by the lyophil process. Mycologia 37:499

Schipper MA, Bekker-Holtman J. 1976. Viability of lyophilized fungal cultures. Anton van Leeuwenhock 42:525

Tesh RB, Schneidau JD, Erwin CA. 1967. The effect of freezing and storage at -24°C on the survival of pathogenic fungi in excised tissue. Am. J. Clin. Pathol. 48: 100

Werhanm CC. 1946. Mineral oil as a fungus culture preservative. Mycologia 38:691

Chapter 4

SUPERFICIAL MYCOSES

The superficial infections include diseases that elicit few complaints, with patients being concerned primarily due to cosmetic effects. The superficial mycoses include otomycosis, black piedra, white piedra, pityriasis versicolor, and tinea nigra. Trichomycosis axillaris, a bacterial infection, is included for comparative purposes.

OTOMYCOSIS

(External otitis, myringomycosis, fungus ear, hot weather ear)

Definition

Otomycosis is a mild or chronic infection of the external ear characterized by itching, inflammation, and an accumulation of large masses of epithelial debris containing either bacteria or fungi, or both. (Figure 33).

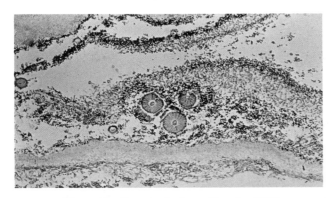

Figure 33. Otomycosis *Aspergillus niger* X200

Etiologic agents

A total of 53 species of fungi have been reported as agents of otomycosis. Probably less than 10% of cases are caused by fungi as the primary invaders. Some of the more frequently reported genera are *Aspergillus, Penicillium, Mucor,* and *Rhizopus.* Bacteria most frequently isolated as the primary cause are species of *Pseudomonas, Micrococcus, Staphylococcus, Streptococcus, Proteus,* and others.

Occurrence

Humans: The disease is worldwide in distribution, especially in tropical and subtropical regions, and is prevalent in the southern and southwestern parts of the United States.

Animals: Otomycosis does occur and probably is due to many of the same organisms as occurs in humans.

Laboratory Procedures

Specimen collection: Use techniques to avoid contamination. Under the supervision of a physician, especially in the case of deep-seated infections, the exudate and debris should be removed and streaked on culture media as soon as possible or placed in a sterile vial for examination as soon as facilities are available.

Direct examination: Place the epithelial debris on a slide in a drop of 10% KOH and examine after adding a coverglass. The exudate should be stained by Gram's method (see staining procedures, page 34) and examined for the presence of bacteria.

Microscopically, fungi should appear in the KOH preparation as fragments of mycelium, with or without branches and septa, and in some cases conidiophores and conidia or sporangiophore and spores may be present. Direct demonstration is diagnostically more accurate than culture, as contaminants may be present.

Microscopically, bacteria present on the stained slide may be *Pseudomonas* or *Proteus* if Gram-negative, or *Streptococcus* or *Micrococcus,* if Gram-positive. Coliforms, bacilli, diphtheroids, and others may be present on the stained slide. Cultures should be made for identification of the organisms.

Cultures: For fungi, the material from the ear should be streaked on Sabouraud glucose agar plates or slants and held for two to three weeks, as most saprophytic fungi develop during this time. Remove a portion of the colony and place on a slide with lactophenol; if too thick, tease apart and place on a coverglass. The cellophane tape coverglass mount will keep more of the reproductive structures of the fungus intact for identification. Look for conidiophores (or sporangiophores) and conidia (or spores), septate or nonseptate hyphae, or any other clues for identification of the saprophytic fungus. Check the section on contaminant fungi in this manual or reference books that contain descriptions of thousands of species in the Deuteromycota (Fungi Imperfecti) for identifications. In many cases, isolates will be species of *Aspergillus, Penicillium, Mucor,* or *Rhizopus.* In some cases, pathogenic fungi causing dermatomycosis have been isolated.

For bacteria, suitable media, such as nutrient agar, tryptose soybean broth, blood agar, should be streaked and incubated at 37°C. The predominant organism or organisms should be identified. If *Staphylococcus* is the predominant organism, a coagulase test should be run; if results are positive, the organism is considered pathogenic. Sensitivity tests to penicillin, streptomycin, terramycin, chloromycetin, erythromycin, sulfanilamide, sulfadiazine, and other antibiotics that are available should be run to determine the proper choice for treatment, as many organisms have become resistant to these therapeutic agents.

Animal inoculation: Not necessary for establishing pathogenicity.

Questions

1. Why is otomycosis an inaccurate description for this disease?

2. Of what value are bacterial sensitivity tests to physicians?

Selected References

Bezjak V, Arya OP. 1970. Otomycosis due to *Aspergillus niger.* E. Afr. Med. J. 47:247

Haley LD. 1952. Etiology of otomycosis. **I.** Mycologic flora of the ear. **II.** Bacterial flora of the ear. **III.** Observations on attempts to induce otomycosis in rabbits. **IV.** Clinical observations. Arch. Otolaryngol. 52:202, 208, 214, 220

Jones EH, McLain PG. 1962. Fungal infections of external ear canal. South Med. J. 55:910

Jones EH. 1965. *External Otitis: Diagnosis and Treatment.* Charles C. Thomas, Springfield, IL

Kingery FA. 1965. The myth of otomycosis. JAMA 191:129

McGonigle JJ, Jillson OF. 1967. Otomycosis: An entity. Arch. Dermatol. 95:45

Rush-Munro FM. 1966. *Allescheria boydii (Monosporium apiospermum)* associated with cases of otomycosis in New Zealand. NZJ Med. Lab. Tech. 20:3

Singer DE, Freeman E, Hoffert WR, et al. 1952. Otitis externa. Bacteriological and mycological studies. Ann Otol. Rhinol. Laryngol. 61:317

Stuart EA, Blank F. 1955. Aspergillosis of the ear. A report of twenty-nine cases. Can. Med. Assoc. J. 72:334

Talwar P, Chakrabarti A, Poonamjit K, Mittal AM, Mehra YN. 1988. Fungal infections of the ear with special reference to chronic suppurative otitis media. Mycopathologia 104(1):47

Thorne E, Fusaro R. 1971. Subcutaneous *Trichophyton rubrum* abscesses. A case report. Dermatologica 142:167

Wolf FT. 1947. Relation of various fungi to otomycosis. Arch. Otolaryngol. 46:361

Yamashita K. 1972. Otomycosis in Japan and Formosa. Jap. J. Med. Mycol. 13:29

PIEDRA

(Black piedra, white piedra, tinea nodosa)

Definition

Piedra is a fungus on the hair in the form of small stony nodules. Black piedra affects the hair of the scalp, while white piedra involves the hair of the beard and mustache. White piedra has lighter brown-colored nodules that are less firmly attached to the hair shaft.

Etiologic Agents

Piedraia hortai (Brumpt) Fonseca et Area Leão, 1928, causes black piedra; *Trichosporon beigelii* (Küchenmeister et Rabenhorst) Vuillemin, 1902, causes white piedra. Synonym: *Trichosporon cutaneum.*

Occurrence

Humans: Black piedra is found chiefly in South America, Central America, southern Asia, and Africa. White piedra is reported in South America, central Europe, Japan, England, the Orient, and in a few cases the United States.

Animals: Black piedra has been reported in monkeys and a chimpanzee. Black piedra caused by *P. quintanilhae* has been found in African subprimates and primates only.

White piedra has been reported in horses, chimpanzee pelts, and a black spider monkey.

Laboratory Procedures

Specimen collection: Where available, hairs with the stony nodules should be cut off and placed in a sterile container or an envelope for examination.

Direct examination: Place infected hair on a slide containing a drop of 10% KOH or lactophenol and add a coverglass. Slides with lactophenol may be sealed with fingernail polish.

Microscopically, the nodules caused by *P. hortai* vary in size and shape. The somatic structure is a tightly formed stroma of dark-brown, dichotomously branched hyphae, four to eight µm in diameter. The presence of numerous septations with thick walls in the hyphae gives the appearance of arthroconidia (Figure 34). If the nodule is broken apart, numerous asci may be seen with two to eight ascospores that are fusiform, slightly curved, with a polar filament at each end, or sometimes the spores are considered banana-shaped.

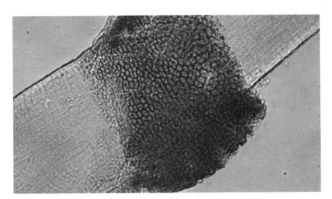

Figure 34. Black piedra, *Piedraia hortai* on hair

Microscopically, the nodules caused by *T. beigelii* (Figure 35) vary in size and are softer and more easily separated from the hair shaft than those caused by *P. hortai*. The somatic structure is a transparent, greenish-brown mycelial mass which forms round to rectangular cells, usually 2 to 4 µm in diameter, in the hyphal strands. Hyphae separate into oval arthroconidia, but no asci are formed.

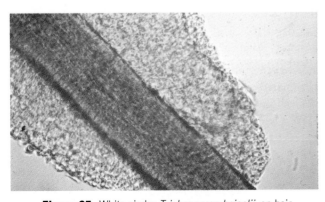

Figure 35. White piedra *Trichosporon beigelii,* on hair

Culture: *P. hortai.* Colonies develop readily from hairs placed into Sabouraud glucose agar with cycloheximide at room temperature. *P. hortai* in culture develops a greenish-brown to black colony, which is raised or flat in the center and is glabrous to cerebriform (Figure 36). Microscopically, the hyphae are dark, thick-walled, closely septate, with numerous chlamydoconidia or enlarged irregular cells. Asci and ascospores may form in culture.

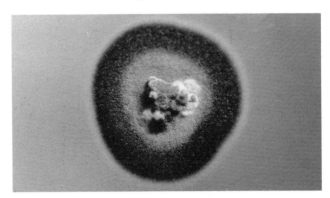

Figure 36. *Piedraia hortai,* colony

T. beigelii. Colonies grow rapidly from hairs placed into Sabouraud glucose agar. The organism is sensitive to cycloheximide. *T. beigelii* in culture develops rapidly as a cream-colored, slimy, soft colony, later becoming finely wrinkled, raised in the center, darker, and more firmly attached to the agar (Figure 37). Microscopically, the presence of hyaline hyphae, arthroconidia, and blastoconidia (Figure 38) is characteristic. No asci are formed.

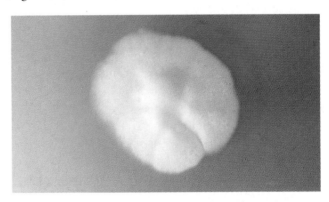

Figure 37. *Trichosporon beigelii,* colony

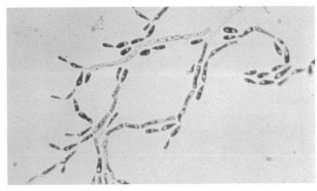

Figure 38. *Trichosporon beigelii,* Arthroconidia and blastoconidia

Biochemical tests necessary for species determination: *T. beigelii* will not ferment sugars. It usually assimilates glucose, galactose, sucrose, lactose, maltose, cellobiose, trehalose, raffinose, L-arabinose, and erythritol. This organism is urease positive, arbutin is split, but potassium nitrate is not assimilated.

Animal inoculation: Laboratory animals are not successfully infected.

Questions

1. How can black and white piedra be differentiated from trichomycosis axillaris on the hair shaft?

2. Compare hairs from cases of black and white piedra with an ectothrix or mosaic hair infection.

Selected References

Adam BA, Soo-Hoo TS, Chong KC. 1977. Black piedra in West Malaysia. Austral. J. Dermatol. 18:45

Chong KC, Adam BA, Soo-Hoo TS. 1975. Morphology of *Piedraia hortae.* Sabouraudia 9:157

Coimbra CEA, Jr, Santos RV. 1989. Black piedra among the Zoro Indians from Amazonia (Brazil). Mycopathologia 107(1):57

Daly JF. 1957. Piedra in Vermont. Arch. Dermatol. 75:584

Horta P. 1911. Sobre una nova forma de piedra. Mem. Inst. Oswaldo Cruz 3:87

Kaplan W. 1959. Piedra in lower animals. J. Am. Vet. Med. Assoc. 134:113

King DS, Jong SC. 1977. A contribution to the genus *Trichosporon.* Mycotaxon 6:391

Lochte T. 1937. Über das Vorkommen der Piedra beim Schimpansen und über die beziehungen der tierischen Piedra zur menschlichen. Arch. Dermatol. Syph. 175:107

Londero AT, Ramos CD, Fischman 0. 1966. White piedra of unusual localization. Sabouraudia 5:132

Stenderup A, et al. 1986. White piedra and *Trichosporon beigelii* carriage in homosexual men. J. Med. Vet. Mycol. 24:401

Takashio M, Vanbreuseghem R. 1971. Production of ascospores by *Piedraia hortai* in vitro. Mycologia 63:612

Walzman M, Leeming JG. 1989. White piedra and *Trichosporon:* the incidence in patients attending a clinic in genitourinary medicine. Genitourin. Med. 65:331.

PITYRIASIS VERSICOLOR

(Tinea versicolor, liver spots)

Definition

Pityriasis versicolor is a superficial infection of the horny layer of the epidermis characterized by irregular fawn-to-brown, or at times achromatic, scaly patches principally on the chest or back, and occasionally on arms, thighs, groin, neck, axillae, or face (page 64, Figures 64 and 65). Some systemic mycoses occur in premature infants and debilitated persons.

Etiologic Agents

Malassezia furfur (Robin) Baillon, 1889. *Pityrosporum orbiculare* is synonymous. Normal flora of humans.

Malassezia pachydermatis (Weidman) Dodge 1935. On animals and normal flora of humans.

Occurrence

Humans: The disease, caused by *M. furfur* comprises not over 5% of the fungus diseases in temperate regions, but frequency increases up to 50% in tropical areas of the world. Cases have occurred after large doses of ACTH or corticosteroids. Fungus also causes catheter-acquired fungemia in adults and fungemia in neonates. Occasionally small embolic lesions develop in the lungs or other organs (see opportunistic infections, page 167). *M. pachydermatis* has been associated with psoriasis or mycosis fungoides on the skin and with febrile systemic syndrome of neonates receiving parenteral lipid nutrition by the central venous catheter.

Animals: *M. pachydermatis* has been isolated from an Indian rhinoceros, hogs, cats, an Indian elephant, and a black bear.

Laboratory Procedures

Specimen collection: The fawn-to-brown patches should be scraped with a scalpel and collected on a slide or in a container for examination. Cellulose tapes may be pressed against the skin to obtain the scales for examination.

Direct examination: To locate all areas of infection on the skin, Wood's light may be used. Infected lesions show a pale-yellow fluorescence under dark conditions. Furfuraceous scales show some fluorescence after removal from the lesions.

Place scales in a drop of 10% KOH, or a drop of calcofluor white on a slide and add a coverglass. Heat gently and examine. A little blue-black ink may be added to the 10% KOH to color the somatic structures of the fungus (see mounting media, page 33).

Thin scales may be mounted in a drop of lactophenol with cotton blue (or Trypan blue) or in a drop of methylene blue, or fixed to a slide and stained with the periodic acid-Schiff method (see page 33). Other stains, including Gram's and acridine orange, may be used.

Specimens can be stained directly on vinyl plastic tape (Keddie, Orr, and Liebes, 1961). Pieces of Scotch brand tape containing infected fragments of the horny layer of the skin can be held with a forceps and transferred through the solutions for staining, the adhesive side being mounted toward the coverglass after staining. Alternatively the adhesive side of the tape may be put up on a slide and drops of the stain placed on it rather than submerging the tape into solutions.

Microscopically, the organisms appear as clusters of thick-walled, round cells, 3 to 8 μm in diameter. Some may be budding forms. Numerous short, straight, or angular hyphae may surround the clusters (Figure 39).

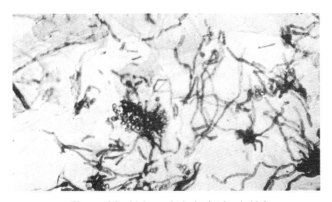

Figure 39. *Malassezia furfur* (stained skin)

Culture: Routine culture of *M. furfur* is not necessary for diagnosis. The organism can be grown at 37°C on Sabouraud glucose agar or malt agar containing strepto-mycin, penicillin, and cycloheximide with a layer of steril-ized olive oil over the surface. The second species, *M. pachydermatis* grows readily on Sabouraud glucose agar incubated at 30° to 35°C for 4 to 5 weeks. The addition of 1% Tween 80 may increase the rate of growth. The colonies contain oval budding cells that have a broad-based isthmus. Elongate hyphae are rarely seen.

Animal inoculation: Laboratory animals are not success-fully infected.

Histopathology: The organism will grow abundantly in the outer layers of the stratum corneum. Histologic sec-tions readily show the organism after staining with hema-toxylin and eosin, Giemsa, methylene blue, or periodic acid-Schiff stain.

Question

How does pityriasis versicolor differ from tinea nigra?

Selected References

Benham RW. 1939. The cultural characteristics of *Pityrosporum ovale*—lipophilic fungus. J. Invest. Dermatol. 2:187.

Boiron GJ, Surleve-Bazeille E, Gauthier Y, et al. 1978. Etude ultrastructurale de divers stades evolutifs de pityriasis versicolor. Ann. Dermatol. Venerol. 105:141

Brooks R, Brown L. 1987. Systemic infection with *Malassezia furfur* in an adult receiving long-term hyperalimentation therapy. J. Infect. Dis. 156:410

Burke RC. 1961. Tinea versicolor: Susceptibility factors and experimental infection in human beings. J. Invest. Dermatol. 36:389

Cohen MM. 1954. A simple procedure for staining tinea versicolor (*M. furfur*) with fountain pen ink. J. Invest. Dermatol. 22:9

Gordon MA. 1951. Lipophilic yeastlike organisms associat-ed with tinea versicolor. J. Invest. Dermatol. 17:267

Keddie F, Shadomy S. 1963. Etiological significance of *Pityrosporum orbiculare* in tinea versicolor. Sabouraudia 3:21

Keddie FM. 1966. Electron microscopy of *Malassezia fur-fur* in tinea versicolor. Sabouraudia 5:134

Keddie R, Orr A, Liebes D. 1961. Direct staining on vinyl plastic tape, demonstrating the cutaneous flora of the epidermis by the strip method. Sabouraudia 1:108

Kreger-van Rij NJW. 1984. General classification of the yeasts. *In* The Yeasts: A taxonomic study. 3rd Ed. Edited by NJW Kreger-Van Rij. Amsterdam, Elsevier Science Publishers, pp. 1-44

Larocco, M, et al. 1988. Recovery of *Malassezia pachyder-matis* from eight infants in a neonatal intensive care nursery: clinical and laboratory features. Pediatr. Infect. Dis. 7:398

Lorenzini R, Bernardis F de. 1987. Studies on the isola-tion, growth and maintenance of *Malassezia pachy-dermatis*. Mycopathologia 99:129

Malassez L. 1874. Note sur le champignon da pityriasis simple. Ecole Prat Hautes Etude Lab d'Histol Coll France Trav. 1:170.

Marcon MJ, Powell DA. 1992. Human infections due to *Malassezia.* spp. Clin. Microbiol. Rev. 5:101

Nazzaro-Porro M, Passi, et al. 1977. Induction of hyphae in culture of *Pityrosporum* by cholesterol and cholesterol esters. J. Invest. Dermatol. 69:531

Salkin IF, Gordon MA. 1977. Polymorphism of *Malassezia furfur.* Can J. Microbiol. 23:471

Sternberg TH, Keddie F. 1961. Immunofluorescence studies in tinea versicolor. Arch. Dermatol. 84:999

TRICHOMYCOSIS AXILLARIS

(Leptothrix, trichomycosis nodosa)

Definition

Trichomycosis axillaris is a bacterial infection of the axillary and pubic hairs. Yellow, red, or black concretions develop around the hair shaft (Figure 40).

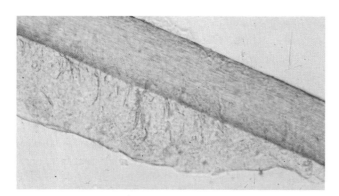

Figure 40. Trichomycosis axillaris
Corynebacterium tenuis on hair

Etiologic Agent

Corynebacterium tenuis (Castellani) Crissey et al, 1952 *(Nocardia tenuis* Castellani, 1912).

Occurrence

Humans: Common in temperate climate, more widespread in the tropics.

Animals: No record of infection.

Laboratory Procedures

Specimen collection: Collect axillary or pubic hairs with nodules scattered along the hair shaft. Note color and lack of luster.

Direct examination: Place infected hairs under Wood's ultraviolet light and note pale-yellow color when concretion is yellow.

Place infected hairs on a slide containing a drop of 10% KOH or lactophenol and add a coverglass. Heat gently for rapid clearing. Slides with lactophenol may be sealed with fingernail polish.

Microscopically, the concretions sometimes show short bacillary forms not over 1 μm in diameter (Figure 40) or, if black, have clumps of cocci mixed with bacillary forms (usually *Micrococcus castellani* and *M. nigrescens*). Crushed material may be Gram stained.

Culture: Culture is not necessary for diagnosis. After immersion of hair with granules in 70% alcohol for one second, the granules are soaked in buffered saline overnight and cultured. Casman's sheep blood agar (Difco) or brain-heart infusion agar with 1% Tween 80 may be used. Incubate for seven days at 37°C. Cultures of diphtheroids should develop.

Animal inoculation: Laboratory animals are not susceptible to an infection.

Question

Compare the microscopic appearance of trichomycosis axillaris with those of white and black piedra. Any differences? Compare with infected hairs from tinea capitis cases.

Selected References

Crissey JT, Rebell GC, Laskas JJ. 1952. Studies on the causative organism of trichomycosis axillaris. J. Invest. Dermatol. 19:187

Freeman RG, McBride ME, Knox JM. 1969. Pathogenesis of trichomycosis axillaris. Arch. Dermatol. 100:90

McBride ME, Freeman RG, Knox JM. 1968. A method for the isolation of the causative organisms of trichomycosis axillaris. Br. J. Dermatol. 80:509

Negroni P. 1978. Estudios sobre la tricomicosis axilar. I. Caracteres microbiologicos del organismo cultivado. Rev Argentina Micologia 1:12

TINEA NIGRA

(Pityriasis nigra, microsporosis nigra)

Definition

Tinea nigra is a superficial fungus infection of the palm of the hands, rarely found on the neck or other parts of the body. It is characterized by brown to black macular lesions on the skin (see Chapter 5, Figures 62 and 63).

Etiologic Agent

Exophiala werneckii (Horta) von Arx 1970 (*Cladosporium werneckii* Horta, *Phaeoannellomyces wernecki* (Horta) McGinnis et Schell, 1985). This organism probably occurs in the soil and on wood or paint in warm climates. There is a close resemblance to *Aureobasidium* (*Pullularia*) *pullulans* in the early stages of colony formation. Infection probably occurs from injection of the skin with contaminated materials.

Occurrence

Humans: The disease has been reported in Central America, South America, Southeast Asia, Africa, Europe, Indonesia, and the United States.

Animals: No record of infection.

Laboratory Procedures

Specimen collection: Scrapings should be taken from pigmented lesions of tinea nigra for examination microscopically, for culture, and for laboratory study.

Direct examination: Place scrapings on a slide with 10% KOH and examine microscopically. The fungus appears in the epithelial cells of the skin as pigmented, light-brown to dark-green, branched, septate hyphae 1.5 to 3 µm in diameter. Swollen cells and chlamydoconidia should be seen.

Culture: Infected material will grow on Sabouraud glucose agar with or without the addition of cycloheximide and chloramphenicol at room temperature. A three-week period should be allowed for growth before the culture is considered negative.

Colonies develop slowly with a moist, shiny-black yeastlike appearance, reaching maximum size after two weeks. These older colonies have less moisture on the surface and become dark green with grayish mycelium on the surface. Transfers develop the yeastlike growth at first, but soon become blackish with aerial mycelium.

Microscopically, the black yeastlike portion of the colony contains blastoconidia or budding cells which have developed laterally from the dark hyphal cells.

Blastoconidia may form clusters along the hyphae (similar to *Aureobasidium* spp. and *Candida* spp.). Short conidiophores on the sides or apices of the hyphae produce chains or clusters of one- to two-celled dark conidia. This simulates spore formation in *Cladosporium* (or *Hormodendrum*). Older hyphae may lack spores, or may have conidiophores of the *Cladosporium* type.

Exoantigen test: This test is useful for differentiation of *Exophiala werneckii* from other black fungi pathogenic in humans.

Animal inoculation: Animal infection is of no value in laboratory diagnosis of the disease. Superficial infection can be produced experimentally in guinea pigs or by intraperitoneal injection of the organism in mice, and recovered a few days later.

Questions

1. What are the differences and similarities in the hyphae and conidia of the genera *Aureobasidium, Candida, Cladosporium* (*Hormodendrum*), and *Exophiala*?

2. Compare the appearance of the hyphae in skin scrapings from tinea nigra and tinea corporis cases. Are there any microscopic differences?

Selected References

Babel DE, Pelachyk JM, and Hurley JP. 1986. Tinea nigra masquerading as acral lentiginous melanoma. J. Dermatol. Surg. Oncol. 12:502

Castellani A, Chalmers AJ. 1919. *Manual of Tropical Medicine.* 3rd ed. Bailliere, Tindall and Cox, London

Espinel-Ingroff A, et al. 1986. Exoantigen test for *Cladosporium bantianum, Fonsecaea pedrosoi,* and *Phialophora verrucosa.* J. Clin. Microbiol. 23:305

Gomez SH, Cardenas JV, Rendon PI. 1968. Tinea nigra. Mycopath. Mycol. Appl. 34:11

Gustafson RA, Hardcastle RV, Szaniszlo PJ. 1975. Budding in the dimorphic fungus *Cladosporium werneckii.* Mycologia 67:942

Keddie F. 1964. *Cladosporium werneckii.* Infection and in vivo culture. Arch. Dermatol. 89:432

Merwin CF. 1965. Tinea nigra palmaris. Review of literature and case report. Pediatrics 36:537

McGinnis MR. 1979. Taxonomy of *Exophiala werneckii* and its relationship to *Microsporum mansonii.* Sabouraudia 17:145

Nishimura K, Miyaji M. 1984. *Hortae,* a new genus to accommodate *Cladosporium werneckii.* Jap. J. Med. Mycol. 23:139

Ritchie EB, Taylor TE. 1964. A study of tinea nigra palmaris. Arch. Dermatol. 89:601

Volcan G, Godoy GA, Battistini F, et al. 1976. Fruiting organs of *Cladosporium werneckii.* Sabouraudia 14:115

Chapter 5

DERMATOPHYTOSES

The dermatophytoses are infections produced in the keratinized tissues, including nails, hair, and stratum corneum of the skin. The fungi that produce dermatophytoses are known as dermatophytes. There are three genera: *Microsporum*, *Epidermophyton*, and *Trichophyton*. When other organisms, such as *Candida* and other fungi, are involved in cutaneous infections, the disease is known as dermatomycosis. The clinical types of dermatophytoses are known as tineas (ringworm). Ringworms are designated by location, such as tinea capitis (ringworm of the scalp) and tinea pedis (ringworm of the foot). The various dermatophytes do not necessarily correlate with location of disease on the body. Granulomatous lesions in subcutaneous tissues have occasionally been reported. Isolation and identification of the species from skin or nail scrapings or from stubs of infected hairs are essential in cases difficult to treat medically .

CLASSIFICATION

Classification of the dermatophytoses is based on two systems: clinical symptoms involving various areas of the body (used before the fungus can be identified, as the same species can produce similar symptoms in different parts of the body) and morphologic characteristics of the fungus to separate genera based on the shape of the macroconidia (fuseaux), (Table 5, page 75); an example is tinea capitis caused by species of *Microsporum* or *Trichophyton* (Table 2, page 60).

MYCOLOGIC CLASSIFICATION OF DERMATOPHYTES

The three genera to which dermatophytes belong— *Microsporum*, *Epidermophyton*, and *Trichophyton* were separated by Emmons in 1934 on the basis of differences in the macroconidia (see section on the genus concerned for details). Ajello (1968) transferred the species *Keratinomyces*

ajelloi from the genus *Keratinomyces* to the genus *Trichophyton* on the basis of macroconidia and the perfect state.

The species in the three genera of the dermatophyte were considered members of the phylum Deuteromycota (Fungi Imperfecti) until the discovery of the perfect state of *T. ajelloi* (Dawson and Gentles, 1961) and *M. gypseum* (Nannizzi, 1927, Stockdale, 1963) as well as others. Species with perfect states, produce asci and ascospores and are now considered in the family Arthrodermataceae, phylum Ascomycota. The two teleomorphic (perfect state) genera of *Microsporum* and *Trichophyton* were *Nannizzia* and *Arthroderma* respectively. After careful study of more species with the perfect state, Weitzman et al (1986) noted little difference between *Nannizzia* and *Arthroderma*, and proposed the genus *Arthroderma* for both genera.

The importance of the sexual stage (Table 3, page 66) has been for identification and genetic studies. Some previously described species, when mated, have developed the perfect state in the laboratory by using the hair-bait technique or the oatmeal tomato-paste agar medium developed by Weitzman (see under laboratory procedures, pages 41-42).

Microsporum and *Trichophyton* are usually separated into three categories on the basis of host preference and natural habitat. Anthropophilic species usually infect humans and rarely animals. Zoophilic species are usually pathogens in animals, with occasional transmission to humans. The geophilic species inhabit the soil and serve as a source of infection in humans and other animals.

The sexual stage species complex for *M. gypseum*, *T. mentagrophytes* and *T. terrestre* will be mentioned in the discussions of species. Table 3 (page 66) shows the Imperfect and Perfect States of the Dermatophytes.

Clinical laboratory identification of the dermatophytes is based on the macroscopic and microscopic characteristics of the asexual state of growth in culture. Biochemical

(continued on page 68)

Table 2. Dermatophyte Infections

DISEASE	DERMATOPHYTE
Tinea capitis (ringworm of the scalp), Figures 42-52	*Microsporum*—any species *Trichophyton*—any species except *T. concentricum*
Tinea barbae (ringworm of the beard) Figure 61	*T. mentagrophytes, T. rubrum, T. violaceum, T. verrucosum, T. megninii, Microsporum canis*
Tinea corporis (ringworm of the body), Figures 52–60, 71, 73	*T. mentagrophytes, T. rubrum, T. concentricum (tinea imbricata). M. audouinii, M. canis* and any of the other dermatophytes may be involved
Tinea cruris (jock itch, gym itch, ringworm of the groin) Figures 69, 70, 72	*Epidermophyton floccosum, T. mentagrophytes, T. rubrum, (Candida albicans* - ringworm-like symptoms)
Tinea pedis (athlete's foot, ringworm of the feet), figure 68	*E. floccosum, T. mentagrophytes, T. rubrum, (C. albicans*—ringworm-like symptoms)
Tinea unguium (ringworm of the nail), Figures 74–75	*E. floccosum, T. mentagrophytes, T. rubrum, (C. albicans*—ringworm-like symptoms) Rare: *T. schoenleinii, T. tonsurans*
Ringworm in animals: attacks skin, hair, feathers, nails, claws, and hooves. Figures 41a, 41b	*M. canis var. canis, M. canis var. distortum, M. cookei, M. gypseum, M. nanum, M. persicolor, M. vanbreuseghemii, T. equinum, T. mentagrophytes, T. verrucosum*
Favus in animals (tinea favosa)	*M. gallinae, T. simii*

Organisms Causing Skin Infections[*]

Tinea capitis
Microsporum audouinii - Figure 42 and 43 (Wood's light)
M. canis - Figure 44 and 45
M. gypseum
M. ferrugineum
Trichophyton violaceum - Figure 49
T. tonsurans - Figures 46 and 47 ("black dot" ringworm)
T. schoeleinii - Figures 48 (favus)
T. rubrum - Figure 50
T. mentagrophytes - Figure 51 (kerion)
T. megninii
T. verrucosum

Tinea imbricata
T. concentricum - Fig 58

Tinea corporis, tinea barbae and tinea manuum
Trichophyton verrucosum - Figure 52 and 73
Microsporum audouinii - Figure 53
M. canis - Figure 54
M. gypseum - Figure 55
M. ferrugineum
Trichophyton violaceum - Figure 49
T. tonsurans - Figures 56 and 57
T. schoenleinii - Figure 48
T. rubrum - Figure 50 and 59
T. mentagrophytes - Figures 60 tinea manuum and 61 (tinea barbae)
T. mentagrophytes - Figure 71
T. megninii
Epidermophyton floccosum - Figure 72

(continued on page 61)

Organisms Causing Skin Infections[*]

Pityriasis versicolor
Malassezia furfur - Figures 64 and 65

Tinea Nigra (palmaris)
Cladosporium werneckii - Figure 62
C. werneckii - Figure 63

Tinea pedis, T. manuum, Tinea cruris, T. unguium
Dermatophytids, etc.
Trichophyton rubrum - Figures 66, 67, 68, 69 and 70

Onychomycosis
Candida albicans - Figure 74

Tinea unguium
Trichophyton rubrum - Figure 75

Tinea in animals
Trichophyton verrucosum - Figures 41a
Trichophyton mentagrophytes - Figure 41b

[*] The genus and species are determined by macroscopic and microscopic characteristics from culture.

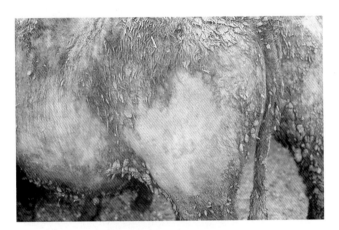

Figure 41a. Tinea on cow
Trichophyton verrucosum

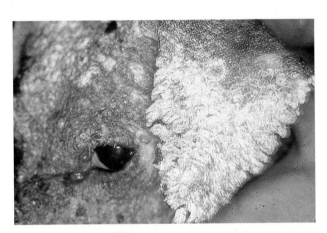

Figure 41b. Dog tinea
Trichophyton mentagrophytes

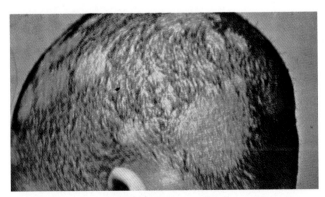

Figure 42. Tinea capitis
Microsporum audouninii

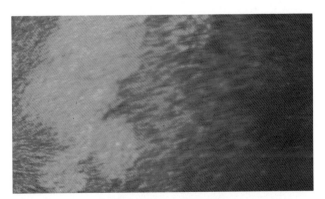

Figure 43. Tinea capitis
Microsporum audouninii

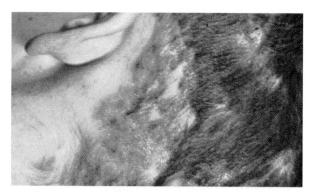

Figure 44. Tinea capitis
Microsporum canis

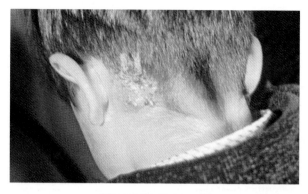

Figure 45. Tinea capitis
Microsporum canis

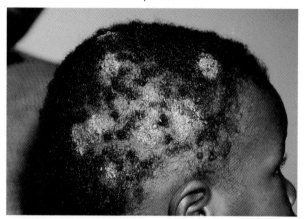

Figure 46. Tinea capitis
Trichophyton tonsurans

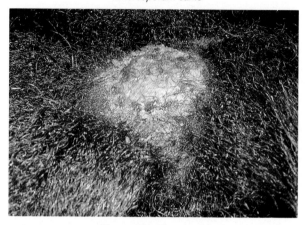

Figure 47. Tinea capitis
Trichophyton tonsurans

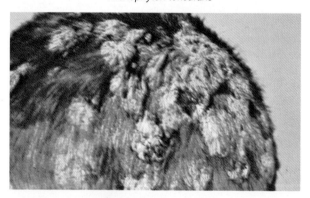

Figure 48. Tinea capitis
Trichophyton schoeleinii

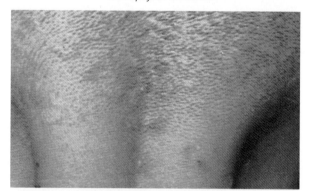

Figure 49. Tinea capitis
Trichophyton violaceum

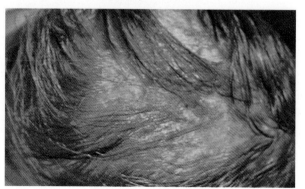

Figure 50. Tinea capitis
Trichophyton rubrum

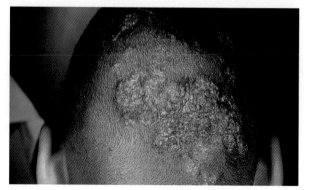

Figure 51. Tinea capitis
Trichophyton mentagrophytes

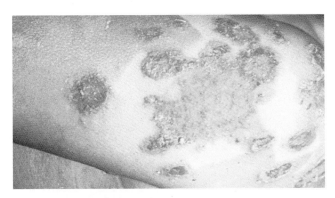

Figure 52. Tinea corporis
Trichophyton verrucosum

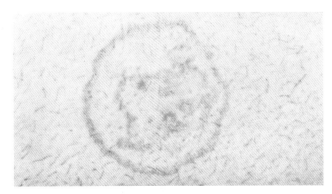

Figure 53. Tinea corporis
Microsporum audouinii

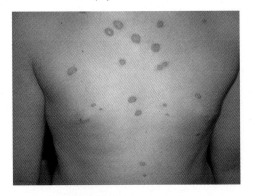

Figure 54. Tinea corporis
Microsporum canis

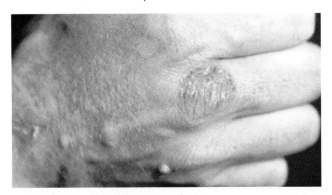

Figure 55. Tinea manuum
Microsporum gypseum

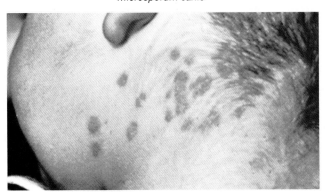

Figure 56. Tinea corporis
Trichophyton tonsurans

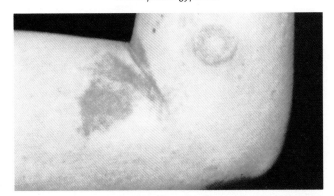

Figure 57. Tinea corporis
Trichophyton tonsurans

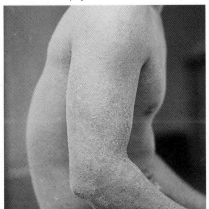

Figure 58. Tinea imbricata
Trichophyton concentricum

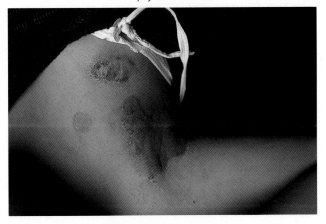

Figure 59. Tinea corporis
Trichophyton rubrum

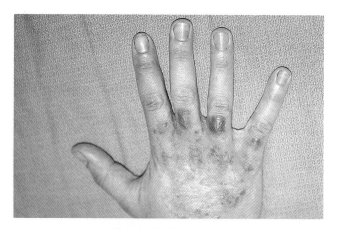

Figure 60. Tinea manuum
Trichophyton mentagrophytes

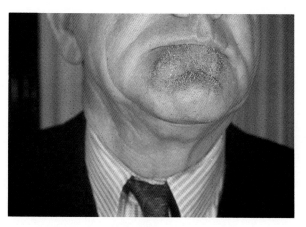

Figure 61. Tinea barbae
Trichophyton mentagrophytes

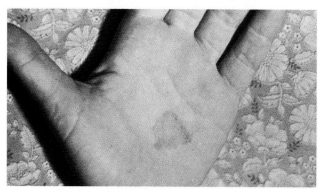

Figure 62. Tinea nigra
Cladosporium werneckii

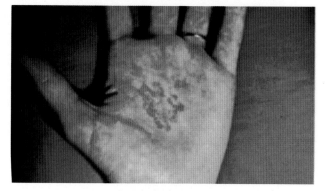

Figure 63. Tinea nigra
Cladosporium werneckii

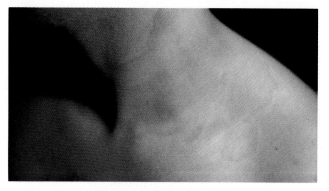

Figure 64. Pityriasis versicolor
Malessezia furfur

Figure 65. Pityriasis versicolor
Malessezia furfur

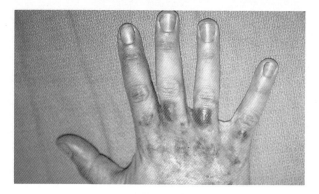

Figure 66. Tinea manuum
Trichophyton rubrum

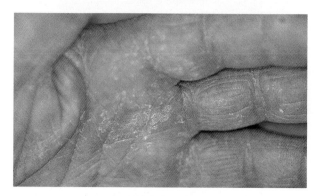

Figure 67. Tinea manuum
Trychophyton rubrum

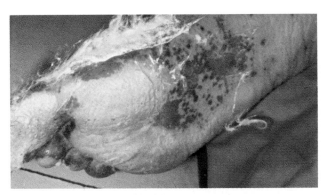

Figure 68. Tinea pedis
Trichophyton rubrum

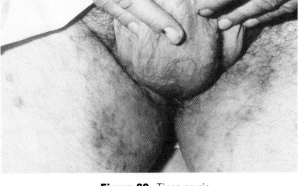

Figure 69. Tinea cruris
Trichophyton rubrum

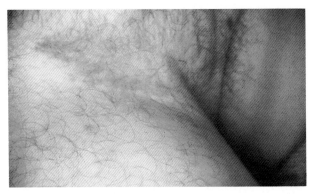

Figure 70. Tinea cruris
Trichophyton rubrum

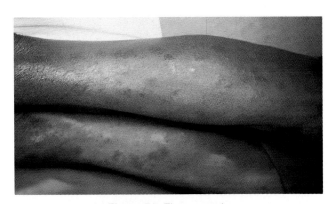

Figure 71. Tinea corporis
Trichophyton mentagrophytes

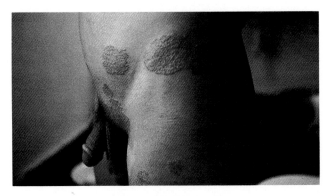

Figure 72. Tinea cruris
Epidermophyton floccosum

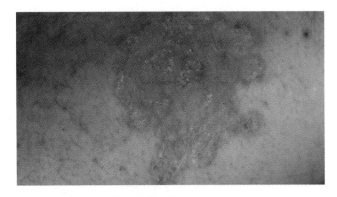

Figure 73. Tinea corporis
Trichophyton verrucosum

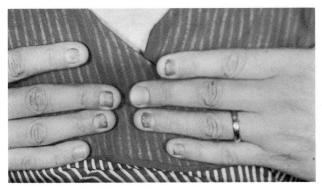

Figure 74. Onychomycosis
Candida albicans

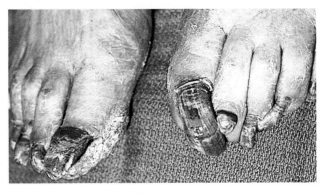

Figure 75. Tinea unguium
Trichophyton rubrum

Table 3. The Known Imperfect and Perfect States of the Dermatophytes

IMPERFECT OR ANAMORPH STATE	PERFECT OR TELEOMORPH STATE
(phylum Deuteromycota) (Class Hyphomycetes)	(phylum Ascomycota) (Class Plectomycetes)
Microsporum Gruby, 1843: attacks hair and skin	
	Arthroderma Currey ex Berkeley emendo Weitzman et al., 1986
M. amazonicum	
	A. borelii (Moraes et al) Padhyeetal et al, 1986
M. audouinii	
M. boullardii	*A. corniculatum* (Takashio de Vroey) Padhye et al, 1986
M. canis var. *canis*	*A. otae* (Hasegawa et Usui) (McGinnis et al, 1986)
M. canis var. *distortum*	*A. cajetani* (Ajello) Ajello et al, 1986
M. cookei	*A. fulvum* (Stockdale) Weitzman et al, 1986
M. fulvum (gypseum)	*A. incurvatum* (Stockdale) Weitzman et al, 1986
M. gypseum	*A. gypseum* (Nannizzi) Weitzman et al, 1986
M. gypseum	
*M. ferrugineum	
M. gallinae	*A. obtusum* (Dawson et Gentles) Weitzman et al, 1986
M. nanum	*A. persicolor* (Stockdale) Weitzman et al, 1986
M. persicolor	
M. praecox	*A. racemosum* (Rush-Monnro et al) Weitzman et al, 1986
*M. racemosum	*A. grubyi* (Georg et al) Ajello et al, 1967
M. vanbreuseghemii	
Epidermophyton Sabouraud, 1910: Attacks skin and nails	
E. floccosum	*Arthroderma* Currey ex Berkeley emendo Weitzman et al, 1986
Trichophyton Malmsten, 1945: Attacks skin, nails, and hair	

* Species not likely to be found in the United States

(continued next page)

Table 3. *(continued)*

IMPERFECT OR ANAMORPH STATE	PERFECT OR TELEOMORPH STATE
Ectothrix—invaded hair	
T. mentagrophytes	*A. benhamiae* Ajello et Cheng, 1967
T. mentagrophytes	*A. vanbreuseghemii* Takashio, 1973
T. equinum	
T. rubrum	
T. verrucosum	
*T. megninii	
Ectothrix—endothrix—invaded hair	
*T. simii	*A. simii* Stockdale et al, 1965
Endothrix—invaded hair	
T. tonsurans	
T. schoenleinii	
*T. violaceum	
*T. gourvilii	
*T. soudanense	
*T. yaoundei	
Hair not invaded	
*T. concentricum	
Saprophytic in soil	
T. ajelloi	*A. uncinatum* Dawson et Gentles, 1961
T. flavescens	*A. flavescens* Padhye et Carmichael, 1971

* Species not likely to be found in the United States

(continued next page)

Table 3. (continued)

IMPERFECT OR ANAMORPH STATE	PERFECT OR TELEOMORPH STATE
T. georgiae	A. ciferrii Varsavsky et Ajello, 1964
T. gloriae	A. gloriae Ajello et Cheng, 1967
T. terrestre	A. quadrifidum Dawson et Gentles, 1961
T. terrestre	A. incingulare Padhye et Carmichael, 1972
T. terrestre	A. lenticularum Pore et al, 1965
T. vanbreuseghemii	A. gertleri Bohme, 1967

* Species not likely to be found in the United States

requirements have been used to identify some of the species of the dermatophytes. Further information on identification of the dermatophytes is given under **Laboratory Diagnosis** on page 70.

SUGGESTIONS FOR LABORATORY STUDY OF DERMATOPHYTES

1. Study young and older colonies of all the dermatophytes periodically to note changes, rates of growth, and morphologic characteristics for differentiation of the individual species.

2. Make slide cultures by the Riddell method or other methods or direct mounts of the different species of the three genera to study the microscopic characteristics (see methods, page 6).

3. Study the procedures for obtaining materials from patients on page 28. If patients with ringworm are available, check the nail, skin, or hair material to see if it is positive. Then try several methods for isolation in culture of the organism.

4. Use Wood's light (filtered ultraviolet light) (see page 28) on the infected hairs to see the characteristic fluorescence. Check fluorescence of some organic substances.

5. Try isolating some unknowns that have been made from spore suspensions of known cultures in saline solution. If more than one organism is placed in the unknown, try to separate the organisms in pure culture.

6. When clinical cases of animal ringworm of the hair become available, such as *Microsporum canis* in a kitten, keep the animal after death in the deep freeze for future use in class. Mosaic hairs on a kitten have remained viable and virulent for 39 years (since 1955) in the deep freeze. The hairs can be readily used for microscopic study and for isolation of the fungus in culture.

7. Isolate contaminated material from ringworm cases on media with and without cycloheximide and antibacterial substances. Note the difference in the rate of colony growth and in the morphologic appearance. Without cycloheximide more fungal contaminants will appear.

8. Grow the dermatophytes on several different media and note the difference in the morphologic appearance of the colonies.

9. Use visual aids, such as film strips, kodachromes of cases, cultures and microscopic characteristics, and movies when available in the study of the dermatophytes.

10. Use hair for isolation of dermatophytes from soil. Use a moat with cans or jars under the legs and mineral oil added to the cans. This will keep mites from entering or leaving the moat.

   a. Collect soil from areas with high organic content, such as flower beds, barnyards, animal pathways, or other selected locations.

b. Fill a petri dish approximately half full with the soil sample, which should be moistened with sterile distilled water containing 500 μg penicillin, 300 μg streptomycin, and 0.5 mg cycloheximide/ml (see page 41).

c. Scatter short pieces of sterilized human hair or horsehair over the surface of the soil and incubate at room temperature.

d. Examine after one to two weeks for the development of hyphae on the surface of the hair. If fungal growth is present, place the hair on Sabouraud glucose agar with cycloheximide and chloramphenicol. Check the identification of the colony in ten days or more. In some cases, nonpathogenic keratinophilic fungi will be isolated.

e. Check the hairs periodically, for about one month, for the development of ascocarp (gymnothecia) or the perfect state of some of the dermatophytes. Use oatmeal tomato-paste (Weitzman and Silva-Hutner) medium for the study of the perfect state (see procedures, page 42). Some commonly isolated species are: *Microsporum gypseum, M. cookei, Trichophyton ajelloi,* and *T. terrestre.*

11. Set up the media for differentiation of the species of *Trichophyton* based on nutritional requirements (see procedures, page 44).

12. The cellophane tape method may be used to pick up conidia and hyphae of dermatophytes from cultures or from material from ringworm cases for staining and slide mounts (see page 5).

13. Use the soil-hair culture technique for the study of the perfect state of the dermatophytes. Several of the dermatophytes will produce ascocarps under suitable culture conditions. The perfect states of the genus *Arthroderma,* related to the imperfect genera *Microsporum* and *Trichophyton* (see list of dermatophytes), can be grown on a soil-hair, or Weitzman's culture medium for the study the ascigerous (perfect) state (see procedures, page 42).

The two compatible strains for each species are inoculated in close proximity on the surface of soil (sterilized or unsterilized) or agar medium. Sterilized horse mane or tail hair, or child's hair, cut short, should be scat-tered over the surface of the soil. Other animal hair may be satisfactory, but human hair is less satisfactory for the best production of gymnothecia (Dawson, Gentles, and Brown, 1964). In approximately three to four weeks mature ascocarps should be formed. Use same procedure for agar medium.

Example: Start with two strains of the heterothallic *Microsporum gypseum.* Inoculate these in close proximity on the soil-hair or agar medium and incubate at room temperature (24°C) for three to four weeks. Where the two strains unite, ascocarps of *Arthroderma incurvatum* will appear. Examine the culture for the presence of asci and ascospores, and for peridial hyphae.

14. Animal inoculation: This technique is useful for laboratory study of the nature of the lesions developed by the organisms and for study of immunity. Normally this technique is not used for identification of the dermatophytes. Guinea pigs, and sometimes mice, are the preferred animals for inoculation. Some species, such as *Microsporum canis, M. gypseum,* or *Trichophyton mentagrophytes,* may be established more readily in laboratory animals. A procedure that is useful is as follows:

a. With a small surgical scissors cut the hair off an area about 2 × 2 cm on the back of the guinea pig. The area may be abraded until reddened.

b. Prepare a heavy sporulation suspension of the fungus by grinding with some water or honey to make a paste.

c. Apply the paste to the area and rub in well.

d. In seven to ten days erythema and desquamation should be evident. Examine the area for the presence of the fungus.

e. If the hairs are not infected, check in 15 days.

f. Reisolate the organisms from the lesions.

NOTE: The animals usually will show no sign of the infection after three to four weeks.

LABORATORY DIAGNOSIS

Collection of Clinical Materials

The specimens of skin, nails and hair from areas of tinea should be removed and examined directly under the microscope after being placed on a slide with KOH or combined wtih calcofluor white (CFW), see procedures on page 32. The CFW nonspecifically binds to the cellulose and chitin in the fungal cell wall to give a bright green to blue fluorescence. A portion of the material should be cultured for presence of the organisms.

Skin scrapings: The area of infection on the skin should be washed in 70% alcohol to remove surface contaminants. Scrapings should be taken from the active border areas of the lesion and placed in a sterile container for laboratory examination. Semipermanent mounts may be made (see procedure, page 83).

Nail scrapings: Scrapings or clippings of nails taken from the inner portion of the nail or nail bed should be collected in sterile containers for examination.

Hair: The basal portion of the hair or hair stubs should be pulled or removed with tweezers as the fungus is usually found in this region. Wood's light (ultraviolet light in the 3,650 angstrom unit range) under darkened conditions is useful for locating infected hairs in the scalp when ringworm is caused by certain species of *Microsporum*. The infected hairs usually fluoresce with a bright yellowish-green color. The hairs should be placed in a sterile container for examination later in the laboratory.

Laboratory Examination of Clinical Materials

Examination of hairs, nails, or skin may give the first clue to a mycotic infection, but cultures must be made in order to determine the etiologic agents. The specimens should be placed in 10% to 20% KOH or KOH with calcofluor white on a slide with a coverglass, heated gently, and observed for the presence of fungal hyphae and arthroconidia. Pieces of hair, skin, or nail should be pressed into the surface of Sabouraud glucose agar with chloramphenicol and cycloheximide (Mycosel, or Mycobiotic agar). Dermatophyte test medium (DTM) is useful. Dermatophytes turn the DTM medium red after the medium becomes alkaline. A few contaminants turn the medium red and must be separated by microscopic examination. The plates should be observed for colony growth for at least two weeks before being considered negative. Table 4 (page 71) summarizes the relationship of clinical specimens of hair, nail, or skin, the fungal elements, and the likely genera of the etiologic agents.

Colony Characteristics

The use of a standard medium, such as Sabouraud glucose agar, will be of value in the development of colonies similar to those described in reference books. The rate of growth, pattern, and changes in color, on the surface and reverse side of the colony, are important to observe for identification purposes. Variations within a species may occur, manifested by changes in color, rate of growth, or other characteristics. Some species very commonly develop white, cottony growths by mutation resulting in sterile mycelium. This growth, incorrectly known as "pleomorphism," appears on the surface of a normally growing colony and may be readily located. If these sterile mycelial forms are isolated from lesions of patients, identification is difficult or impossible.

Physiologic Requirements

Research has improved procedures for identification of the dermatophytes on the basis of nutritional requirements. Routine nutritional tests (Bacto *Trichophyton* agars) may be used to differentiate species of *Trichophyton,* in addition to culture studies and microscopic examination of the colony.

The dermatophytes grow at room temperature (25°C) at a pH of 6.8 to 7.0, although these fungi are tolerant of variation in pH and temperatures.

The use of cycloheximide (antifungal) and chloramphenicol (antibacterial) in the quantities recommended in Sabouraud dextrose agar or the use of Mycosel or Mycobiotic agar is helpful in isolation of dermatophytes, as these media retard the growth of saprophytic fungi and most bacteria. (See media, page 44.)

The dermatophytes are able to utilize keratin, a substance found in epidermal tissues, but do not require it when growing in culture. Many keratinophilic fungi that do not produce diseases in animals or humans may be found in the soil.

Microscopic Characteristics

In addition to variation in size, shape, thickness, and character of the wall of the macroconidia (if present in the genus and species), the microconidia may be arranged along the sides of the hyphae or in grapelike clusters (en grappe) and be oval or pear-shaped. Other structures that may be present are: arthroconidia, chlamydoconidia, nodular bodies, pectinate bodies, racquet hyphae, favic chandeliers and spiral cords or coils (Figures 76-85). The macroconidia when present are the most important aid in identification of *Microsporum* and *Epidermophyton*. Genus differentiation is based on the presence or absence of

(continued on page 73)

Table 4. Laboratory Examination of Clinical Specimens of Hair, Nail, and Stratum Corneum with Genera of Etiologic Agents

Genus	One Possible Species	Disease

Clinical Specimen of Hair, Nail, or Skin (stratum corneum layer).

10–20% KOH—to observe Microscopic morphology

Skin, stratum corneum layer

- Septate hyphae
  - colorless (hyaline) hyphae
    - *Microsporum* / *canis* → tinea corporis
    - *Candida* / *albicans* → candidiasis
  - brown colored (dematiaceous) hyphae
    - *Exophiala* / *spinifera* → phaeohyphomycosis
- Yeast cells Pseudohyphae hyphae
  - colorless (hyaline) → *Candida* / *albicans* → candidiasis
  - brown colored (dematiaceous) → *Exophiala* / *jeanselmei* → phaeohyphomycosis
- Septate hyphae short rods yeasts in clusters → *Malassezia* / *furfur* → pityriasis versicolor

hair

- arthroconidia
  - (+)
    - ectothrix
      - mosaic → *Microsporum* / *audouinii* → tinea capitis
      - parallel → *Trichophyton* / *mentagrophytes* → tinea capitis
  - (−) endothrix → *Trichophyton* / *tonsurans* → tinea capitis
- hyphae in hair shaft → *Trichophyton* / *schoenlenii* → tinea capitis
- nodules
  - hard black — black piedra — *Piedraia* / *hortai* → black piedra
  - soft white — white piedra — *Trichosporon* / *beigelii* → white piedra

nail

- septate hyphae
  - *Trichophyton* / *rubrum* → tinea unguium
  - *Epidermophyton* / *floccosum* → tinea unguium
  - *Microsporum* / *gypseum (rare)* → tinea unguium
  - *Scopulariopsis* / *brevicaulis* → onychomycosis
- yeast cells pseudopyphae → *Candida* / *albicans* → onychomycosis

Inoculate some specimen into media, Mycosel & SAB —— Incubate at 45°C —— Examine every 3–4 days after Day 7. Use Flow Charts for identification. —— Final Report

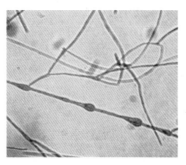

Figure 76. Racquet hyphae X400

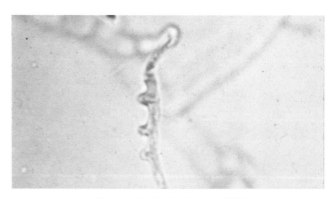

Figure 77. Pectinate body X600

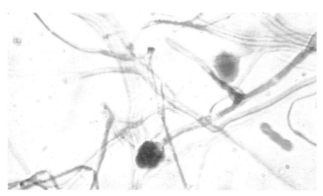

Figure 78. Nodular body X800

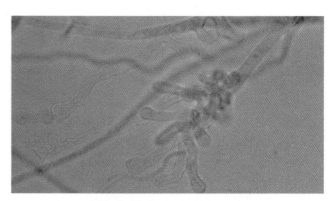

Figure 79. Favic chandelier X600

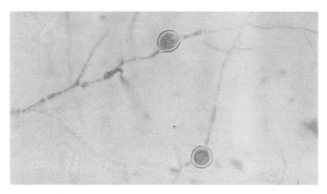

Figure 80. Chlamydoconidia X400

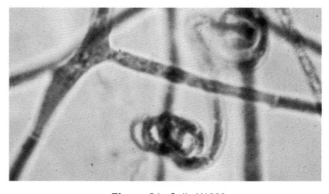

Figure 81. Coils X1600

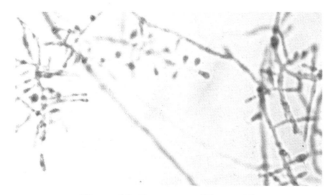

Figure 82. *T. tonsurans,* Microconidia
(borne singly) X400

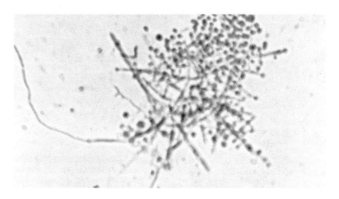

Figure 83. *T. mentagrophytes,* Microconidia
(grapelike clusters) X400

macroconidia and microconidia, their shape, and their distribution along the hyphae.

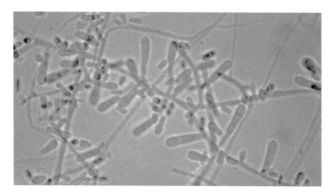

Figure 84. *T. terrestre,* conidia X400

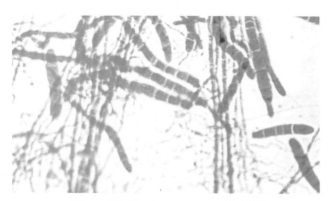

Figure 85. *T. rubrum,* macroconidia X400

The genus *Microsporum* has fusiform, obovate to spindle-shaped macroconidia which usually have pitted, asperulate, echinulate or spiny thick walls. The microconidia may be round, oval, or pear-shaped. Hair invasion is of the mosaic ectothrix type.

The genus *Epidermophyton* produces characteristic multi-celled, clavate macroconidia. Microconidia are absent. Hair is not invaded.

The genus *Trichophyton* develops round, elongate, clavate or pyriform microconidia. The arrangement of microconidia along the hyphae and the shape help in identification of some species. Elongate, clavate to fusiform, thin-walled macroconidia may be present but are not significant for species identification except for two species. Hair invasion is of the ectothrix or endothrix type.

The flow diagram Table 5 (page 75) provides a guide to the more commonly encountered species of the dermatophytes in the clinical laboratory. More detailed descriptions of the species of the three genera are given on the following pages.

MICROSPORUM SPP.

Characteristics

Microsporum consists of a number of species that attack hair and skin of animals and humans. These fungi may cause ringworm of the scalp, beard, or body of humans (tinea capitis, tinea barbae, tinea corporis). In ectothrix hair infections the hyphae fragment into arthroconidia around the hair shaft. Usually the metabolite, a pteridine, produced by the fungus is present in *M. canis, M. audouinii, M. distortum,* and *M. ferrugineum,* giving a bright greenish-yellow fluorescence under Wood's light while on infected hair. Figure 86 illustrates *M. canis* under Wood's light.

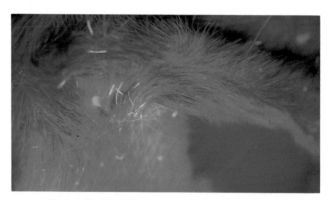

Figure 86. Tinea capitis, *Microsporum*-infected hair under Wood's lamp

The organisms are usually isolated on Sabouraud glucose agar at room temperature with the addition of antibiotics. The colonies vary from moderately slow growing, matted, and furrowed to fast growing, powdery or velvety, and light tan, ferrugineous, yellowish to cinnamon in color. The reverse side of the colony may vary from reddish-brown, ferrugineous, yellowish to reddish-black. Emmon's medium and modified cornmeal agar are useful for production of macroconidia.

The hyphae produce characteristic large, thin to thick, rough-walled, 3- to 15-celled, fusiform to obovate macroconidia. Three species, *M. gypseum, M. fulvum,* and *M. nanum,* have rather thin-walled macroconidia. Small one-celled microconidia are produced on short stalks or are sessile on the hyphae; pectinate hyphae, racquet hyphae, nodular bodies, coils, and chlamydoconidia may be present (Figures 76 through 85).

Etiologic Agents: Asexual, imperfect, anamorph state

Microsporum audouinii is a common cause of tinea capitis, especially in children; *M. canis* is of animal origin, and occasionally causes tinea capitis or tinea corporis in humans; *M. cookei* is a soil-inhabiting organism of little importance as an infective agent in humans; *M. ferrugineum* causes tinea capitis in children (of little importance in North America); *M. gypseum* is a soil-inhabiting fungus occasionally pathogenic in humans; *M. distortum* is a rare cause of tinea capitis and usually causes an inflammatory reaction of the scalp known as kerion. Hairs may or may not fluoresce. *M. nanum* is a rare cause of ringworm in humans; *M. vanbreuseghemii* also is a rare cause of ringworm. Species of *Microsporum* may be geophilic, keratin-utilizing soil saprophytes; zoophilic, with invasion of the cornified substrate in living animals; or anthropophilic, living on humans only.

Etiologic Agents: Sexual, perfect, teleomorph state
The species of *Arthroderma* that produce *Microsporum* asexual state have slight-to-moderate constrictions at each septum on the outer peridial hyphae. Peridial appendages of *Arthroderma* have loosely or tightly coiled spiral hyphae that are long, slender, and tapered. The asci are oval to subglobose with eight smooth, hyaline, oval or lenticular ascospores. In contrast the species of *Arthroderma* that produce *Trichophyton* asexual state have dumbbell-shaped cells making up the outer peridial hyphae.

Laboratory Procedures

Direct examination: Place infected hair and skin if present on a slide containing a drop of 10% KOH and heat the slide gently before examining. Lactophenol may also be used for hair specimens. Slides with infected hairs and lactophenol may be kept by sealing with fingernail polish or other types of cement.

Microscopically, species of *Microsporum* usually form a dense spore sheath, mosaic in pattern around the hair shaft. Note that the growth of the fungus is primarily around the outside of the hair. Hyphae may be seen in the epidermal cells of the skin in some cases (Figure 87).

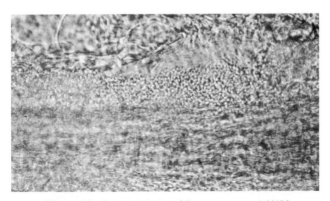

Figure 87. Ectrothrix hair—*Microsporum canis* X400

Culture: All of the species of *Microsporum* can be grown on Sabouraud glucose agar. Add cycloheximide and chloramphenicol or use Mycosel or Mycobiotic agar. At least two or three hair stubs should be placed into the medium and kept for at least two weeks. Other media, such as Dermatophyte Test Medium, may be used for presumptive identification. Emmon's medium and modified cornmeal agar are useful for macroconidia formation.

1. *Microsporum audouinii* Gruby, 1843

Occurrence

Humans: This species, originally endemic in Europe, North America, and other parts of the world, is now rare in children. In the United States this species has been replaced most commonly by *Trichophyton tonsurans*. The ectothrix hairs of *M. audouinii* usually fluoresce.

Animals: *M. audouinii* is not normally found in animals. It has been reported on a dog and a capuchin monkey in the United States and on a dog in England.

Colonies: Colonies on Sabouraud glucose agar develop slowly, forming a matted, velvety surface with straggly edges, and are light tan to brown in color (Figure 88). The reverse side is buff-salmon to orange-brown. Growth on rice grains is poor.

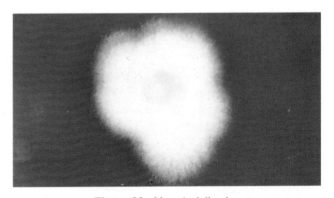

Figure 88. *M. audouinii,* colony

Macroconidia are rarely found on culture medium. Microscopically they are poorly formed and have thick, rough, or smooth walls. Some may be nearly spindle-shaped but are usually very irregular in shape (Figure 89a). The number of cells varies from a few to eight or nine. Microconidia, when present, are sessile or on short stalks along the hyphae, clavate and single-celled. Racquet hyphae, pectinate hyphae, nodular bodies, and chlamydoconidia may be found (Figures 76-80, page 72). Look for these structures in a direct mount or in a slide culture. Terminal beaked chlamydoconidia are characteristic of this species (Figure 89b).

(continued on page 76)

Table 5. Characterization of Certain Dermatophytes
(Grown One to Two Weeks on Sabouraud Plus Antibiotics, Mycosel, or Mycobiotic Agar)

Macroconidia usually rough-walled
Microsporum

- Usually absent, terminal chlamydoconidia, poor growth on rice agar
M. audoinii
- Usually 2 cells
M. namum
- Usually more than 4 cells
  - Elliptical
    - Thick-walled, 4–6 cells
    M. cookei
    - Thin-walled, 4–6 cells
      - *M. gyspseum*
      - More narrow, clavate to elliptical
      M. fulvum
  - Spindle-shaped, thick-walled, 6–12 cells
  M. canis
  - Clavate to elongate
    - Thick-walled, 5–6 cells pink surface, red pigment diffuses
    M. gallinae
    - Thin-walled, 6 cells buff to pink-buff
    M. persicolor
  - Cylindrofusiform
  M. Vanbreuseghemii

Macroconidia clavate, thin, smooth-walled, olive-green colony.
Epidermophyton floccosum
M. Vanbreuseghemii

Microconidia numerous
Trichophyton

- Colonies red, round-clavate microconidia
  - Urease +, cornmeal agar, red color, clavate
  T. rubrum
  - Urease +, cornmeal agar no red color, hair-perforation
  T. mentagrophytes
  - Pink surface
    - Red pigment diffuses no histidine for growth See *M. (T.) gallinae* (usually in fowl)
    - No red pigment diffusion histidine for growth
    T. megninii
    (Europe, Africa)

- Colonies powdery to velvety. white to cream, reverse side yellow to brown
  - Microconidia oval to clavate
    - Urease + microconidia in clusters
      - *T. mentagrophytes*
      - Nicotonic acid required
      T. equinum
  - Microconidia clavate
    - Thiamine, better growth usually sunken or raised center in colony
    T. tonsurans

Microconidia few or absent, only hyphae

- *M. audouinii*
- *Trichophyton*
  - Waxy, folded, slow-growing colonies
    - Violet color
    T. violcaeum
    (rare—USA)
    - Thiamine plus inositol 37°C better growth
    T. verrucosum
    - Cream ro white, favic chandeliers No growth requirements
    T. schoenleinii

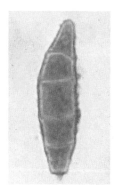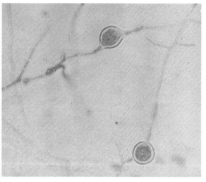

Figure 89. *Microsporum audouinii* X400
a. Macroconidium   b. Chlamydospores

Special comments: Poor growth on rice helps to separate this species from *M. canis.* The addition of yeast extract to the medium may stimulate formation of macroconidia in some strains of *M. audouinii.* Infected hairs usually fluoresce.

2. *Microsporum canis* Bodin, 1902 *M. canis* var. *canis*

Occurrence

Humans: This fungus is the cause of tinea capitis and tinea corporis. The source of infection is usually an animal (the organism is zoophilic). The disease is worldwide in distribution. Infected hairs usually fluoresce.

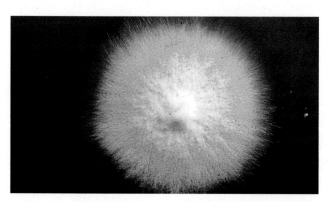

Figure 90. *Microsporum canis,* colony

Animals: *M. canis* has been isolated commonly from ringworm of cats and dogs and less frequently from monkeys, horses, and rabbits.

Soil: Reported from sand beaches in Hawaii and soil in Romania.

Colonies: Colonies on Sabouraud agar develop fairly rapidly, forming cottony or woolly mycelium, white to buff in color, and later becoming buff to brown in the center. The reverse side of the colony is yellow to orange-brown. The bright yellow color occurs when the colonies are five to seven days old. This species grows well on rice grains (Figure 90).

Microscopically, the macroconidia are characteristic of the species, i.e., they are numerous, large, many-celled, and spindle-shaped, with rough thick walls (Figure 91). The macroconidia are 8 to 20 by 40 to 150 µm in size and 6 to 15 celled. A few small, one-celled, clavate to elongate microconidia may be found along the hyphae. Racquet hyphae, pectinate hyphae, nodular bodies, and chlamydoconidia may be seen.

Special comments: *M. canis* grows readily on rice grains (polished) while *M. audouinii* does not. Macroconidia form more readily on Emmons' medium or on modified cornmeal agar.

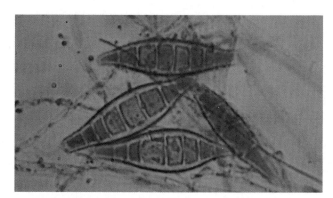

Figure 91. *Microsporum canis,* macroconidiaX800

Perfect state (teleomorph): *Arthroderma otae* (Hasegawa and Usui, 1974) McGinnis et al, 1986. This is the ascomycetous state of *M. canis.* The ascocarps are globose, white changing to buff with age, 280 to 700 µm in diameter. Peridial hyphae are hyaline, septate, echinulate, constricted at cell junction, and usually dichotomous, rarely verticillately branched. The tips of the peridial hyphal branches are usually blunt and often curved toward the ascocarps. The three kinds of appendages are: (1) long (up to 150 µm), straight, slender, smooth-walled and septate hyphae, (2) spiral or long coiled hyphae, and (3) hyphal appendage with thick-walled, echinulate macroconidia. Subglobose, thin-walled, evanescent asci (5 to 7 µm) contain eight smooth, lenticular ascospores (2 to 2.5 by 2.5 to 3.8 µm).

3. Microsporum canis var. *distortum*

Occurrence

Humans: A few reports of tinea capitis in the United States, Australia, New Zealand. Greenish fluorescence in infected hairs.

Animals: *M. canis* var. *distortum* has been reported in monkeys, dogs, horses, and pigs. Hairs usually fluoresce.

Colonies: Colonies develop fairly rapidly, resembling *M. canis* var *canis*. The reverse side of the colony may have no yellow to tan.

Microscopically, macroconidia are like *M. canis* var. *canis* with thick-walled, rough surfaced macroconidia, but bent and distorted (Figure 92). Clavate microconidia are sessile on the hyphae.

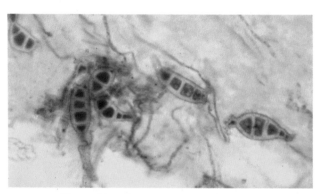

Figure 92. *Microsporum canis* var *distortum* Macroconidia X200

Special comments: *M. canis* var. *distortum* grows well on rice grains (polished) like *M. canis* var. *canis*. Microconidia produced on modified cornmeal agar.

4. Microsporum cookei Ajello, 1959

Occurence:

Humans: Smooth skin infections have been reported in humans.

Animals: Although isolated from dogs, rats, and monkeys, no lesions developed. Usually isolated from soil.

Colonies: Colonies on Sabouraud glucose agar develop rapidly and are flat and spreading, with a rather powdery surface which is yellowish, buff, or dark tan due to the macroconidial mass (Figure 93). The colony resembles a mutant of *M. gypseum* with dark pigments. Reverse side is deep purplish-red.

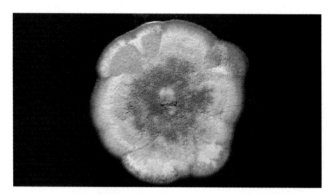

Figure 93. *M. cookei*, colony

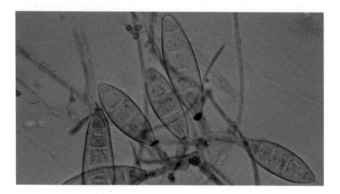

Figure 94. *M. cookei*, macroconidia X400

Microscopically, the numerous macroconidia are oval to ellipsoidal, echinulate, with very thick walls (Figure 94). Macroconidia are 31 to 50 by 50 by 10 to 15µm on Sabouraud or modified cornmeal agars, and similar to *M. gypseum* except for wall thickness.

Special Comments: None.

Perfect State (Teleomorph): *Arthroderma cajetani* Ajello, 1961. The perfect state appears in some strains on hair in culture. The ascocarps are globose, pale buff to yellow in color, 368 to 686µm in diameter; peridial hyphae are slightly constricted, hyaline, septate verticillately branched, and echinulate. Two kinds of appendages are present: elongated, slender tapered hyphae up to 480µm long, and elongated, slender hyphae coiled into spirals. Asci are globose or ovate, golden, smooth-walled, and 3 to 3.6 by 1.8μm in size. Heterothallic.

5. *Microsporum ferrugineum* Ota, 1922 (synonym: *Trichophyton ferrugineum*)

Occurence

Humans: This organism causes tinea capitis in children in middle Europe, Asia, Russia, and Africa. Hairs usually fluoresce.

Animals: Not reported.

Colonies: Colonies are rather slow growing, heaped, with many deep furrows, glabrous and waxy, with a deep yellow-orange color (Figure 95). A white velvety cover may form over the colony. The colonies develop sectors readily with variations in color intensities, at times appearing as non-pigmented forms, resembling *T. verrucosum*.

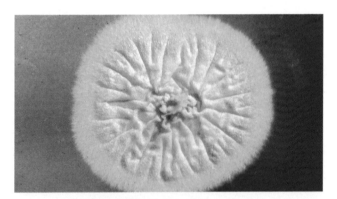

Figure 95. *M. ferrugineum, colony*

Microscopically the only structures seen are hyphae, bamboo hyphae, and chlamydoconidia (Figure 96). The small-spored ectothrix type hair infection similar to *M. canis* is the basis for locating this species in the genus.

Special comments: No special nutritional requirements. Stock cultures should be maintained at room temperature.

6. *Microsporum gallinae* (Megnin) Grigorakis, 1929 (synonym: *Trichophyton gallinae* Silva et Benham, 1952).

Occurrence:

Humans: Very rare in humans as tinea capitis, tinea corporis, and tinea cruris. Ectothrix hair infection, no fluorescence.

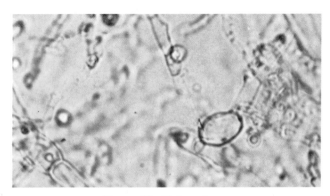

Figure 96. *M. ferrugineum*
hyphae and chlamydoconidia X800

Animals: Occasionally the cause of favus in chickens. Also reported in a cat, mouse, and monkey.

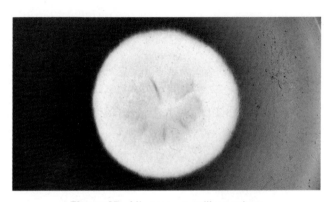

Figure 97. *Microsporum gallinae, colony*

Colonies: Colonies are moderately fast growing, at first flat, then heaped with radial folds. Older folds may show pink color. Edges of colonies may be irregular. Reverse side of colony develops a yellow color at first, then changes to a deep strawberry-red color, diffusable in the medium (Figure 97).

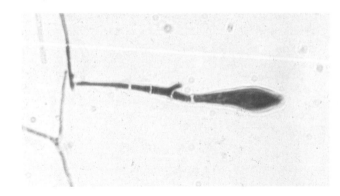

Figure 98. *Microsporum gallinae, macroconidium X400*

Microscopically, a few small pyriform develop. Macroconidia may occur and are thin-walled, smooth or with an echinulate surface at the tips. The macroconidia are two- to ten-celled, club-shaped to elongate to slipper-shaped with blunt tips, 6 to 8 by 15 to 50µm, and frequently curved.

Special comments: The addition of thiamine or yeast extract may may increase sporulation. The presence of echnulations on the macroconidia was the basis for change of the genus from *Trichophyton* to *Microsporum*.

7. *Microsporum gypseum* (Bodin) Guiart and Grigorakis, 1928

Occurrence:

Humans: This species, which is the cause of an inflammatory type tinea corporis or tinea capitis, is worldwide in distribution. Usually no fluorescence of infected hairs.

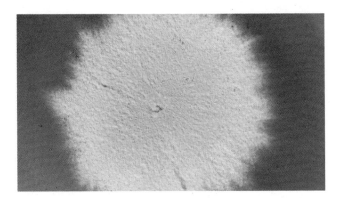

Figure 99. *Microsporum gypseum*, colony

Animals: *M. gypseum* has been reported in dogs, horses, rabbits, squirrels, monkeys, cats, pigs, rats, and mice.

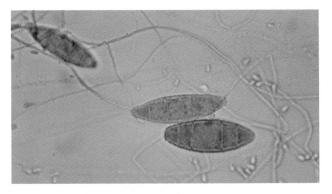

Figure 100. *Microsporum gypseum* microconidia and macroconidia

Soil: Geophilic in soil throughout the world.

Colonies: Colonies grow rapidly on Sabouraud agar,

becoming powdery and buff to cinnamon-brown in color (Figure 99). Some strains may form white aerial mycelium at first and then become matted. In older colonies sterile hyphal growth (pleomorphism) develops rapidly as a cottony growth over the original powdery surface. Reverse side of colony is pale-yellow to tan and occasionaly red in some strains.

Microscopically, a slide culture or on slide containing a portion of the colony will show numerous large, rough, thin-walled, ellipsoid, three-to nine-celled, commonly four- to six-celled macroconidia, 8 to 12 by 30 to 50µm in size, with echinulate walls (Figure 100). Clavate microconidia are usually sessile on the hyphae.

Special comments: None.

Perfect state (Teleomorph): *Arthroderma incurvatum* (Stockdale) Weitzman et al, 1986, and *Arthroderma gypseum* (Nannizzi) Weitzman et al. *A. incurvatum* and *A. gypseum* have similar ascocarp morphology in the sexual state of *M. gypseum*. The ascocarps are globose, light-buff or yellow-buff and 350 to 650µm in size when grown on hair or on oatmeal agar. The peridial hyphae of *A. gypseum* are asperulate, septate (small constrictions), verticillately branched, and the branches curve out, then back. Some branches are spirally coiled at the apex. Asci are globose to ovate, 5 to 7µm in size, with eight smooth, lenticular ascospores, 2.8 to 3.5 by 1.5 to 2.0µm in size. *A. gypseum*, which has similar ascocarps may be differentiated from *A. incurvatum* by the peridial hyphal branches curving back over the ascocarp.

8. *Microsporum fulvum* Uriburu, 1909

Occurrence

Humans: Ringworm in humans similar to that of *M. gypseum*. No fluorescence.

Animals: Reported in dogs, occasionally other animals.

Soil: Geophilic throughout the world.

Colonies: Colonies grow rapidly on Sabouraud agar, becoming dense, downy to floccose, and tawny-buff in color. The advancing edge of the colonies is often fluffy white. Pleomorphic. Reverse side of the colony is usually dark red or colorless, yellow-brown.

Microscopically, the characteristic large, thin-walled macroconidia are clavate to bullet-shaped and measure 24 to 58 by 7.5 to 12µm. Four to six cells are usual. Clavate microconidia are numerous and similar to those of *M. gypseum*.

Special comments: Similar to *M. gypseum* except for shape of macroconidia.

Perfect state (Teleomorph): *Arthroderma fulvum* (Stockdale), Weitzman et al, 1986. The ascocarps are larger (500 to 1,300µm) than *A. gypseum* but otherwise the same. The asci, ascospores, and peridial hyphae are similar to *A. gypseum*. Identification is based on mating with compatible strains.

9. *Microsporum nanum* Fuentes, 1956

Occurrence:

Humans: Tinea capitis has been reported in a boy and tinea corporis was reported in a man. Rare in the United States.

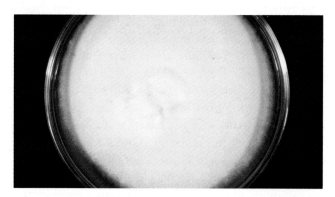

Figure 101. *M. nanum,* colony

Animals: Periodically causes tinea in pigs.

Soil: In the United States, Mexico, Canada, and Australia.

Colonies: Colonies grow rapidly producing a powdery surface. The color of the colony is buff with a granular surface (Figure 101). The colonies may become white and cottony in the pleomorphic form. The reverse side of the colony is frequently red to brown.

Microscopically, the characteristic macroconidia are small, pear-shaped or clavate, rather thin-walled, usually verrucose; the spore two- to three-celled, 12 to 18 by 4 to 7.5µm in size (Figure 102). Numerous microconidia may be formed on hair and soil cultures, while only a few are formed on Sabouraud agar. The hair filaments are perforated *in vitro*. Ectothrix type hair, spores are sparse on animals or humans, with no fluorescence.

Special comments: Some *Chrysosporium* species may produce conidia similar to the macroconidia of *M. nanum*.

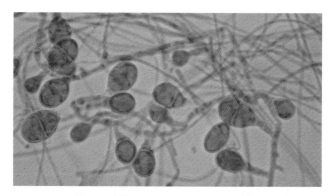

Figure 102. *M. nanum*—macroconidia

Perfect state (Teleomorph): *Arthroderma obtusa* Dawson et Gentles, 1961. The ascocarps are globose, 250 to 450µm in diameter, with pale-yellow peridial hyphae. Peridial hyphae are hyaline, septate, branched dichotomously, at obtuse angle from main hypha, cells thick-walled, echinulate, cylindrical, about 13 by 4 to 7µm, with one to two slight constrictions. Appendages are septate, smoothwalled, with lateral or terminal tightly coiled spirals. Asci subglobose, evanescent, 5.5 by 5 to 6µm in size. Eight ascospores, usually smooth, lenticular, 2.7 to 3.2 by 1.2 to 2µm in size, and yellowish.

10. *Microsporum persicolor* (Sabouraud) Guiart and Grigorakis, 1928.

Occurrence:

Humans: Rare cause of ringworm in Britain, Europe, and the United States.

Animals: Zoophilic, reported on bank voles, field voles, bats, shrews, and mice.

Soil: Reported worldwide.

Colonies: Colonies are fast growing, flat at first, becoming fluffy and folded, yellowish-buff to pink. The reverse is variable from peach, rose, to deep ochre. On sugar-free medium areas of rose to red or deep wine appear.

Microscopically the organism resembles *T. mentagrophytes* due to the abundance of clusters of clavate, fusiform, or globose microconidia. The predominance of stalked, elongate, clavate microconidia is distinctive. Coils are common. The macroconidia are sparce, thin-walled, clavate to fusiform, and six-celled, with some echinulations at the tip.

Special comments: On sugar-free medium (Pablum agar) the surface and reverse of the colonies develop rose to deep wine tints, which helps distinuish it from *T. mentagrophytes*. On this medium long, clavate, stalked microconidia are characteristic.

Perfect state (Teleomorph): *Arthroderma persicolor* (Stockdale) Weitzman et al, 1986. The buff-colored ascocarps are globose, 250 to 900μm in diameter with peridial hyphae asperate, septate, hyaline to buff in color, and dichotomously branched with distal ends curved over the ascocarps. The peridial branches are composed of symmetric cells with one central constriction, and at times terminate with coils. Asci evanescent, subglobose, 4.3 to 6 by 7μm with eight hyaline ascospores yellow in mass, smooth-walled, lenticular, and 2.3 to 3.3 by 1.5 to 2.1 μm in size.

11. *Microsporum vanbreuseghemii* Georg, Ajello, Friedman, and Brinkman, 1962

Occurrence:

Humans: A rare ringworm infection reported in the United States, also in Africa, India, and Russian republics.

Animals: Reported in dogs, squirrels, and cats.

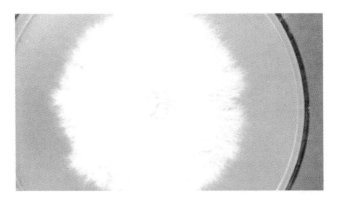

Figure 103. *M. vanbreuseghemii,* colony

Soil: Isolated from soil.

Colonies: Colonies are fast spreading, flat, surface powdery or downy, creamy-yellow to pink in color (Figure 103). The reverse side of the colony is colorless to yellow. Variants or pleomorphism develop readily.

Microscopically, the numerous macroconidia are cylindrofusiform, seven to ten septations, thick-walled with a rough surface (Figure 104). These rough or echinulate macroconidia are 58.8 to 61.7 by 10.4 to 110.6μm in size. Microconidia may be abundant, pyriform to obovate in shape.

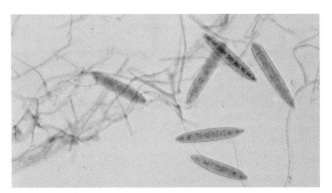

Figure 104. *M. vanbreuseghemii,* macroconidia X400

Special comments: This species differs from *Trichophyton ajelloi* by the lack of a purple pigment, readily infects guinea pigs, and has echinulate macronidia. Little or no fluorescence in infected hairs.

Perfect state (Teleomorph): *Arthroderma grubyi* (George, Ajello, Friedman, et Brinkman) Ajello et al., 1986. The ascocarps are globose, white to pale buff, and 150 to 600μm in diameter. The peridial hyphae are hyaline, septate, branched dichotomously, and branched uncinately, usually curving away from main hyphae. Cells thick-walled, echinulate, phalangiform, 2 to 7.5μm in diameter. Spirals terminal on peridial hyphae. Asci globose, evanescent, 4.8 to 6.0μm in size with eight hyaline, smooth-walled, yellow, oval ascospores, 2.4 by 3.0μm in size. Heterothallic.

Descriptions of rare species of *Microsporum*: *M. praecox* and *M. racemosum* are not included in this manual.

Animal inoculation: *M. gypseum* and *M. canis* and some of the other species will infect kittens, puppies, young rabbits, and other young laboratory animals. In three to five days after inoculation, a severe inflammatory reaction develops, and later a heavy crust. Some of the hair may become involved and drop out as in alopecia. After a month or more the laboratory animals usually recover spontaneously. If laboratory animals are inoculated, observe the course of infection.

Questions

1. What are the important macroscopic and microscopic characteristics used to distinguish the species of the genus *Microsporum?* Select the key characteristics for each species and learn to recognize them (Examples: *M. canis, M. gypseum,* and *M. cookei*).

2. Is it possible to distinguish the species of *Microsporum* causing a tinea capitis case by microscopic examination of an infected hair? Explain.

3. Of what value is Wood's light in the laboratory identification of *Microsporum* spp.? Is there any difference in fluorescence between species of *Microsporum*?

4. What is the value to the physician of specific identification of the fungus in clases of tinea capitis?

Selected References

Ajello L. 1956. Soil as a natural reservoir for human pathogenic fungi. Science 112

Ajello L. 1968. A taxonomic review of the dermatophytes and related species. Sabouraudia 6:147

Ajello L. 1977. Taxonomy of the dermatophytes: A review of their imperfect and perfect states. *In* Iwata, K. (ed.) *Recent Advances ln Medical and Veterinary Mycology.* University of Tokyo Press, Tokyo

Barson WJ. 1985. Granuloma and pseudogranuloma of the skin due to *Microsporum canis.* Arch. Dermatol. 121:895

Benham RW. 1953. Nutritional studies of the dermatophytes: effect on growth and morphology, with special reference to the production of macroconidia. Trans. NY. Acad. Sci. 15:102

Brock JM. 1961. *Microsporum nanum:* A cause of tinea capitis. Arch. Dermatol. 84:504

Brooks BE, Alli JH, Campbell CC. 1959. Isolation of *Microsporum distortum* from a human case. J. Invest. Dermatol. 33:23

Dawson CO, Gentles JC. 1961. The perfect stages of *Keratinomyces ajelloi* Vanbreuseahem, *Trichophyton terrestre* Durie and Frey, *Microsporum nanum* Fuentes. Sabouraudia 1:49

Devroey C, Wuytack-Raes C, Fossoul F. 1983. Isolation of saprophytic *Microsporum praecox* Rivalier from sites associated with horses. Sabouraudia 21:255

Hasegawa A, Usul K. 1975. *Nannizzia oate* sp. nov., the perfect state of *Microsporum canis* Bodin. Jap. J. Med. Mycol. 16:148

Hazen EL. 1957. Effect of temperature and nutrition upon macroconidial formation of *Microsporum audouinii.* Mycologia 49:11

Hill TW. 1975. Ultrastructure of ascosporogenesis in *Nannizzia gypsea.* J. Bacteriol. 122:743

Hironaga M, Nosaki K, Watanabe S. 1980. Ascocarp production by *Nannizzia otae* on keratinous and non-keratinous agar media and mating behavior of *N. otae* and 123 Japanese isolates of *Microsporum canis.* Mycopathologia 722:135

Luedeman GM, LeeBreton E. 1972. Laboratory mill for pulverizing and homogenizing nail specimens as an aid to microscopy and culture confirmation. Appl. Microbiol. 23:814

Onsberg P. 1978. Human infections with *Microsporum persicolor* in Denmark. Br. J. Dermatol. 99:531

Orr GF. 1969. Keratinophilic fungi isolated from soils by a modified hair bait technique. Sabouraudia 7:129

Padhye AA. 1969. Cellophane mounts of ascigerous states of dermatophytes and other keratinophilic fungi. Mycologia 60:1242

Padhye AA, Carmichael JW. 1989. Tinea capitis caused by *Microsporum praecox* in a patient with sickle cell anemia. J. Med. Vet. Mycol. 27:313

Resusta A, Rubio MC, Alejandre MC. 1991. Differentiation between *Trichophyton mentagrophytes* and *T. rubrum* by sorbitol assimilation. J. Clin. Microbiol. 29:219

Sinski JT, Kelley LM. 1991. A survey of dermatophytes from human patients in the United States from 1958 to 1987. Mycopathologia 114:117

Stockdale PM. 1961. *Nannizzia incurvata* gen. nov., sp. nov., a perfect state of *Microsporum gypseum.* Sabouraudia 1:41

Stockdale M. 1963. The *Microsporum gypseum* complex (*Nannizzi incurvata* Stockd., *N. gypsea* (Nann.) comb. nov., *N. fulva* sp. nov.). Sabouraudia 3:114

Tagami H. 1985. Epidermal cell proliferation in guinea pigs with experimental dermatophytosis. J. Invest. Dermatol. 85:153

Wolf FT, Jones EA, Nathan HA. 1958. Fluorescent pigment of *Microsporum.* Nature (London) 182:475

Wright C, Lennox JL, James WD, Oster CN, Tramont EC. 1991. Generalized chronic dermatophytosis in patients with human immunodifficiency virus type 1 infection and CD4 depletion (Correspondence). Arch. Dermatol. 127 (2):265

EPIDERMOPHYTON SPP.

Characteristics

Epidermophyton consists of two species, *E. floccosum* and *E. stockdaleae. Epidermophyton floccosum,* the only pathogenic species in the genus, is a common cause of tinea cruris and tinea pedis.

It may cause epidemics in institutions, camps, and other group settings.

Etiologic Agents

Epidermophyton floccosum (Harz) Langeron and Milochevitch, 1930, is the only pathogenic species in this genus. The second species, *E. stockdaleae* Prochacki and

Engelhardt-Zasada, 1974 has been reported as a soil isolate with some colony variations.

Occurrence

Humans: *E. floccosum* is found throughout the world; it has a higher incidence in the tropics than elsewhere.

Animals: Reported in a dog. Not likely to occur in animals.

Laboratory Procedures

Specimen collection: Skin scrapings or pieces of the inner nail should be placed in a sterile container. A portion of the specimens may be put directly into a suitable medium.

Direct examination: Place infected skin or pieces of nail on a slide containing a drop of 10% to 20% KOH or with a drop of calcofluor white and add a coverglass. Heat gently to speed clearing and softening of the material.

Although there are a number of methods for staining nails and scales for permanent slides, the following method for making semipermanent mounts has been satisfactory for skin or nail material if the washing procedure is carefully followed. With reasonable care, the slides should last for a long period after being sealed with fingernail polish or sealing compounds.

1. Place the material (skin or nail) in a small glass container with 10% to 20% KOH (thin flakes of skin for five minutes and small pieces of nail for 20 minutes or more).

2. Remove the digested material from the KOH solution by decanting.

3. Wash thoroughly with water two or three times for five to ten minutes each time.

4. Wash two or three more times with 1% lactic acid or acetic acid to neutralize the material.

5. Mount small pieces of the material in lactophenol and seal coverglasses with fingernail polish or sealing compounds.

Microscopically, the fungus appears in the material as septate, branching mycelial strands identical to those that may be found in *Microsporum* skin infections. The threadlike hyphae of the fungus may be seen under low power, but more details of the hyphae and arthrconidia, if present, may be seen under higher magnification (Figure 105).

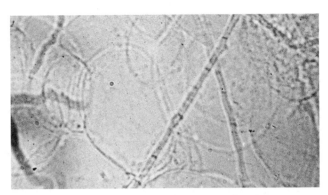

Figure 105. Hyphae in skin, KOH positive X600

Precautions: (1) Do not mistake fat globules or air bubbles for arthroconidia or the crystals of KOH that give a mosaic pattern for the branching mycelium. (2) At least two or more preparations of randomly selected material should be made before a negative microscopic finding is reported. A confirmatory culture must be made.

Culture: The fungus grows slowly at room temperature on Sabouraud glucose agar with the addition of chloramphenicol and cycloheximide to prevent bacterial contamination and overgrowth by saprophytic molds. Three or four pieces of infected material should be placed into the agar medium.

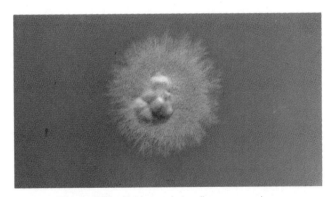

Figure 106. *Epidermophyton floccosum*, colony

Colonies: Colonies develop fairly rapidly with a velvety to powdery surface, khaki-yellow color, and a cottony center (Figure 106). The reverse side of the colony is yellow to tan in color. The khaki-yellow colonies usually develop numerous radiating furrows. In several weeks some strains become covered with the pleomorphic form, which is cottony with mostly white, sterile aerial mycelium.

Microscopically, many large clavate, smooth, thin-walled, two to six-celled macroconidia, 7 to 12 by 20 to 40µm in size, single or in clusters (Figure 107). No microconidia are produced. Chlamydoconidia, usually racquet hyphae, and nodular bodies may he present. Occasionally spirals may be found. Look for these on a slide culture.

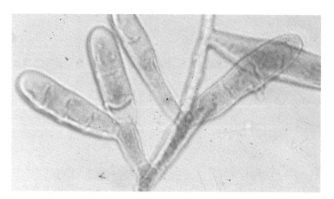

Figure 107. *Epidermophyton floccosum,* macroconidia

Special comments: Stock cultures may be difficult to maintain, as colonies are pleomorphic and low temperature is not favorable. Media with low sugar content or a modified cornmeal agar are better for macroconidial production.

Animal inoculation: Laboratory animals are not successfully infected.

Questions

1. Distinguish the genus *Epidermophyton* from *Microsporum.*

2. Is it posible to distinguish mycelium of *Epidermophyton, Microsporum,* and *Trichophyton* in infected skin or nail material?

Selected References

Ajello L, Getz MD. 1954. Recovery of dermatophytes from shoes and shower stalls. J. Invest. Dermatol. 22:17

Castellani A. 1910. Observations on new species of *Epidermophyton* found in tinea cruris. Br. J. Dermatol. 22:147

Lloyd KM, Greer JE. 1961. Two clinical variations in *Epidermophyton floccosum.* Arch. Dermatol. 84:2

McCormack P, Benham RW. 1952. An unusual finding in *Epidermophyton floccosum.* J. Invest. Dermatol. 19:315

Prochacki H, Engelhardt-Zasada C. 1974. *Epidermophyton stockdaleae* spp. nov. Mycopathologia 54:341

Rippon JW. 1992. Forty-four years of dermatophytes in a Chicago clinic (1944-1988). Mycopathologia 119:(1) 35

Scheklakow ND, Delektorski WW, Babajan KR. 1977. Einige Besonderheiten der Ultrastruktur der *Epidermophyton floccosum* und sein Lagerung in den Geweben der Kranken mit Epidermophytia inquinalis. Castellani 5:131

TRICHOPHYTON SPP.

Characteristics

The genus *Trichophyton* consists of a large number of species which attack the skin, nails, and hair, resulting in a wide variety of symptoms, depending upon the species and the location of the infection. Infected hairs have arthroconidia in parallel rows on the outside of the shaft (ectothrix type) or inside the shaft (endothrix type). This genus is the most likely cause of tinea pedis and tinea unguium in humans. Other types of ringworm in adults and children also may be due to species in this genus. The clinical symptoms vary considerably for this group of organisms so that laboratory identification is necessary for final diagnosis. Usually no fluorescence occurs in hairs infected by *Trichophyton* spp.

Most of the *Trichophyton* species may be isolated on Sabouraud glucose agar at room temperature. The addition of antibacterial substances and antifungal substances for inhibition of saprophytes is desirable. Specific media may be needed for species identification.

Colonies: Colonies of this genus may appear cottony to velvety, granular to powdery, raised or wrinkled and folded with a velvety to waxy surface. Pigmentation varies from white, pink, red, purple, violet, yellow, or orange to brown.

Microscopically some species have numerous microconidia that are small single-celled, spherical, clavate, or pyriform in shape and borne singly on the sides of hyphae (enthryse) or in grapelike clusters (en grappe). Macroconidia, which are rare or lacking in some species, appear as long, thin-walled, many-celled, clavate to fusiform structures, 20 to 50 by 4 to 8μm in size. Racquet hyphae, nodular bodies, coiled hyphae, and chlamydoconidia may be present.

Etiologic Agents

In 1968 there were 20 species that appeared distinct (Ajello, 1968). Ajello (1968) transferred the genus *Keratinomyces* to *Trichophyton* along with the new combination *T. ajelloi* and *T. longifusum.* A new species was described, *T. gloriae,* by Ajello and Cheng (1967). There are six species that invade the hair to produce an ectothrix-type infection. The following four are common in the United States: *T. mentagrophytes* (Robin) Blanchard, 1896; *T. equinum* (Matruchot and Dassonville) Gedoelst, 1902;

Bodin, 1902. The species not likely to be reported in the United States is *T. megninii* Blanchard, 1896.

In the six species that produce an ectothrix-type hair infection, the arthroconidia are formed on the outside of the hair shaft. Seven species have an endothrix-type hair invasion with the hyphae breaking up into arthroconidia inside the hair shaft, except that *T. schoenleinii* is of the "favic type" with less breaking up of hyphae into arthroconidia. Three occur in the united States: *T. tonsurans* Malmsten, 1945; *T. schoenleinii* (Lebert) Lanaeron and Milochevitch, 1930; and *T. violaceum* Bodin, 1902. The endothrix species not likely to occur in the United States are: *T. gourvillii* Catanei, 1933; *T. simii* (Pinoy) Stockdale, Mackenzie, and Austwick, 1965; *T. soudanense* Joyeux, 1912; and *T. yaoundei* Cochet and Doby-Dubois, 1967. The hair is not invaded in the species *T. concentricum* Blanchard, 1896. The following have been isolated from soil: *T. georgiae* Varsavsky and Ajello, 1964 (perfect state: *Arthroderma ciferrii* Varsavsky and Ajello, 1964); *T. terrestre* Durie and Frey, 1957 (perfect state: *Arthroderma quadrifidum* Dawson and Gentles, 1961) and two other perfect states for *T. terrestre* (see page 92) *T. ajelloi* (Vanbreuseghem) Ajello, 1976 (perfect state: *Arthroderma uncinatum* Dawson and Gentles, 1961); *T. gloriae* Ajello and Cheng, 1967; (perfect state: *Arthroderma gloriae* Ajello and Cheng, 1967); *T. vanbreuseghemii* Rioux, Jarry, and Juminer, 1964 (*Arthroderma gertleri* Bohme, 1967).

Laboratory Procedures

Specimen collection: Scrapings of the skin and shavings of the nails should be collected from the active border of the lesions where the fungus is more likely to be found. Infected hairs should be depilated. The specimens should be collected in a sterile container or paper packets or inoculated directly into the proper medium.

Direct examination: Place the infected hair, skin, or nail on the slide with 10% KOH or with a drop of calcofluor white and add a coverglass. Heat gently to clear and soften the material. If hair is put in lactophenol, the slide may be sealed and kept for future reference. Positive skin or nail material may be preserved by the semipermanent mount method (see laboratory procedure under *Epidermophyton*). The nail and skin material also may be stained with periodic acid-Schiff stain for skin material. The addition of blue-black ink to the KOH solution without the addition of calcofluor white will aid in differentiation of the fungal elements.

Microscopically, these fungi appear as septate, branching mycelial strands similar to *Microsporum* and *Epidermophyton* mycelial strands in the skin or nail. Older hyphae may have arthroconidia. Be sure to differentiate any artifacts from the fungus hyphae in the determination of positive material. Let slide stand until artifacts appear and compare with hyphae, if KOH is used (see photograph of a positive skin Figure 105, page 83).

Microscopically, the infected hairs will show rows of arthroconidia inside the hair shaft (endothrix type) or outside the hair shaft (ectothrix type). *T. schoenleinii* and *T. violaceum* may show cupshaped crusts (scutula) at the base of the hair shaft. The former also will have air spaces in the areas left by the degenerate hyphae and few or no arthroconidia inside the hair shaft.

Culture: All of the species of *Trichophyton* can be grown at room temperature: *T. verrucosum* grows better with the addition of yeast extract to Sabouraud glucose agar. At least two or three pieces of skin, nail, or hair stubs should be placed into the agar medium and kept for two weeks or more before the culture is considered negative. The addition of cycloheximide and chloramphenicol to the medium is desirable for the isolation of these species from clinical materials. Other media, such as dermatophyte test medium, may be used for presumptive identification (see page 36 for media preparation).

Table 5 (page 75) is a flow diagram of the characteristics microscopically and of the colonies in culture for the different species of *Trichophyton*.

Nutritional tests for differentiation of *Trichophyton* species: Acid-cleaned glassware should be used for the nutritional tests. The basal medium consists of casein or ammonium nitrate agar, plus the addition of thiamine, inositol, nicotinic acid, or histidine added singly or in combination to one of the basal media. It is important to take a very small amount of the fungal colony for each transfer to avoid a carry-over of the nonvitamin free medium. The use of these media is especially helpful in differentiation of *T. equinum* from *T. mentagrophytes*, *T. tonsurans* from *T. mentagrophytes*, *M. gallinae* from *T. megninii*, and *T. verrucosum* from some strains of *T. schoenleinii*. Expected results are shown in Table 6 (page 87). These media are commercially available. For preparation of the media, see page 44.

Ectothrix Hair Invasion

1. *Trichophyton mentagrophytes* (Robin) Blanchard, 1896

Occurrence

Humans: This species is a common cause of an inflammatory-type ringworm on the feet (athlete's foot or tinea pedis), hands, smooth-skin area (tinea corporis), and nails (tinea unguium). It also occurs on the beard (tinea barbae) and scalp (tinea capitis). Infections occur throughout the world.

Animals: This organism may cause ringworm in cattle, horses, dogs, cats, sheep, pigs, rabbits, squirrels, monkeys, chinchillas, silver foxes, laboratory rats, and mice and at times in other animals.

Soil: Occasionally isolated.

Colonies: Colonies develop rather rapidly, having a powdery to granular surface and being light buff (Figure 108) to rose-tan in color. Some isolates may have a deep wine color (Figure 109) instead of the light buff color on the reverse side (Figure 110). On subsequent transfers or in older colonies a fluffy, cottony, white mycelium may appear (pleomorphic).

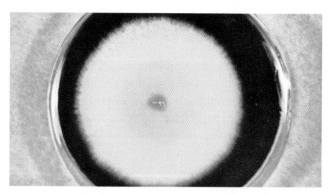

Figure 110. *T. mentagrophytes* var. *erinacei*, colony

Microscopically, a lactophenol slide mount of a powdery or granular culture will show numerous microconidia singly and in clusters along the hyphae (en grappe). Note the clusters in Figure 111. The microconidia are round, thin-walled, one-celled. Characteristic spirals, nodular bodies, chlamydoconidia, and racquet hyphae may be present. The cottony colonial forms should have fewer conidia and other structures present. The macroconidia may be rare or numerous in different strains, clavate to variable in shape, three- to five-celled, thin-walled, aand 4 to 7 by 20 to 50µm in size.

Special comments: No special nutrients needed. On autoclaved hair *T. mentagrophytes* will perforate it and *T. rubrum* will not. On cornmeal agar the red strains of this species produce no color while *T. rubrum* produces a deep rose-red color. Urease test is positive in seven days for *T. mentagrophytes,* but negative for *T. rubrum.* Typical colonies of *T. mentagrophytes* var. *mentagrophytes* are flat, cream to buff and powdery on the surface. *T. mentagrophytes* var. *quinckeanum* may produce deeply pigmented colonies while *T. mentagrophytes* var. *erinacei* is likely to produce yellow granular forms. *T. mentagrophytes* var. *interdigitale* produces downy to cottony colonies with a cream center and white margins.

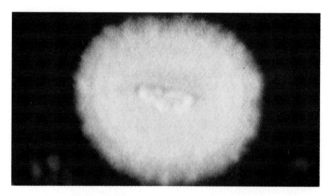

Figure 108 *Trichophyton mentagrophytes* colony

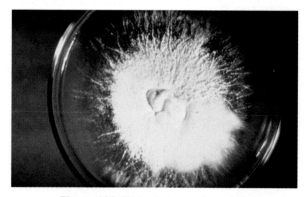

Figure 109 *Trichophyton mentagrophytes* colony

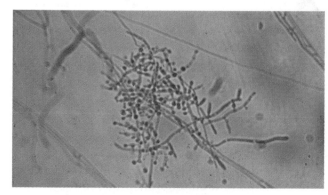

Figure 111. *T. mentagrophytes*, microconidia (grape-like clusters) X400

Table 6. Nutritional Patterns for *Trichophyton* spp.

Species	Test Media*	
	Casein (#1)	Casein + Nicotinic Acid (#5)
T. equinum	0	4+
T. mentagrophytes	4+	4+
	Casein (#1)	Casein + Thiamine (#4)
T. mentagrophytes	4+	4+
T. rubrum	4+	4+
T. tonsurans	± to 1+	4+
T. violaceum	±	4+
Microsporum ferrugineum	4+	4+
	NH_4NO_3 (#6)	NH_4NO_3 + Histidine (#7)
M. gallinae	4+	4+
T. megninii	0+	4+

	Casein (#1)	Inositol (#2)	Casein + Thiamine (#4)	Casein + Thiamine + Casein + Inositol (#3)
T schoenleinii	4+	4+	4+	4+
T. verrucosum	84% 0	±	0	4+
	15% 0	0	4+	4+
T. concentricum	50% 4+	4+	4+	4+
	50% 2+	2+	4+	4+

* 4+ indicates maximum growth for the series of test tubes as compared with growth in other tubes. ±indicates a trace of growth around the inoculum. Little or no growth indicates biochemical deficiencies.

Perfect state (Teleomorph): *Arthroderma benhamiae* Ajello and Cheng, 1967. Ascocarps globose, 400 to 500μm in diameter, white. Peridial hyaline hyphae, interwoven, asperulate, dumbbell-shaped with spiral appendages. Asci globose, thin-walled, hyaline, evanescent, with eight ascospores, 1.2 to 2.8μm in size. *A. vanbreuseghemii* Takashio, 1973, is a second perfect state of *T. mentagrophytes* species complex. The differences are larger ascospores, 2 to 3.5μm in diameter, and no interspecific crosses.

2. *Trichophyton equinum* (Matruchot and Dassonville) Gedoelst, 1902

Occurrence

Humans: Usually does not occur in humans.

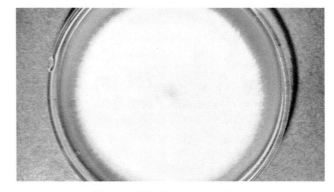

Figure 112. *T. equinum,* colony

Animals: Commonly a cause of ringworm in horses, occasionally in dogs. Worldwide except in Africa.

Colonies: Colonies grow rapidly, flat, developing folds when older. Surface white, cottony with yellow color in the edge around the new growth. Later the colony becomes velvety and cream-tan in color. The reverse side of the colony is bright yellow at first, becoming dark pink to brown in time. Nicotinic acid (niacin) is usually required for growth. *T. equinum* colony, Figure 112.

Microscopically, a few to many spherical to pyriform, short stalked microconidia along the hyphae or in clusters. The macroconidia, clavate and thin-walled, are rare. Nodular bodies and other structures may be present.

Special comments: Nicotinic acid (niacin) is a diagnostic, special nutritional requirement for most strains. Isolates from Australia and New Zealand require no growth factors.

3. *Trichophyton rubrum* (Castellani) Sabouraud, 1911

Occurrence

Humans: A frequent cause of tinea corporis, tinea pedis, tinea cruris and tinea unguium. Lesions with marked reddened margins and central clearings. Distributed throughout the world.

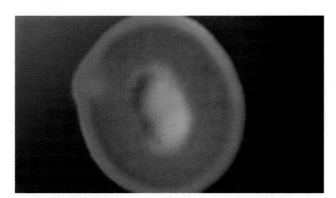

Figure 113. *Trichophyton rubrum*, colony

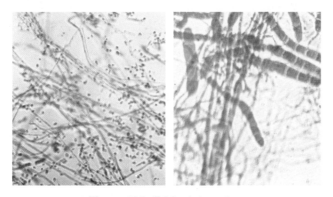

Figure 114. *Trichophyton rubrum*
a) microconidia X200 b) macroconodia X400

Animals: Rare in animals, but reported in a dog, cat, rabbit, monkey, sheep, and cow.

Colonies: Colonies that are primary isolates are cottony to velvety and white. The reverse side of the colony develops reddish to rose-purple pigmentation which may appear on the top surface of marginal hyphae (Figure 113).

Microscopically, numerous clavate microconidia (2 to 3 by 3 to 5μm) are clusters and along edges of the hyphae on slides made from primary cultures, or slide cultures. Usually few macroconidia, chlamydoconidia, racquet hyphae, and nodular bodies are produced in some cultures. Numerous long, thin-walled, three to eight-celled macro conidia are formed in cultures on heart infusion tryptocase agar. Observe as many of these structures as possible under the microscope (Figures 114a and 114b).

Special comments: No special nutrients are needed. On autoclaved hair, *T. rubrum* will not perforate it *in vitro*. On potato dextrose agar and cornmeal agar the pigment formation for some strains is very marked for this species, while *T. mentagrophytes* produces no red color. Urease test is negative in seven days.

4. *Trichophyton verrucosum* Bodin, 1902

Occurrence

Humans: A highly inflammatory infection involving areas of the scalp (tinea capaitis), the beard (tinea barbae), and exposed areas of the body (tinea corporis). This species occurs throughout the world.

Animals: This species is most likely to be the cause of ringworm in cattle, donkeys, dogs, goats, sheep, and horses.

Colonies: Colonies develop best on enriched media such as Sabouraud glucose agar plus yeast extract, or modified cornmeal agar with yeast extract. Thiamine and inositol may be substituted for yeast extract. The colonies are slow growing, heaped, deeply folded, glabrous and waxy or with a fine white velvety surface. Colors vary in isolations from white to bright yellow. Study the growth rate of this species and compare with other *Trichophyton* species. Some strains require both thiamine and inositol for growth. Most rapid growth occurs at 37°C (Figure 115).

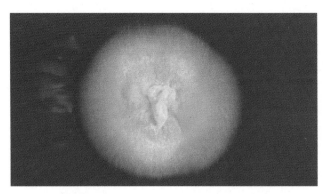

Figure 115. *Trichophyton verrucosum,* colony

Microscopically, only chlamydoconidia are seen in the hyphae on Sabouraud glucose agar. On media enriched with thiamine, microconidia are usually produced, and on rare occasions "rattained" three- to five-celled macroconidia, varying in size and shape, may be seen.

Special comments: Special nutrients are needed, thiamine, and for many strains, inositol. Stock cultures should be kept at room temperature and not in the refrigerator.

5. *Trichophyton megninii* Blanchard, 1896

Occurrence

Humans: This fungus is the primary cause of tinea barbae and occasionally the cause of tinea corporis and tinea capitis in Europe and Africa.

Animals: Reported on dogs.

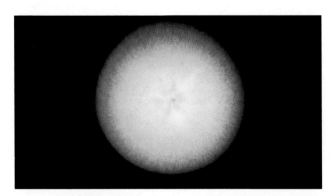

Figure 116. *Trichophyton megninii,* colony

Colonies: Colonies are slow growing, cottony to velvety and white at first, becoming pink later. A nondiffusable rose to red pigment develops on the reverse side (Figure 116). The addition of L-histidine to the medium or the use of trypticase dextrose agar stimulates growth. Compare with *M. gallinae,* Figure 97, page 78.

Microscopically numerous small, pyriform to clavate microconidia may be seen singly or in clusters along the hyphae. Macroconidia, which are rare, develop as clavate, two- to ten-celled, with thin, smooth walls.

Special comments: Special nutrients needed. This species requires L-histidine for growth on a NH_4NO_3 basal medium.

Ecto-endothrix Hair Invasion

Trichophyton simii (Pinoy) Stockdale, Mackenzie, and Austwick, 1965

Occurrence

Humans: Several cases from contact with animals. Hair invasion of the neoendothrix type.

Animals: Ringworm infection, originating in or from India, has been found in monkeys, poultry, and a dog. Infected hairs in animals fluoresce.

Soil: Occurs as a saprophyte.

Colonies: Colonies are fast growing, 75 to 84 mm in diameter in 14 days at 25°C, with a conical, velvety, umbo center, finely granular. The surface is white to pale buff or rosy buff, and the reverse side is colorless at first, later vinaceous. In three or four weeks the vinaceous color may diffuse into the medium and onto the surface, if on 2.5% malt extract agar. On glucose peptone agar the surface is pale buff with the reverse side straw to salmon colored.

Microscopically, there are numerous smooth-walled, cylindrical to fusiform macroconidia on complexly branched hyphae with four to seven (sometimes up to ten) septa. Microconidia are rare at first, more numerous later, clavate to pyriform with a narrow base. Spirals may be present.

Special comments: No special nutrients needed. Colonies grow more rapidly than *T. mentagrophytes,* are thinner and more granular. On malt extract agar *A. simii* produces a vinaceous color, while *T. simii* shows ecto-endothrix infections. *T. simii* produces more macroconidia.

Perfect state (Teleomorph): *Arthroderma simii* Stockdale, Mackenzie, and Austwick, 1965. Ascocarps globose, pale buff, 200 to 750 μm in diameter. Peridial hyphae hyaline, pale buff, septate, verrucose walls. Some peridial hyphae have spirals, loosely or tightly coiled. Asci subglobose, evanescent, 5 to 7.7µm in diameter, with eight hyaline, smooth-walled, lenticular ascospores 2.9 to 3.3 by 1.7 to 2.1µm, yellow in mass. Heterothallic.

Endothrix Hair Invasion

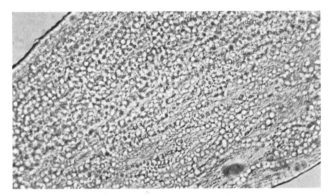

Figure 117. Endothrix hair
Trichophyton violaceum X400

1. *Trichophyton tonsurans* Malmsten, 1945

Occurrence

Humans: This species usually causes tinea capitis with a black dot appearance from broken and crumbled hair shafts on the scalp due to abundant sporulation inside the hair. Occasionally tinea corporis, tinea pedis, or tinea unguium may occur. Worldwide.

Animals: Rare, but cases reported in a horse and a dog.

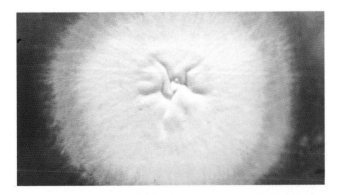

Figure 118. *Trichophyton tonsurans*, colony

Colonies: Colonies develop fairly slowly on Sabouraud glucose agar, forming raised or sunken centers and a folded surface with yellowish color in the depressions. The surface of the colony is velvety to powdery with a variation in color from creamy white, yellow, or rose to brown. (Figure 118). Compare with other species.

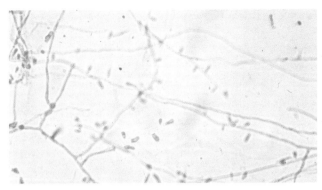

Figure 119. *Trichophyton tonsurans*, microconidia X400

Microscopically, numerous varied length, clavate microconidia (2 to 5 by 3 to 7µm) are attached along the sides of the hyphae or on short stalks (Figure 119). The thin-walled, club-shaped macroconidia are rare. Numerous chlamydoconidia and racquet hyphae may be seen.

Special comments: *T. tonsurans* grows better with the addition of thiamine, which helps to separate this species from *T. mentagrophytes* and *T. rubrum*. The narrow clavate microconidia are also characteristic.

2. *Trichophyton schoenleinii* (Lebert) Langeron and Milochevitch, 1930

Occurrence

Humans: Primarily a favus infection of tinea capitis, at times causing tinea corporis, and at times tinea unguium. The hairs typically have degenerate hyphae or air spaces and hyphae present, with cup-like crusts in the hair follicles (scutula). More common in Eurasia and North Africa than in North or South America.

Animals: Cases have been reported in dogs, cats, hedgehogs, mice, cows, horses, rabbits, and guinea pigs.

Colonies: Colonies are very slow growing, heaped with many irregular folds, waxy smooth, later or upon subsequent transfers becoming velvety white. The color varies from yellowish white to to light brown (Figure 120). This species grows well at room temperature or 37°C without the addition of vitamins to the medium.

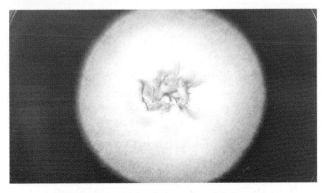

Figure 120. *Trichophyton schoenleinii*, colony

Microscopically, the characteristic structures are the "favic chandeliers" (Figure 121), even though other species in this group may have these same structures. Chlamydoconidia or hyphal swellings are commonly found, but no macroconidia have been reported. Microconidia may be formed in rare cases, especially on rice grains.

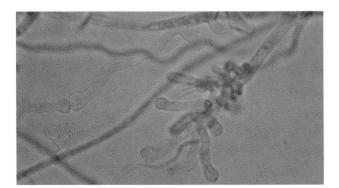

Figure 121. Favic chandeliers X600

Special comments: No special nutrients needed. *T. schoenleinii* is readily differentiated from *T. verrucosum* which grows well at 37°C and *T. schoenleinii* needs no thiamine.

3. *Trichophyton violaceum* Sabouraud, apud Bodin, 1902

Occurrence

Humans: Usually a cause of ringworm of the scalp and body (tinea capitis and tinea corporis), at times causes tinea unguium and favus-like symptoms. Present in Europe, North Africa, Russia, Eastern Europe, United States, and Brasil. Hair invasion is of the endothrix type with many arthroconidia inside the shaft (Figure 117).

Animals: Reported to have infected a calf, dog, cat, horse, mouse, and pigeon.

Colonies: Colonies are slow growing (up to three or four weeks required), forming a heaped, folded, glabrous, waxy surface with a violet color. Later, a velvety, aerial mycelium may appear. More vigorous growth occurs with the addition of trypticase and thiamine to Sabouraud glucose agar (Figure 122). Loss of pigment may occur in variants when transfers are made. Compare colony characteristics with those of *T. schoenleinii.*

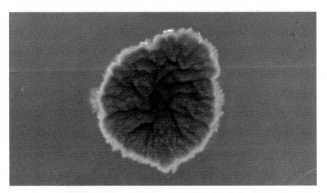

Figure 122. *Trichophyton violaceum,* colony

Trichophyton concentricum Blanchard, 1896

Occurrence

Humans: This organism is the chief cause of tinea imbricata (tinea corporis with concentric rings of scales on the skin), occurring commonly in South Pacific islands and also in Guatemala, southern Mexico, and central Brasil. **Animals:** No reported cases.

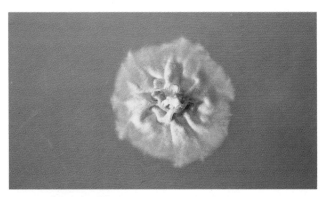

Figure 123. *Trichophyton concentricum,* colony

Colonies: Colonies are raised, deeply folded, smooth and white at first, becoming cream to amber or brown, and covered with short gray hyphae (Figure 123). The reverse side of the colony is cream to brown in color. Slow growing, 5 to 20 mm in diameter after ten days.

Microscopically, this organism is similar to strains of *T. schoenleinii.* The swollen hyphae with chlamydoconidia and aborted hyphal branches are typical. Macroconidia and microconidia are lacking.

Special comments: About 50% of the strains grow better with thiamine in the medium.

Saprophytes Found in Soil

1. *Trichophyton georgiae* Varsavsky and Ajello, 1964

Occurrence

The habitat of this nonpathogenic species is soil or hairs of the oppossum in the United States.

Colonies: Colonies are flat with an umbonate, grayish vinaceous center. The periphery is more granular, pale brownish to vinaceous with a fringed edge. Reverse side of colony is brown, spotted with dark red or vinaceous brown.

Microscopically, microconidia are abundant, variable in size and shape, elongate-clavate or at times pyriform to subglobose, one-celled, up to three-celled on occasions, 4.2 to 6.4 by 2.0 to 2.4μm in size.

Special Comments: None.

Perfect state (Teleomorph): *Arthroderma ciferrii* Varsavsky and Ajello, 1964. Ascocarps globose, 500 to 800μm in diameter with appendages, ochraceous-salmon becoming brownish-vinaceous with age. Peridium has uncinately branched hyphae with curled ends. Peridial hyphae dumbell-shaped, asperulate. Appendages two types: smooth-walled, spiralled hyphae, or smooth-walled, tapered hyphae. Asci subglobose, evanescent, with eight ascospores. Heterothallic.

2. *Trichophyton terrestre* Durie and Frey, 1957

Occurrence

This nonpathogenic species is found in soil throughout the world and has been isolated from hair of wild rats and horses.

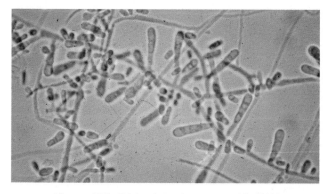

Figure 124. *Trichophyton terrestre,* colony

Colonies: Colonies are moderately fast growing, 50 to 30μm in diameter after ten days, powdery to velvety, resembling *T. mentagrophytes* at times, with a pale lemon-yellow to buff surface color (Figure 124). The reverse colony color may be yellow or reddish.

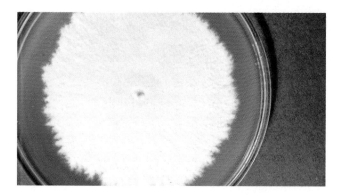

Figure 125. *Trichophyton terrestre,* conidia X400

Microscopically, microconidia are peglike to clavate with a flat base. Transitional forms from microconidia to several-celled macroconidia may be present (Figure 125). Spiral coils may form.

Special comments: No special nutrients needed.

Perfect state (Teleomorph): *Arthoderma quadrifidum* Dawson and Gentles, 1961. Ascocarps globose, pale buff, 400 to 700μm, average 580μm in diameter without appendages. The peridial hyphae are pale yellow, hyaline, septate, incinately branched with cells that are thick-walled, strongly echinulate, dumbbell-shaped when young, maturing into short humerus bonelike forms with condyles on one side. The appendages are septate with spirals of varying length. Subglobose, evanescent asci produce eight hyaline ascospores that are smooth or finely roughened, lenticular, 1.8 to 2.7 by 0.9 to 1.8μm and yellow in mass. Heterothallic. Two other perfect states are known: *A. lenticularum* Pore, Twao et Plunkett, 1965; and *A. incingulare* Padhye et Carmichael, 1972.

3. *Trichophyton ajelloi* (Vanbreuseghem) Ajello, 1967

Occurrence

Humans: A few cases of tinea corporis have been reported. Usually no evidence of infection.

Animals: A few rare cases reported in cattle, a dog, a horse, and a squirrel.

Soil: Frequently isolated from soil.

Culture: This organism grows readily at room temperature on Sabouraud glucose agar (with the addition of antibiotics if material is contaminated).

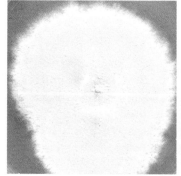 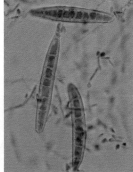

Figure 126. *Trichophyton ajelloi*
a. colony   b. macroconidia X200

Colonies: Colonies grow rapidly, with a flat surface varying from finely powdered to downy, and cream, tan or orange-tan in color (Figure 126a). The reverse side of the colony varies from no pigmentation to to reddish or deep bluish-black.

Microscopically, macroconidia are numerous, cylindro-fusiform (cylindric with tapering ends), thick, smooth-walled, with 5 to 12 cells, 20 to 65 by 5 to 10µm in size (Figure 126b). Microconidia usually abundant, pyriform to ovate in shape, sessile.

Special comments: White cottony areas (pleomorphic) develop readily in the colonies.

Perfect state (Teleomorph): *Arthroderma uncinatum* Dawson and Gentles, 1961. Ascocarps globose, white to buff, 300 to 900µm in size. The peridial hyphae are hyaline, septate, uncinately branched usually away from the main branch of the main hyphae. Cells are thick-walled, echinulate, dumbbell-shaped, and 4 to 5µm in diameter. The spirals are smooth-walled, borne terminally or laterally of peridial hyphae. The asci are globose, evanescent, 4.9 by 7.2µm in size, with yellow ascospores.

4. *Trichophyton gloriae* Ajello and Cheng, 1967

Occurrence

No reports of infection in humans or animals. Isolated from soil in California, New Mexico, and Arizona.

Culture: These develop a flat, downy to powdery surface with a variation in color from white, cream, yellow to cinnamon (resembles *T. ajelloi*). Reverse side a chrome-yellow.

Microscopically, chlamydoconidia and hyphal swellings are the usual mycelial structures seen on Sabouraud agar. Microconidia may occur in small numbers on media enriched with thiamine.

Special comments: All strains are partially dependent on thiamine for growth. Stock culture should be kept at room temperature in preference to refrigerated.

5. *Trichophyton gourvillii* Catanei, 1933

Occurrence

Humans: This endothrix species is the cause of tinea capitis and tinea corporis in Africa.

Animals: No known cases.

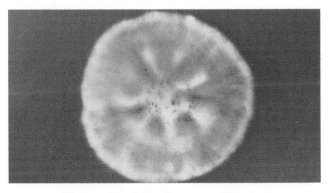

Figure 127. *Trichophyton gourvillii*, colony

Colonies: Colonies are somewhat similar to those of *T. violaceum* and *T. soudanense*. The surface is folded, heaped, and waxy, later becoming velvety with light lavender to deep garnet-red pigmentation. (Figure 127)

Microscopically, microconidia and macroconidia have been reported in some isolates.

Special comments: No special nutritional requirements. In contrast, *T. violaceum* needs thiamine and *T. megninii* requires histidine.

6. *Trichophyton soudanense* Joyeux, 1912

Occurrence

Humans: This endothrix species primarily causes ringworm of the scalp (tinea capitis) and tinea corporis. Occurs primarily in Africa and occasionally in Brasil, the United States, and Great Britain through immigration of individuals.

Animals: No known cases.

Colonies: Colonies are slow growing (5 to 20 mm in diameter after ten days), flat, later raised or at times folded in center. Surface is smooth to velvety, lemon-yellow to apricot in color (Figure 128). Reverse side of colony is yellow to orange. Variants (pleomorphisms) develop readily.

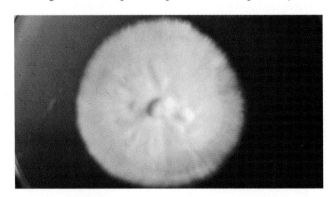

Figure 128. *Trichophyton soudanense*, colony

Microscopically, the hyphae separate readily into arthroconidia. Numerous or occasional microconidia occur and are ovoid or clavate to pyriform in shape. Reflexive or right angle branching of hyphae are bunched into a bushlike bundle.

Special Comments: No special nutrients needed. Stock cultures survive better at room temperature than in refrigerator.

7. *Trichophyton yaoundei* Cochet and Dubois, 1957

Occurrence

Humans: This endothrix species causes tinea capitis and is found primarily in the Cameroon and Congo areas of Africa.

Animals: No known cases.

Colonies: Colonies are slow growing, very glabrous, raised and folded, and white to cream in color at first, later becoming tan to chocolate brown in a few weeks with some diffusion of the pigment in the medium. There may be some submerged hyphal growth in the medium. Pleomorphic changes or sectors develop. Subcultures may lose the characteristic brown color.

Microscopically, numerous chlamydoconidia form on the irregular hyphae. No macroconidia; microconidia are rare, when present pyriform in shape along the hyphae.

Special comments: No special nutritional requirements. Young colonies may resemble *T. verrucosum* but do not require thiamine for growth.

8. *Trichophyton vanbreuseghemii* Rioux, Jarry, and Juminer, 1964
    Occurrence

Humans: Reported as a hand infection.

Animals: No infections.

Soil: Worldwide.

Colonies: Colonies are powdery to fine velvety, buff in color. The center has folds. Microscopically, the microconidia are club-shaped, with broad attachment scars, and are along the hyphae. The macroconidia are club-shaped to cylindrical with round ends and are thin-walled. In older macroconidia the cells may separate.

Special comments: None.

Perfect state (Teleomorph): *Arthroderma gertleri* is heterothallic, with peridial hyphae developing a row of oval beadlike cells.

Questions

1. Distinguish *Trichophyton* from *Microsporum* and *Epidermophyton.*

2. How are the *Trichophyton* species separated?

3. Compare the mode of growth of species of *Trichophyton* with *Microsporum* in the hair.

4. Describe the technique for isolation of a dermatophyte, beginning with a lesion on a patient.

5. Compare the appearance of *Malassezia furfur* with *Trichophyton* in the skin.

6. Differentiate hair infections with *Corynebacterium tenuis,* black or white piedra, *Microsporum* spp., and *Trichophyton* spp. Can the genus be distinguished, in all cases should cultures be made?

7. After reading some of the current literature on physiologic studies of growth of the dermatophytes, compare the effects of various compounds upon the growth of these fungi.

8. Where do the perfect states (teleomorph) of some of the dermatophytes usually occur?

9. Explain why the species in the former genus *Keratinomyces* were were transferred to the genus *Trichophyton.*

Selected References

Ajello L. 1968. A taxonomic review of the dermatophytes and related species. Sabouraudia 6:147

Ajello L. 1977. Taxonomy of the dermatophytes: A review of their imperfect and perfect states. *In* Iwata K (ed). *Recent Advances in Medical and Veterinary Mycology,* University of Tokyo Press, Tokyo

Ajello L, Georg LK. 1957. In vitro hair cultures for differentiating between atypical isolates of *Trichophyton mentagrophytes* and *Trichophyton rubrum.* Mycopathologia 8:3

Badillet G, Rush-Munro F, Augsburger J. 1975. Interet du milieu lactritmel de Borelli dans l'identification des dermatophytes. Bull. Soc. Mycol. Med. 4:55

Benham RW. 1948. Effect of nutrition on growth and morphology of the dermatophytes. I. Development of macroconidia in *Trichophyton rubrum.* Mycologia 40:232

Bibel DJ, Crumrine DA, Yee K, et al. 1977. Development of arthrospores of *Trichophyton mentagrophytes* Infect Immunol. 15:958

Catanei A. 1933. Description de *Trichophyton gourvilli* n. sp., agend k'une teigne del'homme. Bull. Soc. Path. Exot. 25:377

Connole MD. 1965. Keratinophillic fungi on cats and dogs. Sabouraudia 4:45

Cox DR, Blank F. 1977. Tinea capitis due to *Trichophyton soudanense* Arch. Dermatol. 13:1600

Dawson CO. 1963. Two new species of *Arthroderma* from the soil from rabbit burrows. Sabouraudia 2:185

Dawson CO, Gentles CJ. 1961. The perfect state of

Keratinomyces ajelloi Vanbreuseghem; *Trichophyton terrestre* Durie and Frey, and *Microsporum nanum* Fuentes. Sabouraudia 1:49

Druhet E. 1953. Recherches sur la nutrition des dermatophytes III. L'histidine, facteur de croissance des *Trichophyton* du groupe *rosaceum*. Ann. Inst. Pasteur. 85:791

Dyson JE Jr, Landay ME. 1963. Differentiation of *Trichophyton rubrum* from *Trichophyton mentagrophytes*. Mycopathologia 22:6

Emmons CW. 1934. Dermatophytes. Arch. Dermatol. Syph. 30:337

English MP, Gibson MD. l959. Studies in the epidemiology of the tinea pedis. II. Dermatophytes on the floors of swimming-baths. Br. Mycol. J. 1:1446

English MP, Stockdale PM. 1968. *Trichophyton proliferans* sp. nov., a human pathogen. Sabouraudia 6:267

Fischman 0, De Camargo ZP, Grinhlat M. 1976. *Trichophyton mentagrophytes* infection in laboratory white mice. Mycopathologia 59:113

Georg LK. 1956. Studies on *Trichophyton tonsurans* II. Morphology and laboratory identification. Mycologia 48:354

Georg LK. 1960. Epidemiology of the dermatophytes: Sources of infection, modes of transmission and epidemicity. Ann. NY. Acad. Sci. 89:69

Georg LK, Camp LB. 1957. Routine nutritional tests for the identification of dermatophytes. J. Bacteriol. 74:113

Georg LK, Doupagne P, Pattyn SR, et al. 1963 *Trichophyton yaoundei* a dermatophyte indigenous to Africa. J. Invest. Dermatol. 41:19

Georg LK, Kaplaǹ W, Camp LB. 1957. *Trichophyton equinum* reevaluation of its taxonomic status. J. Invest. Dermatol. 29:27

Gip L. 1964. Isolation of *Trichophyton gallinae* from two patients with tinea cruris. Acta Derm-venereal 44:251

Gordon MA, Little GN. 1968. *Trichophyton* (*Microsporum gallinae*) ringworm in a monkey. Sabouraudia 6:207

Grappel SF. 1976. Role of keratinases in dermatophytosis. IV. Reactivities of sera from guinea pigs with heat-inactivated keratinase II. Dermatologica 153:157

Gugnani HC, Shrivastav JB, Gupta NP. 1967. Occurrence of *Arthroderma simii* in soil and on hair of small mammals. Sabouraudia 6:77

Hejtmanek M, Kunert J. 1965. A dwarf form of *Keratinomyces ajelloi*. Sabouraudia 4:3

Hironaga M, Nozaki K, Watanabe S. 1983. *Trichophyton mentagrophytes* granulomas. Arch. Dermatol. 119:482

Hsu YC, Volz PA. 1975. Penetration of *Trichophyton terrestre* in human hair. Mycopathologia 55:179

Kaaman T, Forslind B. 1985. Ultrastructural studies on experimental hair infections in vitro caused by *Trichophyton mentagrophytes* and *Trichophyton rubrum*. Acta. Derm. Vereol. 65:536

Kane J, Smitka C. 1978. Early detection and identification of *Trichophyton verrucosum*. J. Clin. Microbiol. 8:740.

Kane, J, editor. 1996. *Laboratory Handbook of Dermatophytes*. Star Publishing Co. Belmont, CA

Klein DT. 1964. Time-temperature interaction in the indication of pleomorphism in *Trichophyton mentagrophytes*. J. Gen. Microbiol. 34:125

Londero AT. 1962. The geographic distribution and prevalence of dermatophytes in Brazil. Sabouraudia 2:108

Padhye AA, Ajello L. 1977. The taxonomic status of the hedgehog fungus *Trichophyton erinacei*. Sabouraudia 15:103

Padhye AA, Carmichael JW. 1971. The genus *Arthroderma* Berkeley. Can. J. Bot. 49:1525

Padhye AA, Carmichael JW. 1972. *Arthroderma insingulare* sp. nov. gymnoascaceceous state of the *Trichophyton terrestre* complex. Sabouraudia 10:47

Philpot C. 1967. The differentiation of *Trichophyton mentagrophytes* from *T. rubrum* by a simple urease test. Sabouraudia 5:189

Raubitschek F, Maoz R. 1957. Invasion of nails in vitro by certain dermatophytes. J. Invest. Dermatol. 28:261

Rebell G, Taplin D. 1970. *Dermatophytes, Their Recognition and Identification*. Revised Edition. University of Miami Press. Coral Gables, FL

Rees RG. 1967. *Arthroderma flavescens* spp. nov. Sabouraudia 6:206

Rezusta A, Ribio MC, Alejandre, MC. 1991. Differentiation between *Trichophyton mentagrophytes* and *T. rubrum* by sorbitol assimilation. J. Clin. Microbiol. 29:219

Rioux JA, Jarry DT, Juminer B. 1964. Un nouveau dermatophyte isole du sol: *Trichophyton vanbreuseqhemii*, n. spp. Naturalia Monspel. Ser. Bot. 16:153

Rippon JW, Medenica M. 1964. Isolation of *Trichophyton soudanense* in the United States. Sabouraudia 3:301

Rippon JW, Eng A, Malkinson FD. 1968. *Trichophyton simii* infection in the United States. Arch. Dermatol. 98:615

Rippon JW. 1985. The changing epidemiology and emerging patterns of dermatophyte species. In *Current Topics in Medical Mycology* Vol. 1. Edited by MR McGinnis. New York, Springer-Verlag p. 208

Rosenthal SA, Wapnick H. 1963. The value of Mackenzie's "hair brush" technique in the isolation of *T. mentagrophytes* from clinically normal guinea pigs. J. Invest. Dermatol. 41:5

Sabouraud R. 1894. *Les Trichophyties Humaines*. Rueff et Cie, Paris

Schechter Y, Landau JW, Dabrowa N, et al. 1968. Disc

electrophoretic studies of intraspecific variability of proteins from dermatophytes. Sabouraudia 6:133

Seale ER, Richardson JB. 1960. *Trichophyton tonsurans.* Arch. Dermatol. 81:87

Seeliger HPR. 1985. The discovery of *Achorion schoenleinii:* facts and "stories." Mykosen 28:161

Silva M. 1953. Nutritional studies of the dermatophytes. Factors affecting pigment production. Trans. NY. Acad. Sci. 15:106

Smith JM, Marples MJ. 1963. *Trichophyton mentagrophytes* var. *erinacei.* Sabouraudia 3:1

Stockdale PM. 1967. *Nannizzia persicolor.* spp. nov., the perfect state of *Trichophyton persicolor* Sabouraud. Sabouraudia 5:355

Stockdale PM, Mackenzie DW, Austwick PK. 1965. *Arthroderma simii* spp. nov., the perfect state of *Trichophyton simii* (Pinoy) comb. nov. Sabouraudia 4:112

Sudman MS, Schmitt JA, Jr. 1965. Differentiation of *Trichophyton rubrum* and *Trichophyton mentagrophytes* by pigment production. Appl. Microbiol. 13:290

Summerbell RC. 1987. *Trichophyton kanei* sp. nov., a new anthropophilic dermatophyte. Mycotaxon 28:409

Swartz HE, Georg LK. 1955. The nutrition of *Trichophyton tonsurans.* Mycologia 47:475

Tagami H. 1985. Epidermal cell proliferation in guinea pigs with experimental dermatophytosis. J. Invest. Dermatol. 85:153

Takashio M. 1972 Is *Arthroderma benhamiae* the perfect state of *Trichophyton mentagrophytes?* Sabouraudia 10:122

Takashio M. 1979. Taxonomy of dermatophytes based on their sexual states. Mycologia 71:968

Takatori K, Ishijo S. 1985. Human dermatophytosis caused by *Trichophyton equinum.* Mycopathologia 90:15

Tanaka S, Summerbell RC, Tsuboi R, Kaaman T, Sohnle PG, Matsumoto T, Ray TL. 1992. Advances in dermatophytes and dermatophytosis. J. Med. and Veter Mycology 30, Supplement 1, 29-39

Taplin D, Zaias N, Rebell G, et al. 1969. Isolation and recognition of dermatophytes on a new medium (DTM). Arch. Dermatol. 99:203

Torres G, Georg LK. 1956. A human case of *Trichophyton gallinae* infection. Disease contracted from chickens. Arch. Dermatol. 74:191

Vanbreuseghem R. 1952. Technique biologigue pour l'isolement des dermatophytes du sol. Ann. Soc. belg. Med. Trop. 32:173

Vanbreuseghem R, DeVroey C, Takashio M. 1970. Production of macroconidia by *Microsporum ferru-* *gineum* Ota 1922. Sabouraudia 7:252

Varsavsky E, Ajello L. 1964. The perfect and imperfect forms of a new keratinophillic fungus *Arthroderma ciferri* sp. nov., *Trichophyton georgiae* sp. nov. Riv. Pat. Veg. 4:351

Weigl E. 1976. Simple technique of epicutaneous inoculation guinea pigs with dermatophytes. Mycopathologia 59:149

Weitzman I, Silva-Hutner M. 1967. Non-keratinous agar media as substrates for the ascigerous state in certain members of the Gymnoascaceae pathogenic for man and animals. Sabouraudia 5:335

Weitzman I, Rosenthal S. 1984. Studies in the differentiation between *Microsporum ferrugineum* Ota and *Trichophyton soudanense* Joyeux. Mycopathologia 84:95

Wright DC, et al. 1991. Generalized chronic dermatophytosis in patients with human immunodeficiency virus Type I infection and CD4 depletion. Arch. Dermatol. 127:265

Zaias N. 1972. Onychomycosis. Arch. Dermatol. 105:263

DERMATOMYCOSIS

Dermatomycoses have occasionally been isolated from human skin and nails. The first valid skin infection from a soil organism was described as *Hendersonula toruloidea* Nattras 1933 by Gentles and Evans (1970). *Scytalidium hyalinum* Campbell and Mulder 1977 has been isolated periodically from skin and nail infections. *Scytalidium* is a conidial anamorph of *Hendersonula.* In Jamaica nearly 40 per cent of the population carries this infection on their skin. Some yeastlike fungi due to *Candida* species develop a dermatophytelike disease. A few cases of skin infection by continued contact include *Saccharomyces cerevisiae* (Bakers' yeast), and *Trichosporon capitatum. Scopulariopsis brevicaulis* has occasionally been isolated from skin and nail infections. Some erythematous lesions have been associated with *Fusarium moniliforme,* and *Aspergillus flavus.*

Scytalidium hyalinum Campbell and Mulder 1977, a conidial anamorph of *Hendersonula,* has pale brown one-to two-celled arthroconidia and is hyaline in culture. *Hendersonula toruloidea* Nattrass 1933 is a dematiaceous pycnidial forming hyphomycete. These organisms do no grow in the presence of cycloheximide in the medium.

Selected References

Bereston ES, Keil H. 1941. Onychomycosis due to

Aspergillus flavus. Arch. Derm. Syph. 44:420

Carruthers JA, Stein L, Black WA. 1982. Persistent skin and nail infection by an exotic fungus *Hendersonula toruloidea.* Can. Med. Assoc. J. 127:608

DiSalvo AF, Fickling AM. 1980. A case of nondermatophytic toe onychomycosis caused by *Fusarium oxysporum.* Arch. Dermatol. 116:699

Gentles JC, Evans EGV. 1970. Infection of the feet and nails with *Hendersonula toruloidea.* Sabouraudia 8:72

Moore MK. 1986. *Hendersonula toruloidea* and *Scytalidium hyalinum* infections in London, England. J. Med. Vet. Mycol. 24:219

Onsberg P. 1980. *Scopulariopsis brevicaulis* in nails. Dermatologica 161:259

Summerbell RC, Kane J, and Krajden. 1989. Onychomycosis, tinea pedis and tinea manuum caused by nondermatophytic filamentous fungi. Mycoses 32:609

Chapter 6

SUBCUTANEOUS MYCOSES

The subcutaneous mycoses include a varied group of infections characterized by a lesion developing at the site of inoculation. In contrast, the organisms causing the systemic mycoses primarily enter by the pulmonary route. In most cases the subcutaneous fungal infections are the results of traumatic implantation into the skin. The ensuing disease either remains localized or slowly spreads to the surrounding tissue as is the case with the mycetomas. Some of these infections may spread via the lymphatic channels as frequently is the situation for sporotrichosis. In rare cases hematogenous and lymphatic dissemination have occurred for chromoblastomycosis.

The agents of the subcutaneous mycoses vary in relative virulence, are soil saprophytes, and are extremely variable in ability to adapt to the host tissue which results in variations in the disease development. The agent of sporotrichosis is temperature dependent with limited virulence. Most of the soil isolates are nonpathogenic. In chromoblastomycosis the causative agents usually form sclerotic cells rather readily. However in debilitated patients the same organisms may be mycelial in tissue. Other dematiaceous fungi are mycelial and restricted to opportunistic infections in severely compromised patients. This latter group of fungi with mycelium in tissue belong in the phaeohyphomycosis. Two other diseases included in the heterogeneous subcutaneous mycoses are Lobo's disease (keloid blastomycosis) and rhinosporidiosis.

In the study of the subcutaneous mycoses in class or in the laboratory, the following general procedure is suggested for each disease:

1. Transfer culture and observe time required for colony development. Compare with older cultures or other strains. It is *strongly* recommended that a hood or safety cabinet be used for transfer of these fungi.

2. Prepare a slide culture wherever possible or a direct mount of the fungus in a safety hood. Seal the mounted slides of the mature fungus with fingernail polish or another cement and retain for future study.

3. Inoculate laboratory animals with *Sporothrix schenckii* sufficiently in advance for autopsy at the time the disease is being studied in the laboratory. This will establish the pathogenic form which is entirely different from the saprophytic form. This fungus is known as dimorphic.

4. Smears or direct mounts of materials from the lesions of the laboratory animal should be made for study of the tissue form of the fungus. Histologic sections may be made for tissue study. Stain the smears or histologic sections.

5. Study the physiology and immunology for each disease where possible.

6. Study prepared slides from cases for tissue form characteristics.

7. Use audiovisual aids that are available for study.

8. Study the literature.

See Table 7. This flow diagram will aid in determination of the diseases and causative agents from specimens taken from subcutaneous and deep mycoses cases.

MYCETOMA

(Madura foot, maduromycosis)

Definition

Mycetoma is a chronic granulomatous infection usually involving the feet (Figure 129) and occasionally the hands or other areas of the body. The disease is characterized by enlargement, deformity, sinus drainage, and bone destruc-

Table 7. Laboratory Examination of Clinical Specimens from Subcutaneous and Deep Mycosis with Corresponding Genera and an example of a species of the Etiologic Agents

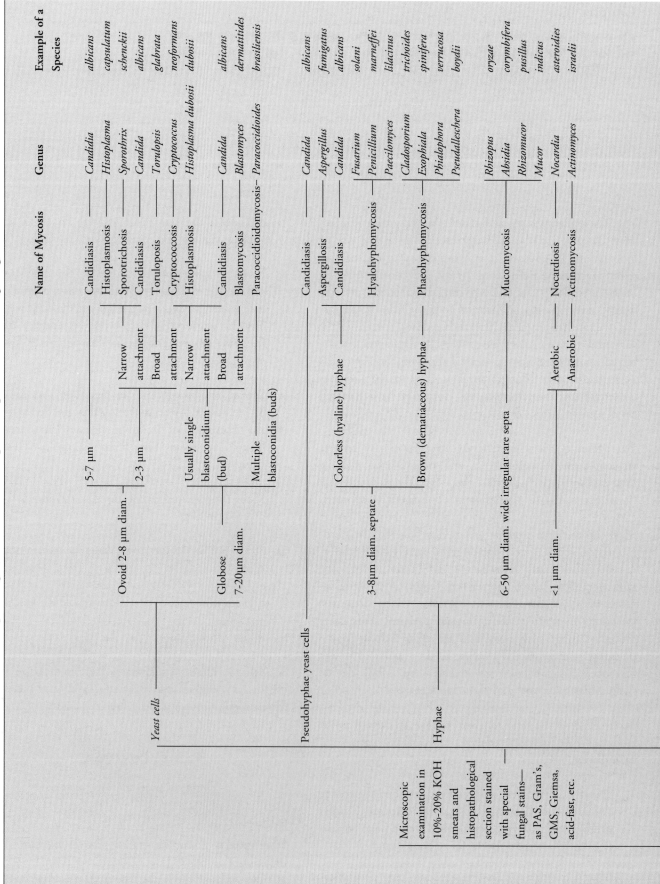

Name of Mycosis	Genus	Example of a Species
Microscopic examination in 10%–20% KOH smears and histopathological section stained with special fungal stains—as PAS, Gram's, GMS, Giemsa, acid-fast, etc.		
Yeast cells — Ovoid 2–8 μm diam. — 5–7 μm		
Candidiasis	*Candida*	*albicans*
Histoplasmosis	*Histoplasma*	*capsulatum*
Ovoid 2–8 μm diam. — 2–3 μm — Narrow attachment		
Sporotrichosis	*Sporothrix*	*schenckii*
Candidiasis	*Candida*	*albicans*
Toruloposis	*Torulopsis*	*glabrata*
Broad attachment		
Cryptococcosis	*Cryptococcus*	*neoformans*
Histoplasmosis	*Histoplasma dubosii*	*dubosii*
Globose 7–20 μm diam. — Usually single blastoconidium (bud) — Narrow attachment		
Candidiasis	*Candida*	*albicans*
Blastomycosis	*Blastomyces*	*dermatitides*
Broad attachment		
Paracoccidioidomycosis—	*Paracoccidioides*	*brasiliensis*
Multiple blastoconidia (buds)		
Pseudohyphae yeast cells		
Candidiasis	*Candida*	*albicans*
Hyphae — 3–8 μm diam. septate — Colorless (hyaline) hyphae		
Aspergillosis	*Aspergillus*	*fumigatus*
Candidiasis	*Candida*	*albicans*
Hyalohyphomycosis	*Fusarium*	*solani*
	Penicillium	*marneffei*
	Paecilomyces	*lilacinus*
Brown (dematiaceous) hyphae		
Phaeohyphomycosis	*Cladosporium*	*trichoides*
	Exophiala	*spinifera*
	Phialophora	*verrucosa*
	Pseudallescheria	*boydii*
6–50 μm diam. wide irregular rare septa		
Mucormycosis	*Rhizopus*	*oryzae*
	Absidia	*corymbifera*
	Rhizomucor	*pusillus*
	Mucor	*indicus*
<1 μm diam. — Aerobic		
Nocardiosis	*Nocardia*	*asteroides*
Anaerobic		
Actinomycosis	*Actinomyces*	*israelii*

Clinical specimen

- Spherules
  - 30-80 μm diam. ——— Coccidioidomycosis ——— *Coccidioides* — *immitis*
  - 100-350 μm diam. ——— Rhinosporidiosis ——— *Rhinosporidium* — *seeberi*
- Filamentous
  - <1 μm diam. ——— Actinomycotic mycetoma — *Nocardia* — *brasiliensis*
    - *Actinomadura* — *madurae*
  - 3-5 μm diam. swollen cells ——— Eumycotic mycetoma — *Acremonium* — *falciforme*
    - *Madurella* — *grisea*
    - *Pseudallescheria* — *boydii*
- Granules
  - Globose cells, dark hyphae ——— Eumycotic mycetoma — *Exophiala* — *spinifera*
  - Bacillary or coccoid cells—1 μm diam. ——— Botryomycosis — *Actinobacillus* — *ligiereresii*
    - *Streptococcus* — *pyogenes*
    - *Staphylococcus* — *aureus*
    - *Proteus* — *vulgaris*
    - *Escherichia* — *coli*
    - *Pseudomonas* — *aeruginosa*
- Sclerotic bodies ——— Chromoblastomycosis — *Fonsecaea* — *pedrosoi*
  - *Cladosporium* — *trichoides*
  - *Phialophora* — *verrucosa*
  - *Exophiala* — *spinifera*
- Chain of hyaline globose cells ——— Lobomycosis — *Loboa* — *laboii*

Examine macroscopically ——— Inoculate 1 tube each SAB, Mycosel. BHIA, and 1 plate of Smith's medium ——— Incubate at 24 or 30°C / 4-6 weeks, if possible *Histoplasma*, 12 weeks ——— Convert to yeast at 37°C if necessary ——— Identify ——— Report tion. The pus usually contains white, light yellow, red, or black grains (Figure 130). Mycetomas are caused by both filamentous fungi and actinomycetes. These involved organisms may cause other diseases which include actinomycosis, mycotic granuloma, and phaeohyphomycosis when the criteria for mycetoma is not met.

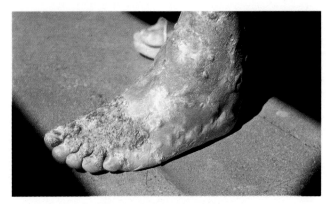

Figure 129. Mycetoma, Foot

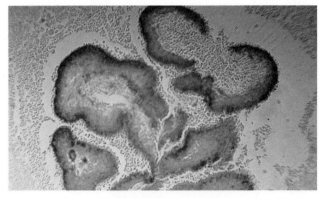

Figure 130. Mycetoma
Granule from mycetoma pedis, Gridley stain X400

Etiologic Agents

Various saprophytic fungi have been isolated as causative agents in mycetoma. There are two forms of mycetomas or tumorlike infections: (1) eumycetic mycetoma caused by species of the higher fungi, and (2) actinomycotic mycetoma caused by members of the actinomycete group.

The important isolates causing eumycotic mycetoma are:

Genus	Grain
Acremonium falciforme	White
Acremonium kiliense	White
Acremonium recifei	White
Aspergillus nidulans	White
Corynespora cassicola	Black
Curvularia geniculata	Black
Curvularia lunata	Black

Cylindrocarpon destructans	White
Exophiala jeansellmei	Black
Fusarium moniliforme	White
Fusarium solani	White
Leptosphaeria senegalensis	Black
Leptosphaeria tompkinsii	Black
Madurella grisea	Black
Madurella mycetomatis	Black
Neotestudina rosatii	White
Polycytella hominis	White
Pseudallescheria boydii	White
Pseudochaetosphaeronema larense	White
Pyrenochaeta romeroi	Black

The following actinomycetes are the most common causes of actinomycotic mycetoma. These organisms are discussed under nocardiosis (page 211), and actinomycosis (page 205).

Agent	Grain
Actinomadura madurae	White-yellow
Actinomadura pelletieri	Garnet-red
Nocardia asteroides	White
Nocardia brasiliensis	White to Yellow
Streptomyces somaliensis	Yellow

Occurrence

Humans: The disease is most common in tropical and subtropical regions, where shoes are not frequently worn. Mycetoma has been reported in Africa, India, Europe, South America, Mexico, and North America and occasionally in other parts of the world. In the United States *Pseudallescheria boydii* is the most likely etiologic agent.

Animals: Cases reported include a dog, a cat, cattle, and horses.

Soil: Most of the organisms have been found in soil and in some cases in plants.

Laboratory Procedures

Specimen collection: Pus should be taken from draining fistulas, or in nondrainage areas pus may be aspirated by a sterile needle and syringe for laboratory studies. Pus, curettings, or biopsy tissues should be collected in sterile shallow bottles or Petri dishes. Use sterile gauze compresses to collect granules.

Direct examination: Gross examination of the pus, curettings, or biopsy material should be made for the presence of small, oval, irregularly formed grains 0.5 to 2 mm in diameter and white, yellow, red, or black in color.

Place some of the grains in water or 10% KOH solution or lactophenol-cotton blue, on a slide, crush and examine under the microscope.

Microscopically, the granules produced by higher fungi often contain colorless or pigmented septate hyphae 2 to 4 μm in diameter with many swellings or chlamydoconidia throughout the structure, including the periphery. Distinguish between granules developed by actinomycetes and higher fungi, noting the difference in width of the hyphae (about 1 μm in diameter for actinomycetes). Eumycotic granules have septate hyphae 2 to 5 μm in diameter with chlamydoconidia in some cases. This finding is important and should be reported immediately to aid in specific treatment, since actinomycotic mycetomas can be treated, and eumycetic mycetomas pose difficult and unique treatment problems. A stained section of a mycetoma is illustrated in Figure 130.

Culture: Colonies of the various fungi develop readily on Sabouraud glucose agar at room temperature. The addition of antibacterial antibiotics is desirable if the granules have true septate hyphae. If the granule has small filaments of an actinomycete, Sabouraud glucose agar without antibiotics or BHI agar is recommended.

Aspirated material may be placed directly on the medium, while granules from draining fistulas should be washed in sterile saline solution of antibiotics to reduce contamination and put on a medium containing antibiotics. Cultures should be incubated both at room temperature and at 37°C. Morphologic and physiologic characteristics are used to identify the etiologic agents.

Etiologic agents: All of the fungal agents causing mycetomas are either in the Deuteromycota or the Ascomycota. Identification is based on morphology and physiologic reactions. Some of these agents are slow growing and should be held 3 to 4 weeks at 30° and 37°C. The actinomycetes as causative agents are under the section on Nocardiosis.

1. *Acremonium (Cephalosporium) falciforme* Carrion, 1951 (white grains)

Colonies: Colonies rather slow growing, cottony or tufted, lavender, buff, or pinkish. Reverse is currant-red in color, occasionally producing a soluble pigment (Figure 131).

Microscopically, hyphae are colorless, 3 to 4 μm in diameter. Conidia are elliptical-shaped, borne in clusters at the tips of simple conidiophores (phialides), one or two-celled, 7-8 × 2.7 to 3.2 μm in size (Figure 132).

Proteolytic activity±; Amylolytic activity-; Glucose+; galactose+; lactose 0; maltose+; sucrose+.

The asexual conidia of *A. kiliense* are one-celled, elliptical and 3 to 6 × 1 to 1.6 μm. Those of *A. recifei* are one-celled, crescent-shaped, and 4 to 7 × 1.3 to 2.0 μm.

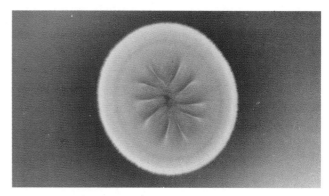

Figure 131. *Acremonium falciforme,* colony

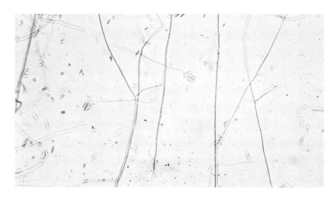

Figure 132. *Acremonium falciforme,* conidia

2. *Aspergillus nidulans:* see section on Aspergillosis (page 169) for more information (**white grains**).

3. *Curvularia geniculata* (**Tracy et Earl**) **Boedigin, 1933.** Sexual state: *Cochliobolus geniculatus,* Nelson 1964 (**black grains**).

Colonies: The colonies are black, typical of dematiaceous hyphomycetes in appearance.

Microscopically, the conidiophores have three to five-celled, curved conidia with an enlarged center cell. *C. lunata* conidia are three-celled.

4. *Exophiala (Phialophora) jeanselmei* (Langeron) McGinnis and Padhye, 1977 (black grains).

Colonies: Colonies slow growing, brown-black, smooth, skinlike and moist on the surface at first, later covered with velvety aerial hyphae. Reverse side of colony is black.

Microscopically, hyphae are at first long rows or chains of budding cells sometimes described as toruloid-like, later developing regular hyphae. *Aureobasidium* like spore formation may be present at first. Later conidia are produced in cuplike or tubelike phialides with a series of annellations.

Proteolytic activity -; Amylolytic activity -.
Carbon assimilation: glucose +; galactose +; lactose 0; maltose +; sucrose +.

5. *Fusarium moniliforme* and *F. solani.* See section on hyalohyphomycosis (page 178) for culture and microscopic characteristics (**white grains**)

6. *Leptosphaeria senegalensis* Segretain, Bayletf, Darasse, et Camain, 1959 (**black grains**)

Colonies: Rapidly growing, producing a downy-grayish colony with the reverse side black usually along with a rose tint in the agar.

Microscopically, no conidia or ascocarps are produced on Sabouraud glucose agar. On cornmeal, ascostroma are produced in several months. In the cavities or locules the asci are interspersed with paraphyses. The eight ascospores in the elongate asci are elongate, five to six cells, with the second cell from the apex enlarged. A second species, *L. tompkinsii,* is similar to *L. senegalensis* except for larger ascocarps and five to eight cells in the ascospores, with the third cell from the apex enlarged.

7. *Madurella mycetomatis* (Laveran) Brumpt, 1905 (**black grains**)

Colonies: Colonies slow growing, cottony to membranous, flat or folded, white, ochraceous, or yellow-brown. Colonies grow best at 37°C or up to 40°C, which distinguishes this species from *M. grisea.*

Microscopically, hyphae are 1 to 6 μm in diameter with many chlamydoconidia. Flask-shaped phialides with round to pyriform conidia 3 to 4 μm in diameter may be produced in some strains when cultured on soil or water agar. Black sclerotia up to 750 μm in diameter may form on media without sugar.

Proteolytic activity: ±; Amylolytic activity +
Carbon assimilation: Glucose +; galactose +; lactose +; maltose +; sucrose -.

8. *Madurella grisea* (Mackinnon, Ferrada, and Montemayer, 1949 (**black grains**)

Colonies: Colonies slow growing, velvety tan or gray aerial mycelium over a cerebriform center and radially folded colony. Older colonies may develop a red to brownish diffusible pigment.

Microscopically, hyphae may be thin, branched, septate, 1 to 3 μm in diameter or larger moniliform, 3 to 5μm in diameter with occasional chlamydoconidia. Both types of hyphae are brownish to black in color. No conidia or sclerotia present.

Proteolytic activity: ±; Amylolytic activity:+.
Carbon assimilation: Glucose +; galactose +; lactose -; maltose +; sucrose +. The lactose and sucrose reactions separate this species from *M. mycetomatis.*

9. *Neotestudina rosatii* Segretain et Destombes, 1961 (**white to brownish white grains**)

Colonies: The organism develops slowly in culture with a more rapid growth at 30° to 37°C. The colonies are tan to brown with radial grooves and a dark brown reverse side.

Microscopically, carbonaceous, scattered ascostroma (ascocarps) are produced with the interior filled with hyaline mycelium containing asci. The asci are nearly spherical, becoming 25 to 30μm long as ascospores mature. The ascospores are dark, curved, and two-celled.

10. *Pseudallescheria boydii* (Schear) **McGinnis, Padhye, and Ajello, 1982 (white grains)**. Imperfect state name: *Scedosporium apiospermum* (Saccardo) Castellani et Chalmers, 1919 (synonym: *Monosporium apiospermum*)

Colonies: Colonies develop rapidly with cottony white, aerial mycelium at first, becoming grey with conidial production, and later brown. Older colonies turn gray with a gray to black pigment on the reverse side (Figure 133a,b). Many isolates produce brown cleistothecia on cornmeal or potato dextrose agar.

Microscopically, a slide mount from the colony or a slide culture should show moderately large, septate hyphae with long or short conidiophores, each terminated by a single oval-to-pyriform conidium, 5 to 7 by 8 to 10μm in size (Figure 134). Occasionally some strains produce a *Graphium* asexual state, known as synnema (clusters of conidiophores) with conidia at the ends of the conidiophores. The conidiogenous cells may show annellations.

Slide mounts from some strains of *P. boydii,* which produce the ascigerous stage, show brown cleistothecia, 50 to 200 μm in diameter. When crushed, evanescent subglobose asci should be seen with eight elliptical, light-brown colored ascospores, 4.5 to 5 by 5.7 to 7 μm in size.

Proteolytic activity +; amylolytic activity -;
Carbon assimilation: glucose+; galactose±; lactose-; maltose -; sucrose ±.

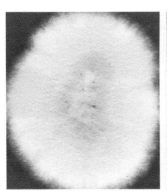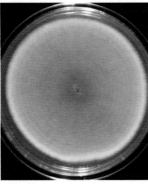

Figure 133. *Pseudallescheria boydii*
a. Colony   b. Reverse of colony

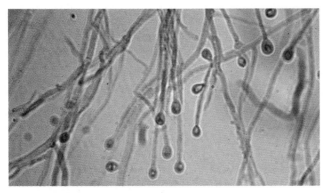

Figure 134. *Pseudallescheria boydii,* conidia

Pathologic studies: Although the granules may be seen readily in sections stained with hematoxylin and eosin, they should also be Gram-stained to aid in differentiation of bacterial masses and fungus granules. The latter stain also aids in distinguishing the filaments of *Nocardia* in granules in case this is the causative organism. The hyphae and chlamydoconidia in the granules developed from higher fungi may be illustrated very well if the pigments are not too dark by the periodic acid-Schiff stain.

Animal inoculations: Most laboratory animals are not suitable for injection with the higher fungi that cause mycetoma. Hamsters (by IP injections) and athymic nude mice (by foot pad) have been shown to develop granules after injections of conidial suspensions.

Questions

1. How are the granules which have developed from infection of an individual with higher fungi distinguished from those developed by the actinomycetes?

2. Explain the origin of the names maduromycosis and mycetoma. Distinguish between eumycetic mycetoma and actinomycotic mycetoma.

Selected References

Ajello L. 1952. The isolation of *Allescheria boydii* Shear, an etiologic agent of mycetomas, from soil. Am. J. Trop. Med. Hyg. 1:227

Ajello L, et al. 1985. *Fusarium moniliforme,* a new mycetoma agent: restudy of a European case. Eur. J. Epidermiol. 1:5

Borelli D. 1962. *Madurella mycetomi y Madurell agrisea.* Arch. Venez. Med. Trop. Parasit. Med. 4:195

Borelli D, Zamora R, Senabre G. 1976. *Chaetosphaeronema larense* nova specie-agente de micetom. Gaceta Medica de Caracas. 84:307

Carrion AL. 1951. *Cephalosporium falciforme* n. sp., a new etiologic agent of maduromycosis. Mycologia 43:522

Cazin J, Decker DW. 1964. Carbohydrate nutrition and sporulation of *Allescheria boydii* J. Bacteriol. 88:1624

Emmons CW. 1944. *Allescheria boydii* and *Monosporium apiospermum.* Mycologia 36:188

Emmons CW. 1945. *Phialophora jeanselmei* comb. n. from mycetoma of the hand. Arch. Pathol. 39:364

Etta LL, Van Peterson LR, Gering D. 1983. *Acremonium falciforme (Cephalosporium falciforme)* mycetoma in a renal transplant patient. Arch. Dermatol. 119:707

Hay RJ, Collins MJ. 1983. An ultrastructural study of pale eumycetoma grains. Sabouraudia 21:261

Lichtman DM, Johnson DC, Mack GR, et al. 1978. Maduromycosis (*Allescheria boydii*) infection of hand. A case report. J. Bone. Joint. Surg. 60:546

Lupan DM, Cazin J Jr. 1977. Serological diagnosis of *petriellidiosis (allescheriosis).* II. Indirect (passive) hemagglutination assay for antibody to polysaccharide antigens of *Petriellidium (Allescheria) boydii* and *Monosporium apiospermum.* Mycopathologia 62:87

Luque AG, Mujica MT, D'Anna ML, Alvarez DP. 1991. Micetoma podal por *Fusarium solani* (Mart.) Allel & Wollenweber. Boletín Micológico 6:1

Mahgoub ES. 1978. Experimental infection of athymic nude New Zealand mice nu nu strain with mycetoma agents. Sabouraudia 16:21

Mariat F, Destombes P, Segretain G. 1977. The mycetomas: Clinical features, pathology, etiology and epidemiology. Contr. Microbiol. Immunol. 4:1

Montes LF, Freeman RG, McClarin W. 1969.

Maduromycosis due to *Madurella grisea.* Report of the fifth North American case. Arch. Dermatol. 99:74

Rippon JW, Carmichael JW. 1976. Petriellidiosis (allescheriosis): Four unusual cases and review of literature. Mycopathologia 58:117

Sanyal M, Thammayya A, Basu N. 1978. Actinomycetoma caused by organisms of the *Nocardia asteroides* complex and closely related strains. Mykosen 21:109

Winston DJ, Jordan MC, Rhodes J. 1977. *Allescheria boydii* infections in the immunosuppressed host. Am. J. Med. 63:830

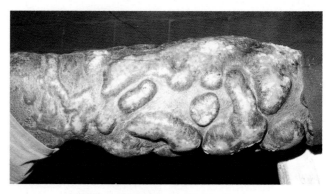

Figure 136. Chromoblastomycosis, Leg

CHROMOBLASTOMYCOSIS

(Chromomycosis)

Definition

Chromoblastomycosis is localized, chronic skin and subcutaneous tissue disease characterized by the development of warty or tumorlike lesions which may ulcerate. The cauliflower-like growths usually develop on the lower extremities and occasionally on the hands, face, ear, neck, chest, shoulders, and buttocks (Figure 135 and 136). The degree of dimorphism exhibited by these organisms depends on the amount of resistance of the host. Some of the dematiaceous fungi (dark brown) can adapt easily to the sclerotic cells of classic chromoblastomycosis. In debilitated patients the same organisms are usually mycelial in morphology. Some of the dematiaceous fungi are usually restricted to opportunistic infections in the severely compromised host. All of the dematiaceous fungi that remain hyphal in the host belong with the disease phaeohyphomycosis (see page 116). These fungi are in contaminated soil and are usually introduced into the tissue or skin by a splinter or abrasion of the skin.

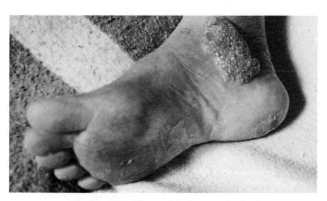

Figure 135. Chromoblastomycosis, Foot

Etiologic Agents

A variety of dematiaceous fungi may be the cause of chromoblastomycosis. There are five principal agents: (a) *Fonsecaea pedrosoi* (Brumpt, 1922) Negroni, 1936 (synonym: *Phialophora pedrosi* Emmons in Binford et al, 1944); (b) *Fonsecaea compacta* Carrion, (*Phialophora compacta* Emmons in Binford et al, 1944); (c) *Phialophora verrucosa* Thaxter in Medlar, 1915; (d) *Cladosporium carrionii* Trejos, 1954; (e) *Rhinocladiella aquaspersa* (Borelli) Schell, McGinnis et Borelli, 1983.

For more detailed discussion of the organisms, the taxonomic position, and nomenclature, reference should be made to the publications of Emmons (1966), Carrion and Silva-Hutner (1971), Al-Doory (1972), McGinnis (1978), and Ajello (1979).

Occurrence

Humans: Worldwide in distribution, including cases in North, Central, and South America, Dominican Republic, Cuba, Costa Rica, Puerto Rico, Jamaica, Africa, Australia, Russia, and occasionally in other parts of the world.

Animals: Reported in several horses and dogs, and frequently in frogs and toads.

Laboratory Procedures

Specimen collection: Crusts from warty lesions or exudates may be isolated directly on the proper agar medium or put in a sterile container for subsequent examination.

Direct examination: Place crusts from the lesions on a slide with 10% KOH, add a coverglass and examine. Exudates may be examined directly on a slide with a coverglass or may be placed in lactophenol and the slide sealed with nail polish. Histologic sections of biopsy specimens may be made and stained.

Microscopically, the organisms are single-celled or clustered, round, with thick-walled sclerotic bodies and black pigment. They multiply by cross-wall formation (splitting), not budding. The size varies from 6 to 12 µm in diameter. Note the thick-walled structure (Figure 137). All the organisms causing chromoblastomycosis have the same appearance in tissue except in the early development of the lesions there are dark hyphae. Hyphae are present in disseminated and cerebral cases.

Culture: All of the organisms can be isolated on Sabouraud glucose agar at room temperature. Inoculated material should be retained in culture for at least three to six weeks before the plates are considered negative. Cycloheximide or chloramphenicol may be added for the selective isolation of these organisms. However, Sabouraud glucose agar without cyclohexamide should be used for isolation of opportunistic dematiaceous organisms. Identification of the cultures is based on their morphologic and physiologic characteristics. The specific identification is difficult as there is no clear delineation taxonomically. Speciation is dependent upon the percentage of the three general types of conidiation.

1. *Fonsecaea Pedrosoi* (Brumpt, 1922) Negroni, 1936

Colonies: Colonies are slow growing, dark green to brown or black on Sabouraud glucose agar, with a feltlike aerial mycelium (Figure 138). Strains of the organism show variation in rate of growth and colony characteristics.

Microscopically, three different methods of conidial formation may be seen, depending upon the strain. Look for these three types in a slide culture or direct slide mount under the microscope.

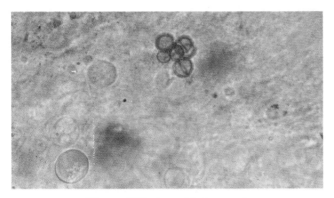

Figure 137. chromoblastomycosis, sclerotic bodies X500

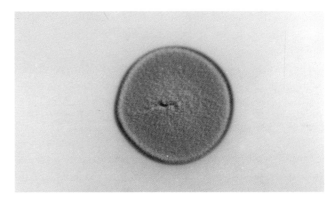

Figure 138. *Fonsecaea pedrosoi,* colony

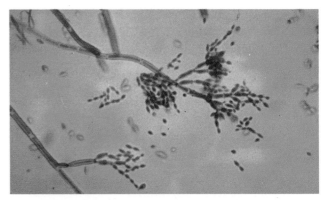

Figure 139. *Fonsecaea pedrosoi,* conidiophores X400

a. The *Cladosporium* type is characterized by branching conidiophores with shield-shaped cells bearing chains of conidia borne terminally. The single-celled conidia are 3 to 6 µm in length and 1.5 to 3 µm in diameter. Separate conidia are brown to green in color, with projections on the ends which represent the previous junction of one conidium with another (Figure 139). The *Cladosporium* type conidial formation usually predominates for *F. pedrosoi*. This type of conidiation is lost when the culture is maintained for a long period.

b. The *Rhinocladiella* type (*Acrotheca*) has conidia formed along the sides of swollen, knotted, club-shaped conidiophores (sympodial conidiophores) that developed terminally or laterally on the hyphae.

c. The *Phialophora* type has conidia developed endogenously or cut off from the base of a terminal cuplike structure on a flask-shaped conidiophore (Figure 143). The phialides have a collarette and lip with a cluster of conidia accumulating.

This type of conidiophore is seen more often in slide cultures and on corn meal medium.

Biochemically, this organism does not hydrolyze starch, coagulate milk, or liquefy gelatin.

2.   *Fonsecaea compacta* Carrion, 1940

Colonies: Colonies of this fungus grow extremely slowly on Sabouraud glucose agar, forming a heaped, brittle colony, dark green to black in color with short aerial mycelium. After a month, tufts of brown-colored mycelium develop in the center of the colony containing conidiophores (Figure 140). *Phialophora*-type conidiophores may form on cornmeal agar cultures.

Microscopically, a slide mount from the mycelial tufts in the center of the colony or a slide culture should show terminal and lateral conidiophores with chains of nearly spherical conidia formed close together as compact heads (Figure 141). The conidia are 1.5 to 2 by 2 to 3 µm in size. Slide mounts from cornmeal agar cultures may show the *Phialophora*-type conidiophores.

Biochemically, this organism does not hydrolyze starch, coagulate milk, or liquefy gelatin.

3.   *Phialophora verrucosa* Thaxter in Medlar, 1915

Colonies: Colonies develop slowly and become greenish brown to black in color with olive to gray-colored mycelium closely matted to the surface (Figure 142).

Microscopically, conidia are produced in clusters from vase-shaped phialides with distinct collarettes, while a direct mount on a slide will frequently disperse the clusters of conidia, and consequently the conidia may appear separate. The phialides are about 3 to 4 µm wide and 4 to 7 µm in length, while the conidia are thin-walled oval cells about 1.5 by 4 µm in size. Higher magnifications should be used to observe these structures (Figure 143).

Biochemically, this organism does not hydrolyze starch, coagulate milk, or liquefy gelatin.

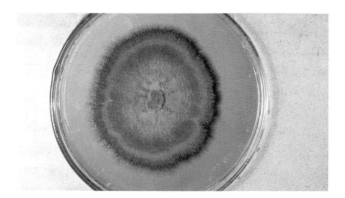

Figure 142. *Phialophora verrucosa,* colony

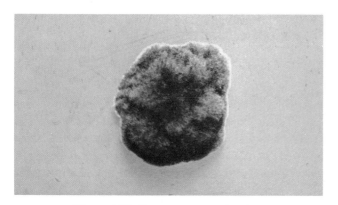

Figure 140. *Fonsecaea compacta,* colony

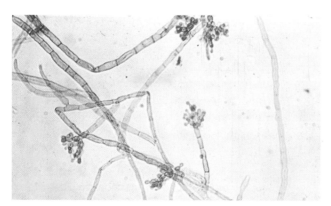

Figure 141. *Fonsecaea compacta,* conidiophores X800

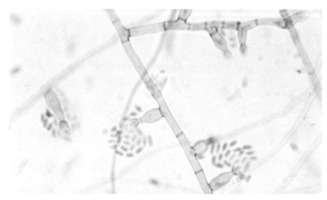

Figure 143. *Phialophora verrucosa,* conidiophores X400

4. *Cladosporium carrionii* Trejos, 1954

Colonies: Colonies of this organism grow slowly, reaching a diameter of 2 to 4 cm in about one month. The colonies are flat with a slight rise in the center covered with short mycelium on the surface and a velvety gray-green to brown color.

Microscopically, the *Cladosporium*-type lateral and terminal conidiophores are seen with long, branched chains of smooth-walled, oval to lemon-shaped conidia that separate readily on a slide mount. The *Acrotheca*-type conidiophore and *Phialophora*-type of phialides are lacking. This fungus appears similar to the saprophytic *Cladosporium* species except conidial chains do not separate readily.

Biochemically, this organism does not hydrolyze starch, coagulate milk, or liquefy gelatin.

5. *Rhinocladiella aquaspersa* (Borelli) Schell, McGinnis et Borelli, 1983

Colonies: This fungus produces colonies with rather rapid growth, floccose, and dark olive-gray in color.

Microscopically, the conidiophores are thick-walled, well defined, dark brown and erect. The conidia are on the upper portion near the tip of the conidiophore, elliptical to clavate, 2 by 5 μm, palebrown, and one or rarely two-celled. Occasionally annellides and phialides develop with balls of one-celled conidia.

6. *Cladosporium* species

Colonies: Colonies of the saprophytic forms vary from flat to irregularly heaped and folded; they are moderately fast growing, have a velvety surface, and are olive green to grayish green with a greenish-black undersurface.

Microscopically, the hyphae are brown to olive in color, with branched conidiophores of varied lengths containing branching chains of conidia. New conidia form by budding at the tips of the chains, but later two-celled conidia may form.

Biochemically, these organisms hydrolyze starch, coagulate milk, and liquefy gelatin. Compare these reactions with the pathogens of chromoblastomycosis.

Animal inoculation: Intraperitoneal or intravenous injection of a spore and hyphal suspension has produced systemic infection involving many internal organs in mice, rabbits, guinea pigs, dogs, and in the frog. The kidneys enlarge greatly in the frog. Brain abscesses develop after injection with *C. trichoides, F. pedrosoi,* and *F. compacta.* Injection of *Exophiala dermatitidis* produces a neurotropic response.

Serology: Serologic tests demonstrate the presence of circulating antibodies and hypersensitivity to the agents of chromoblastomycosis. Standardized antigens are not available. Antigens have extensive cross-reactions among species in this group. Serodiagnosis has not been as useful as diagnosis by biopsy or slide mounts of pus.

Table 8. Chief Characteristics of the Agents of Chromoblastomycosis and some Phaeohyphomycosis.

Organism	Conidial and Colony Charateristics
Fonsecaea pedrosoi	*Cladosporium* type, short chains, at times from tips and sides of conidiophore. *Rhinocladiella* type conidia may prevail.
F. compacta	*Cladosporium* type heads like *F. pedrosoi* only smaller and compact.
Exophiala dematitidis	Yeast colony at first, abstrictions on tip and sides of conidiophores, peg-like phialides (annellide), grows at 40°C.
Phialophora verrucosa	Vase-shaped phialides, other types of conidiation rare.
P. richardsiae	Phialoconidia semiendogenously, phialides long, saucer-shaped lips or collarettes.
Rhinocladiella aquaspersa	Primarily Rhinocladiella type conidiophores with elliptical conidia near the tips.
P. aquaspersa	Primarily Rhinocladiella type conidiophores with ellipticl conidia near the tips
Exophiala jeanselmei	Yeast colony at first, semiendogenously from elongate annellides, abstrictions from tips and sides. No growth at 40°C.
E. spinifera	Abstrictions from sides, tips and along hyphae, conidiophores spikelike, bears conidia semiendogenously.
Cladosporium carrionii	Chains of conidia from branched conidiophores, acropetalous, phialides develop on some media.

Xylohypha bantiana Similar to above. Thermotolerance at 43°C, neurotopism, varied conidia, occasional branching of conidial chains of at least 35, elliptical conidia.

Cladosporium Like *C. carrionii,* not thermotolerant or species pathogenic.

Questions

1. Distinguish in the form of a table or chart between the different fungi causing chromoblastomycosis.

2. What is the meaning of the term chromoblastomycosis? Why is chromoblastomycosis used currently for this disease?

3. Under what family and order would these organisms be placed in the deuteromycota?

Selected References

Ajello L. 1979. Chromoblastomycosis, chromomycosis, and phaeohyphomycosis—a confusion of terms. In International Congress Series No. 480, Human and Animal Mycology. Proceedings of International Society of Human and Animal Mycology. Jerusalem, p. 187

Alviano CS, Farbiarz SR, Travassos LR, Angluster J, de Souza W. 1992. Effect of environmental factors on *Fonsecaea pedrosoi* morphogenesis with emphasis on sclerotic cells induced by propranol. Mycopathologia 119(1):17

Aravysk RA, Aronson VB. 1968. Comparative histopathology of chromomycosis and cladosporiosis in experimental infections. Mycopathologia 36:322

Beneke ES. 1978. Dematiaceous fungi in laboratory-housed frogs. *In* Proc. Fourth International Conference on the Mycoses. Publ. No. 356, Panamerican Health Organization, Washington, DC

Borelli D. 1972. A method for producing chromomycosis in mice. Trans. Roy. Soc. Trop. Med. Hyg. 66:793

Borelli D. 1980. Causal agents of chromoblastomycosis (chromomycetes). *In* Proceedings of the Fifth International Conference on the Mycoses: Superficial, Cutaneous and Subcutaneous Infections. Caracas Panamerican Health Organization Sci. Pub. 396:334

Carrion AL, Silva-Hutner M. 1971. Taxonomic criteria for the fungi of chromoblastomycosis with reference to *Fonsecaea pedrosoi.* Int. J. Dermatol. 10:35

Cole GT, Kendrick B. 1973. Taxonomic Study of *Phialophora.* Mycologia 65:661

Conant NF, Martin DS. 1937. The morphologic and serologic relationships of the various fungi causing dermatitis verrucosa (chromoblastomycosis). Am. J. Trop. Med. 17:553

Emmons CW. 1966. Pathogenic dematiaceous fungi. Jap. J. Med. Mycol. 7-233

Fuentes CA, Bosch ZE. 1960. Biochemical differentiation of the etiological agents of chromoblastomycosis from non-pathogenic *Cladosporium* species. J. Invest. Dermatol. 36:419

Gordon MA, Al-Doory Y. 1965. Application of fluorescent-antibody procedures to the study of pathogenic dematiaceous fungi. Serological relationships of the genus *Fonsecaea.* J. Bacteriol. 89:55

Lane CG. 1915. Cutaneous disease caused by new fungus (*Phialophora verrucosa*). J. Cutan. Dis. 33:840

McGinnis MR. 1978. Human pathogenic species of *Exophiala, Phialophora. In* Proc Fourth International Conference on the Mycoses. Publ No 356 Panamerican Health Organization, Washington, DC

Medlar EM. 1915. A cutaneous infection caused by a new fungus *Phialophora verrucosa* with a study of the fungus. J. Med. Res. 32:507

Nielsen HS Jr, Conant NF. 1968. A new human pathogenic *Phialophora.* Sabouraudia 6:228

Rush HG, Anver MR, Beneke ES. 1974. Systemic chromomycosis in *Rana pipiens.* Lab. An. Sci. 24:646

Silva M. 1960. Growth characteristics of the fungi of chromoblastomycosis. Ann. NY. Acad. Sci. 89: 17

Simpson JF. 1966. A case of chromoblastomycosis in a horse. Vet. Med. Small Anim. Clin. 61: 1207

Szaniszlo PJ, Hsieh PH, Mariowe JD. Induction and ultrastructure of the multicellular (sclerotic) morphology in *Phialophora dermatitidis.* Mycologia 68:117

Trejos A. 1955. *Cladosporium carrionii* n. sp. and the problem of Cladosporia isolated from chromoblastomycosis. Rev. Biol. Trop. 2:75

Uribe J, et al. 1989. Histopathology of chromoblastomycosis. Mycopathologia 105:1

Villalba E, Yegres JF. 1988. Detection of circulating antibodies in patients affected by chromoblastomycosis by *Cladosporium carrionii* using double immunodiffusion. Mycopathologia 102:17

Vollum DL. 1977. Chromomycosis: A review. Br. J. Dermatol. 96:454

SPOROTRICHOSIS

Definition

Sporotrichosis is a chronic infection characterized by nodular lesions and ulcers in the lymph nodes, skin, or subcutaneous tissues and occasionally in internal organs. The disseminated form may involve the skeleton and visceral areas. Primary pulmonary sporotrichosis may occur. The localized lesions are usually found on the hands, arms, or legs (Figure 144). The infection may involve the bones, joints, skin, central nervous system, eyes, or genitourinary tract through hematogenous dissemination.

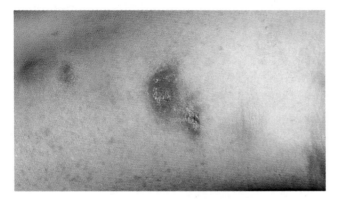

Figure 144. Sporotrichosis, Arm

Etiologic Agent

Sporothrix schenckii Hektoen and Perkins, 1900 (synonym: *Sporotrichum schenckii* Matruchot, 1910).

Occurrence

The fungus has been isolated from soil, wood, and vegetation. The organisms may be injected through wounds from infected splinters or thorns or the conidia inhaled.

Humans: Sporotrichosis is worldwide in distribution. It became less frequent in France after 1920 than prior to this date. It periodically occurs in South, Central, and North America. Subcutaneous and deep sporotrichosis are more common in Mexico than elsewhere. Epidemics have occurred in gold mining workers in South Africa.

Animals: Infections have been reported in horses, cattle, cats, dogs, fowl, camels, rats, mice, mules and donkeys.

Laboratory Procedures

Specimen collection: Pus should be aspirated from unruptured nodules; swabs, scrapings, or biopsies of ulcerated lesions or sputum from suspected cases of pulmonary disease should be collected in a sterile container for laboratory study.

Direct examination: Pus or other infected material may be put on a slide smeared and stained for examination of the usually scarce "cigar bodies." The addition of amylase on the slide is helpful before staining (William Cooper, personal communication). The use of PAS, calcafluor white preparation, or methenamine-silver stains may be of value,

as the few organisms probably present will stand out in sharp contrast.

For better results the fluorescent antibody staining technique is useful for staining of material from lesions, histologic slide preparations, and hyphae and conidia.

Culture: Pus from open lesions or from unopened nodules should be streaked or placed on Sabouraud glucose agar containing cycloheximide and chloramphenicol, brain-heart infusion agar and blood agar with antibiotics may also be streaked and incubated at 37°C. The organism is thermodimorphic. Colonies, cream to white in color, will appear in three to five days and in most cases will later develop a brown-black pigment. Cultures should be held for four weeks before discarding as negative. Sputum from suspected cases of pulmonary disease should be plated on yeast extract phosphate medium.

Colonies: Colonies at room temperature are white at first and leathery and wrinkled. They become smooth as the colonies become older. Strains vary from cream to black in color (Figure 145).

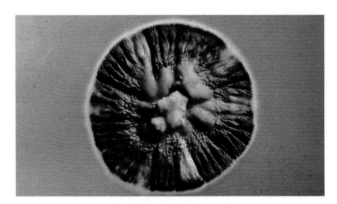

Figure 145. *Sporothrix schenckii*, colony 24°C

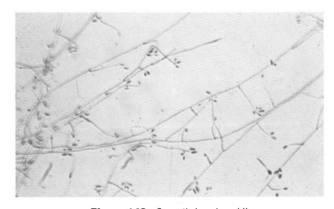

Figure 146. *Sporothrix schenckii*, conidia X400

The organism should be converted into the tissue form by growth on media rich in protein and vitamins at 37°C. Brain-heart infusion agar with or without blood or blood agar is a satisfactory medium for conversion to the yeast or tissue form after one or two serial transfers. The medium should be kept moist during the conversion.

The colonies appear soft, white to cream in color with an irregular surface, and are yeastlike (Figure 147). The conversion to the yeast form is necessary for identification of *S. schenckii.*

Microscopically, slide cultures or mounts from colonies grown at room temperature show fine branching, septate hyphae (2 μm in diameter) with pyriform to spherical conidia borne at the ends of minute sterigmata on the tips of conidiophores resulting in a floral-like arrangement or on the sides of hyphae. The conidia are 2 to 4 by 2 to 6 μm in size (Figure 146). Compare these with the saprophytic fungus *Acremonium* spp.

Microscopically, a slide mount of a portion of a colony grown at 37°C should show round, oval, and fusiform budding cells, commonly called "cigar bodies," varying in size from 1 to 3 by 3 to 10 μm (Figure 148). These are similar to those seen in stained smears from infected laboratory animals. The "cigar bodies" are Gram positive when stained. Prepare a Gram-stained slide of the yeast form. When conversions are made at 37°C, some hyphae may be found along with the cigar bodies.

Perfect state (not verified): Mariat (1968, 1971) presented evidence that *Sporothrix schenckii* and *Ceratocystis stenoceras* (Robak) Moreau (an ascomycete) are closely related. In the conidial form, *S. schenckii* produces both hyaline and dematiaceous conidia while *C. stenoceras* produces only hyaline conidia. Until the perfect state is established *S. schenckii* should remain in the Deuteromycota.

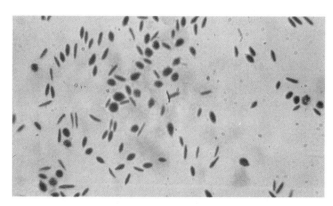

Figure 148. *Sporothrix schenckii,* yeast cells X1000

Special nutritional requirements:

Yeast form: Important factors are: thiamine, biotin (stimulatory), organic nitrogen source (amino acids), CO_2 tension of 5%, and 37°C for conversion and growth of the yeast phase of *S. schenckii.*

Mycelial form: Thiamine is required, organic nitrogen is stimulatory, while inorganic nitrogen can be utilized in culture media.

Histopathologic studies: Routine H and E stained sections from human tissue rarely show "cigar bodies." The sections may show a nonspecific, inflammatory process or appear granulomatous with infiltration of lymphocytes, giant cells, fibrosis, or other changes. As previously indicated, the use of PAS or Gomori methenamine-silver stain or the FA technique will show the organisms, when present, both within and outside the leukocytes or giant cells. In addition to cigar-shaped bodies (See Figure 149), asteroid bodies are occasionally seen in tissue sections.

Serology: The sporotrichin skin test is useful for detection of prior contact with the fungus. The standard sporotrichin preparation is injected intradermally with 1:1,000 dilution of heat-killed, packed yeast cells. A reaction of 5 mm induration after 24 hours is positive.

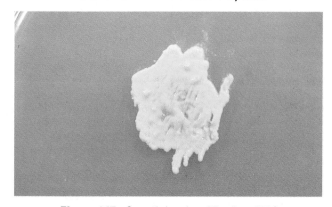

Figure 147. *Sporothrix schenckii,* colony 37°C

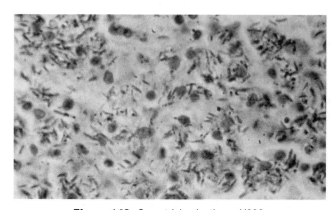

Figure 149. Sporotrichosis, tissue X800

Serologic tests can be used in the diagnosis of sporotrichosis, especially the extracutaneous or systemic forms. Two tests, the slide latex agglutination (LA) and the tube agglutination (TA), are highly sensitive and specific. The LA test has a sensitivity of 94% and can provide results quickly. The TA test is comparable in sensitivity but may show false positives (at 1:8 and 1:16) with sera from patients with leishmaniasis. The immunodiffusion test is 80% positive in tests, and is the easiest serologic procedure to perform. The ID test along with the latex agglutination (LA) are recommended in pulmonary, articular, osseous, and disseminated sporotrichosis.

For more details see references: Blumer et al, 1973; Casserone et al, 1983, and Karlin and Nielson,1970

Animal inoculation: Rats, mice, male hamsters, cats, dogs, and monkeys are susceptible to the disease. Pus or 0.5 to 1.0-ml saline suspensions of the cells from the yeast form (37°C), or mycelial fragments and conidia from the filamentous cultures (24°C), should be inoculated intraperitoneally into white mice or rats. Autopsy should be done after three weeks. Look for peritonitis and granulomas in the mesentery of the infected animal. Male animals should show severe orchitis. Animal inoculation is not necessary for identification of the fungus.

The male mouse or other laboratory animal may be inoculated intratesticularly with 0.2 ml of the fungal suspension to produce orchitis in two to three weeks. Prepare smears from pus or granular material from the animal and Gram stain. The cigar-shaped cells should be evident under the immersion oil lens (Figure 149). The cells are about 1 to 2 μm in diameter and 4 to 5 μm in length, while the round forms are 2 or 3 μm in diameter. Look for budding forms.

Questions

1. Where is *Sporothrix* spp. found in nature?

2. Are there any genera of saprophytic fungi that resemble *Sporothrix?* How can these genera be distinguished?

Selected References

Albornoz MB, Mendoza M, Torres ED. 1986. Growth temperatures of isolates of *Sporothrix schenckii* from disseminated and fixed cutaneous lesions of sporotrichosis. Mycopathologia 95:81

Baker RD. 1947. Experimental sporotrichosis in mice. Am J. Trop. Med. 27:749

Benham RW, Kesten B. 1932. Sporotrichosis: Its transmission to plants and animals. J. Infect. Dis. 50:437

Blumer SO, Kaufman L, Kaplan W, et al. 1973. Comparative evaluation of five serological methods for the diagnosis of sporotrichosis. Appl. Microbiol. 26:4

Casserone SIA, Conti-Diaz E, Zanettza ME. Penade Pereira. 1983. Serología de la esporotrichosis cutanea. Sabouraudia 21:317

Dickerson CL, Taylor RL, Drutz DJ. 1983. Susceptibility of congenitally athymic (nude) mice to sporotrichosis. Infect. Immun. 40:417

Dixon D, et al. 1991. Isolation and characterization of *Sporothrix schenckii* from clinical and environmental sources associated with the largest US epidemic of sporotrichosis. J. Clin. Microbiol. 29:1106

Chuang TY, Deng JS et al. 1975. Rapid diagnosis of sporotrichosis by immunofluorescent methods. Chinese J. Microbiol. 8:259

Fishburn F, Kelley DC. 1967. Sporotrichosis in a horse. J. Arm. Vet. Med. Assoc. 151:45

Hektoen L, Perkins CF. 1900. Refractory subcutaneous abscesses caused by *Sporothrix schenckii,* a new pathogenic fungus. J. Exp. Med. 5:77

Kaplan W, Ochoa AG. 1963. Application of the fluorescent antibody technique to the rapid diagnosis of sporotrichosis. J. Lab. Clin. Med. 62:835

Kaufman L. 1992. Serodiagnosis of fungal diseases. *In* Rose NR, Friedman H (eds). Manual of Clinical Immunology. Am Soc Microbiol, Washington, DC

Kennedy MJ, Bajwa PS, Volz PA. 1982. Gastrointestinal inoculation of *Sporothrix schenckii* in mice. Mycopathologia 78:141

Lane JW, Garrison RG. 1970. Electron microscopy of the yeast to mycelial phase conversion of *Sporothrix schenckii.* Can. J. Microbiol. 16:747

Lipstein-Kresch E. et al. 1985. Disseminated *Sporothrix schenckii* infection with arthritis in a patient with acquired immunodeficiency syndrome. J. Rheumatol. 12:18-5

Lurie HL, Still WF. 1969. The "capsule" of *Sporotrichium schenckii* and the evolution of the asteroid body. A light and electron microscopic study. Sabouraudia 7:64

Mariat F, Drouhet E. 1954. Sporotrichose experimentale du hamster. Observation de formes asteroides de *Sporotrichum.* Ann. Inst. Pasteur. 86:485

Mariat F. 1971. Adaptation de ceratocystis ala vie parasitaire chez l'animaletude de l'aquisition d'un pouvoir pathogene comparable a celui de *Sporothrix schenckii.* Sabouraudia 9:191

Palmer DF, Kaufman L, Kaplan W, et al. 1977.

Serodiagnosis of Mycotic Diseases. Charles C. Thomas, Springfield, Ill

Satterwhite TK, Kageler WV, Conklin BH, et al. 1978. Disseminated sporotrichosis. JAMA 240:771

Simson FW. 1947. Sporotrichosis Infection on Mines of the Witwatersrand. A symposium. Proc. Mine. Med. Off. Assoc., Transvaal Chamber of Mines, Johannesburg, South Africa

Wallk S, Bernstein G. 1964. Systemic sporotrichosis with bony involvement. Arch. Dermatol. 90:355

LOBOMYCOSIS

(Lobo's disease, Keloidal blastomycosis)

This disease is characterized by keloidal, verrucoid skin lesions from exaggerated fibrous hyperplasia. The lesions are composed of granulomatous inflammatory tissue containing many yeast-like globose to lemon-shaped or branched chains. These yeast-like organism are referred to as *Loboa loboi.* There is no systemic spread.

Occurrence

Humans: Most cases are in the Amazon region of Brazil and in Surinam. A few cases have occurred in Colombia, Venezuela, French Guiana, Panama, Costa Rica, Mexico, Guyana, Peru, Bolivia, Ecuador, Honduras, and Europe. The diseases occur in patients working outdoors in rural, hot, humid locations.

Animals: Dolphins.

Laboratory Procedures

Specimen collections: Material is obtained from curettage, surgical excision, or biopsy.

Direct examination: Small pieces of the specimen should be mounted in KOH on a slide for observation under the microscope. Histologic sections of the specimens should be made and stained.

Microscopically, the characteristic globose to lemon-shaped cells about 9 μm in diameter developed singly or in short chains should be seen. Some cells have multiple budding which resemble *Paracoccidioides brasiliensis.* The buds may be attached to the mother cell with a narrow tubular connection similar to *P. brasiliensis.*

Culture: The causative agent of lobomycosis has not been successfully grown in culture. All fungal isolates grown out in culture have been found to be contaminants.

Selected References

Almeida F, Lacaz CS. 1948. Blastomicose tipo Jorge Lobo. An. Fac. Med. Univ. Sao Paulo 24:5

Borelli D. 1962. Lobomycosis experimental. Dermatol. Venez. 1:286

Caldwell DK. et al. 1975. Lobomycosis as a disease of the bottlenosed dolphin. Am. J. Trop. Med. Hyg. 24:l05

Conant NF, Howell A, Jr. 1942. The similarity of the fungi causing South American blastomycosis (paracoccidioidal granuloma) and North American blastomycosis (Gilchrist's disease). J. Invest. Dermatol. 5:353

Landman G, et al. 1988. Crossed-antigenicity between the etiologic agents of lobomycosis and paracoccidioidomycosis evidence by an immunoenzymatic method (PAP). Allergol. Immunopathol. (Madr). 16:215

Lisboa Miranda J. 1972. Lobomicose. Ann. Brazil Dermatol. 47:273

Lobo J. 1931. Um caso de blastomicose produzida poruma especie nova, encontrada em Recife. Rev. Med. Pernambuco. 1:763

Marques de Abreu W, Losbos Miranda J. 1972. Microscopia electronica scanning agente de micose de Jorge Lobo. An. Bras. Dermatol. 47:115

Sesso A, Baruzzi RG. 1988. Interaction between macrophage and parasite cells in lobomycosis: the thickened cell wall of *Paracoccidioides loboi* exhibits apertures to the extracellular milieu. J. Submicrose. Cytol. Pathol. 20:573

Woodard JD. 1972. Electron microscopic study of lobomycosis. (Loboa loboi). Lab. Invest. 27:606

RHINOSPORIDIOSIS

Definition

Rhinosporidiosis is a chronic granulomatous infection producing polypoid tumors of pedunculated and sessile polyps in the mucous membranes of the nose, eyes, ears, larynx, and rarely on other parts of the body.

Etiologic Agent

The disease is caused by *Rhinosporidium seeberi* (Wernicke) Seeber. 1912.

Occurrence

Humans: The fungus is apparently found in water or possibly as a fish disease. It may be transmitted by water or dust or where individuals bathe in muddy or stagnant pools of water. Rhinosporidiosis is found most often in India, Ceylon, and Brazil, with occasional reports of occurrence in the United States (50+ cases), Mexico, Cuba, Argentina, Ecuador, Paraguay, Russia, Iran, Africa, the

Philippines, the Malay States, Europe, England, and Scotland. Over 2,000 cases have occurred in India and Ceylon, and more than 200 cases have been reported in Brazil.

Animals: The disease has been found in horses, mules, cattle, and dogs, especially in India, South America, Africa, Australia, and the United States.

Laboratory Procedures

Specimen collection: Material from the polyps that have been removed surgically should be brought to the laboratory under sterile conditions for examination.

Direct examination: The surface of the polyp may show small white dots indicating the presence of sporangia. Some tissue or nasal discharge from the polyp may be macerated and examined in a KOH preparation on a slide (or sectioned for better results).

The cell wall has been studied by Ashworth (1923) and found to contain cellulose and stored nutrients (fatty material). Nuclear division occurs prior to spore production. Rao (1966) also found chitin in the cell wall. These are all characteristics of the lower fungi of the order Chytridiales.

Microscopically, the direct slide mount or stained tissue sections, if positive, should show round or oval spores 7 to 9 µm in diameter as well as sporangia up to 300 µm in diameter filled with spores (Figure 150). This is similar in appearance to the spherules and endospores of *Coccidioides immitis*.

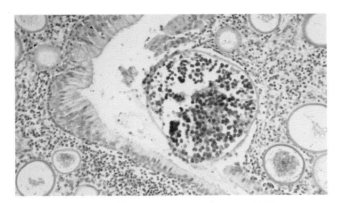

Figure 150. Rhinosporidiosis, Tissue X150

The life cycle, as described by Ashworth (1923) and others consists of:

1. The round, thickened chitinous spore wall, 6 to 7 µm in diameter, contains a nucleus with four chromosomes.

2. The infecting spore enlarges up to 50 or 60 µm in diameter, along with many nuclear divisions.

3. Further nuclear divisions and enlargement occur until the cell is 100 µm in diameter. A thick layer of cellulose is deposited inside the chitinous membrane except at one point where a pore begins to appear.

4. Further nuclear divisions occur with cleavage and rounding up of the cytoplasm which eventually result in a sporangium with nearly 4,000 protoplasmic units.

5. Two more nuclear divisions result in approximately 16,000 spores, 7 to 9 µm in diameter at maturity in an enlarged sporangium up to 300 µm in diameter.

The organism has not been grown in culture media. Levy et al, 1986 have reported the causative agent has been cultivated *in vitro* in an epithelial carcinoma cell culture line. Continuous cultivation was not successful by subculturing.

Pathologic studies: If prepared stained slides are available for demonstration, study the stages in the life cycle of the fungus and pathologic changes. Note that ruptured sporangia may be seen. Released spores from the sporangia incite a polymorphonuclear inflammatory reaction and abscess formation. Further changes commonly are chronic inflammation with conspicuous plasma cells and lymphocytes. For further details see references.

Animal inoculation: There are no reports of successful infection of laboratory animals.

Questions

1. Diagram the life cycle of the organism.

2. Compare and contrast the tissue form of *Rhinosporidium seeberi* with *Coccidioides immitis*. Are there any differences in location of the infection and laboratory procedures for identification of these two etiological agents?

Selected References

Ashworth JH. 1923. On *Rhinosporidium seeberi* (Wernicke, 1903) with special reference to its sporulation and affinities. Trans. Roy. Soc. Edinb. 53(2):301

Caldwell GT, Roberts JD. 1938. United States. JAMA 110:1641

Grover S. 1970. *Rhinosporidium seeberi:* A preliminary study of the morphology and life cycle. Sabouraudia 7:249

Ho MS, Tay BK. 1986. Disseminated rhinosporidiosis. Acad. Med. Singapore 15:80

Kameswaran S. 1966. Surgery in rhinosporidiosis: Experience 293 cases. Int. Surg. 46:602

Kannan-Kutty M, Teh EC. 1974. *Rhinosporidium seeberi:* cell wall formation in sporoblasts. Pathology 6:183

Myers DD, Simon J, Case MT. 1964. Rhinosporidiosis in a horse. J. Am. Vet. Med. Assoc. 145:345

Rao SN. 1966. *Rhinosporidium seeberi:* A histochemical study. Ind. J. Exp. Biol. 14:10

Vanbreuseghem R. 1973. Ultrastructure of *Rhinosporidium seeberi.* Int. J. Dermatol. 12:20.

Woodard BH, Hudson J. 1984. Rhinosporidiosis: ultrastructural study of an infection. South. Med. J. 77:1587

PHAEOHYPHOMYCOSIS

Definition

Phaeohyphomycosis is a collection of a wide variety of clinical diseases caused by a large number of dematiaceous fungi. This group is characterized by melanin-like pigmentation in the hyphal wall and/or conidia. Ajello (1974) proposed the term "phaeohyphomycosis" for the cutaneous, subcutaneous, and systemic infections that form dark-walled dematiaceous septate hyphal elements. Currently since some of the cutaneous dematiaceous infections do not fit the original proposed name, phaeohypomycosis is limited to the subcutaneous and systemic infections caused by the dark-walled hyphae usually in the tissue. In some cases the dematiaceous nature is not revealed until cultured or a melanin stain is used.

Etiologic agents

In recent years numerous dematiaceous fungi have been reported as etiologic agents of phaeohyphomycosis. This list will likely increase as more opportunistic infections occur among immunosuppressed and other debilitated patients. The following etiological agents (Table 9) are the more frequent causes of subcutaneous and systemic phaeo-hyphomycosis.

Table 9. Chief characteristics of the more frequently isolated etiological agents of phaeohyphomycosis

Genera	Chief characteristic of the genera
Alternaria	Conidiophores dark, septate, branched or unbranched with muriform, dark pigmented, beaked tip conidia on single or branched chains.
Aureobasidium	Colonies white at first, turning black and shiny. Hyphae hyaline, with blastoconidia, older hyphae thick-walled, dark with elliptical blastoconidia.
Bipolaris	Cottony, black colony, conidiophores sympodial, dark with thick-walled, multiseptate, cylindrical conidia.
Cladosporium	Conidiophores dark, septate, branched chains of blastoconidia, one to two-celled, with lemon-shaped ends.
Curvularia	Conidiophores dark, sympodial with multi-septate, curved conidia, central cell larger and darker.
Dactylaria	Conidiophores hyaline, sympodial with conidia two-celled, cylindrical-oblong, One-celled, globose phialoconidia may occur.
Exophiala	Conidiophores hyaline, cylindrical to lagenform conidiogenous cell annelids with hyaline to brown balls of conidia at apex.
Exserohilum	Conidiophores dark, sympodial with conidia multiseptate, cylindrical to oblong, dark with protruding hila at the tips.
Fonsecaea	Conidiophores (*Cladosporium* type) light brown, swollen apically from sympodial development, with one- celled light brown conidia in chains. Other types: *Phialophora* and *Rhinocladiella* may develop.
Phaeoannellomyces	Conidiophores and hyphae lacking, one to two-celled yeast cells, brown to black, annellides. May have pseudohyphae. May occur as a synanamorph with *Exophiala.*
Phaeococcomyces	Conidiophores and hyphae lacking. Yeast cells brown to black, may have pseudohyphae. May occur as synanamorph with *Wangiella.*

Phialophora   Conidiophores present or absent, light brown. Conidiogenous cells, phialides with collarettes. One-celled, hyaline or brown conidial balls at apexes of phialides.

Rhinocladiella   Conidiophores light brown, sympodial, may show distinct scars. Conidia one-celled, fusiform to obovate, light brown, basal scar.

Scedosporium   Conidiophores hyaline, varied length, annellides on conidiogenous cells, conidia one-celled, obovate, truncate, single or in balls, nearly hyaline to pale black.

Scytalidium   Hyphae develop one to two-celled arthroconidia, light to dark brown, ellipsoidal to subglobose.

Wangiella   Conidiophores hyphal-like, near hyaline to light brown. Phialides with no distinct collarettes, cylindrical with rounded apices. Conidia one-celled, light brown, in balls that slip down the conidiogenous cells. Annellides may occur on sympodial conidiophores. Considered by some mycologists to be synonymous with Exophiala.

The second list of etiological agents (Table 10) are the less frequent causes of subcutaneous and systemic phaeohyphomycosis. The dematiaceous fungi in both tables are difficult to identify to species without extensive experience of medical mycologists in the larger clinical laboratories or by mycologists specializing in the dematiaceous fungi.

Most of the dematiaceous fungi isolated from human phaeohyphomycosis are found in soil and on dead plant material or as plant pathogens. At times these dematiaceous fungi are recovered from clinical specimens as contaminants. It is important to find the dark hyphal form in clinical specimens as well as in culture. If the culture isolates are the same from different clinical specimens then the fungus is not likely to be a contaminant. The dematiaceous fungus isolated from tissue should grow at 37°C. Many of these dematiaceous organisms will need the assistance of a specialist familiar with species identification.

Table 10. List of the less frequently isolated etiological agents of phaeohyphomycosis

Genera	Species Reported	References
(Ascomycota)		
Arnium	*A. leporinum*	Restrepo, A. et al., 1984
Chaetomium	*C. funicolum*	Koch, F. A., Haneke, H., 1965
	C. cochliodes	Hoppin, E. C. et al., 1983
	C. globosum	Anandi, V., et al., 1989
(Hyphomycetes)		
Anthopsis	*A. deltoidea*	Kwon-Chung, K. J., 1983
Hormonema	*H. dematioides*	Coldiron, B. M., et al., 1990
Lecythophora	*L. mutabilis*	Slifkin, M. L., Bowers, H. M. 1975
	L. hoffmannii	Rinaldi, M. G., et al., 1982
Mycocentrospora	*M. acerina*	Deighton, F. C., et al., 1977
Nigrospora	*N. sphaerica*	Prichard, R. C., et al., 1987
Oidiodendron	*O. cerealis*	Blomquist, Salonen, A., 1969
Phialemmonium	*P. obovatum*	McGinnis, M. R., et al., 1986
Ramichloridium	*R. schulzeri*	Rippon, J. W., et al., 1985
Sarcinomyces	*S. phareomuriformis*	Matsumoto, T., et al., 1986
Taeniolella	*T. stilbospora*	Pietrina, P., et al., 1977
Tetraploa	*T. arilstata*	Markham, W. D., et al., 1990
Ulocladium	*U. chartarum*	Altmeyer, P., Schov, K., 1981
Coniothyrium	*C. fuckelii*	Kiehn, T. C., et al., 1987
Hendersonula	*H. toruloidea*	Elewski, B. E., Greer, D. L., 1991
Phoma	*P. eupyrena*	Bakerspigel, A. D., et al., 1981
	P. hibernica	Bakerspigel, A. D., 1970
	P. Phoma sp.	Young, N. A., et al., 1968
	P. minutella	Baker, J. G., et al., 1987

Laboratory Procedures

Specimen collection: The clinical specimens should be collected aseptically and transported in a labeled sterile container. The type of specimens from phaeohyphomycosis cases include aspirates, surgical specimens, biopsies, scrapings and curettage of plaques and nodules. The specimens should be kept moist.

Direct examination: Aspirates from cysts, curettage of plaques and nodules and abscesses should be put in 10% KOH mounts, heated gently, and examined microscopically. The presence of dark brown septate hyphae should be evident. At times some hyphae are nearly hyaline. The hyphae are 3 to 4 μm in diameter, with variation in shapes. Cyst cells may be up to 25 μm in diameter.

Culture: Clinical specimens should be plated on Sabouraud glucose agar with cycloheximide and chloramphenicol as well as only Sabouraud glucose agar at 30°C and 37°C for four or more weeks before discarding. For better sporulation a transfer should be made from the colony to a modified cornmeal or potato-dextrose agar. In cases of cerebral phaeohyphomycosis it has been difficult to isolate the causative agent, *Cladosporium*, in culture. Colonies of phaeohyphomycotic agents are gray, dark olive gray, or dark brown to black with a yeast-like to woolly surface.

Clinical grouping of types of dematiaceous infections and etiological agents.

1.   **Superficial dematiaceous infections:** See discussion of these infections in Chapter 4, superficial infections.

Black Piedra	**Tinea nigra**
Piedraia hortae	*Exophialia werneckii* *Stenella araguata*

2.   **Cutaneous dematiaceous infections:** These represent the dematiaceous fungi that keratinize cutaneous tissue. See chapter 5, page 97.

Dematiaceous dermatomycosis	**Onychomycosis**
Scytalidium	*Scytalidium* (*Hendersonula*)
Taeniolella	*Phyllosticta* *Pyrenochaeta*

3.   **Keratomycosis:** Colonization of injured lens for infection of the cornea and adjacent structures by the following dematiaceous fungi. Refer to chapter 10 on Keratomycosis (Mycotic Keratitis).

Botryodiplodia	*Lasiodiplodia*
Cladorrhinum	*Phialophora*
Colletotrichum	*Phoma*
Curvularia	*Rhizoctonia*
Exerophilum	*Tetraploa*
Exophiala	

4.   **Subcutaneous phaeohyphomycosis:** These infections are cystlike lesions (phaeomycotic cysts) that develop in the site of the traumatic implantation of soil fungi. The following genera have been reported as etiological agents:

Exophiala (frequent)	*Lecythophora*
Phialophora (frequent)	*Mycocentrospora*
Alternaria	*Oidiodendron*
Amium	*Phoma*
Anthopsis	*Ramichloridium*
Aureobasidium	*Scytalidium*
Bipolaris	*Taeniolella*
Cladosporium	*Ulocladium*
Curvularia	
Dactylaria	
Exserohilum	
Hendersonula	

5.   **Invasive, systemic, and cerebral phaeohyphomycosis:** Patients are usually immunosuppressed with the site of infection usually being the lungs, sinuses, skin (trauma), and occasionally organisms enter during surgery or by injection.

Etiologic agents causing cerebral phaeohyphomycosis: *Cladosporium trichoides* (*Xylohypha emmonsii*) is most likely; others less common are: *Exophiala dermatitidis, Fonsecaea pedrosoi, Dactylaria gallopava, Chaetomium globosum,* and *Bipolaris hawaiiensis.* A number of cases report only brownish hyphae.

Phaeohyphomycosis of the paranasal sinus: Many new dematiaceous fungi are being reported as etiologic agents. The following have been reported: *Drechslera biseptata, Bipolaris spicifera, B. australiensis, B. hawaiiensis, Exserohilum rostratum, E. mcginnisii, Curvularia lunata, Alternaria* species, and *Cladosporium trichoides.*

The following etiologic agents are dematiaceous fungi that may be isolated from patients with phaeohyphomycosis. In many cases speciation of the genus is difficult and will need to be referred to a specialist in medical mycology familiar with the dematiaceous fungi, or reference books should be consulted.

1.   *Alternaria.* Infections involve bone, cutaneous tissue, paranasal sinuses, urinary tract, and patients with immunosuppressive conditions. *Alternaria alternata* is the most frequently reported species. Six other species have been reported.

A. alternata (FR.) Keissler. 1912. Colonies grows rapidly, gray to olive-black with a cottony surface, and no cycloheximide in the medium.

Microscopically, conidiophores are smooth-walled, brown, simple or branched, and straight or flexuous. Conidia are muriform, short or long beaked, pyriform or oblong, light to yellow-brown, verrucose or smooth-walled (20 to 63 by 9 to 18 μm in size), and in long chains. See the contaminant section (page 18) for illustrations.

The determination of *Alternaria* species are difficult. Identification to species should be sent to a specialist.

2. *Anthopsis* is a rare dematiaceous soil fungus. *A. deltoidea* was reported in a case of a bursa cyst with fungal hyphae in the center of granulomata (2 to 3 μm in diameter), branched and septate. The fungus grows slowly on different media at 30°C (no growth at 37°C).

Microscopically, phialidic conidiogenous cells develop from swollen, oval, subglobose to elliptical cells that are terminal for intercalary on hyphae. The phialides are oval to ampullar in shape with or without prominent collarettes.

The phialides appear to be upside down as the conidiogenous areas are at the base of the ampule. The olive-gray conidia are triangular to nearly diamond-shaped and 2 to 3 μm in size.

3. *Aureobasidium pullullans* (de Bary) Arnand, 1918. This species is very common in soil, air, food decay, shower curtains, and other substrates. The fungus has been isolated in cases of visceral infections, in a splenic abscess, and in blood in acute myeloid leukemia.

Colony and microscopic characteristics are under the section on Common Contaminant Fungi, page 18.

4. *Bipolaris*. Three species of *Bipolaris B. australiensis, B. hawaiiensis,* and *B. spicifera* have been recognized as causative agents. Half of the cases are opportunistic infections while the rest were healthy individuals. The types of human infections vary from cutaneous ulceration, osteomyelitis, sinusitis, bronchopulmonary infections, and meningoencephalitis. The three species of *Bipolaris* are commonly found on grasses and other plant substrates. The hyphae in tissue are septate with large, globose, to varied shapes, and hyaline to brown in color.

Two other genera *Exserohilum* and *Drechslera,* are closely related to *Bipolaris*. The distinguishing characteristics are listed in Table 11. No isolates of *Helminthosporium* have been documented as a pathogen in humans or animals.

Table 11. Chief characteristics of *Bipolaris, Drechslera,* and *Exserohilum**

Genus	Conidial Shape	Hilum	Origin of Germ Tube *Conidium*	*Basal Cell*	Orientiation of Germ Tube
Bipolaris	Oblong, ellipsoidal, fusoid (see Figs. 151, a, b)	Continuous with conidial wall, protrudes slightly truncate (see Figures 151, a-d)	One or both ends; rarely others cells (see Figures 151, a-d)	Arising adjacent to or through hilum	Along conidial axis
Drechslera	Cylindrical (see Figures 151, d, e)	Continuous with conidial wall (see Figures 151 d, e)	Intermediate and end cells	Arising midway between conidium and septum (see Figure 151, e)	Perpendicular to conidial axis
Exserohilum	Ellipsoidal to fusoid (see Figures 151, f, g)	Protruding; strongly trucate (see Figure 151, f)	One or both ends; often other cells	Arising adjacent to the hilum (see Figure 151, g)	Along conidial axis

*Modified from McGinnis, M. R., Rinaldi, M. C. and Winn, R. E.. 1986. J. Clin. Microbiol., 106.
All three genera have sympodial (continuously growing) conidiosphores, *Helminthosporium* has a determinate conidiophore (does not extend). *Bipolaris* and *Drechslera* have rounded contour of basal cell of conidium. *Exserohilum* has rounded or conical base of basal cell. In *Drechslera* the first formed septum in a conidium delimits the basal cell. In *Bipolaris* and *Exserohilum* the first septum is in the middle of the conidium. The second septum is near the base in *Bipolaris,* near the apex in *Exserohilum,* and in the middle in *Drechslera*.

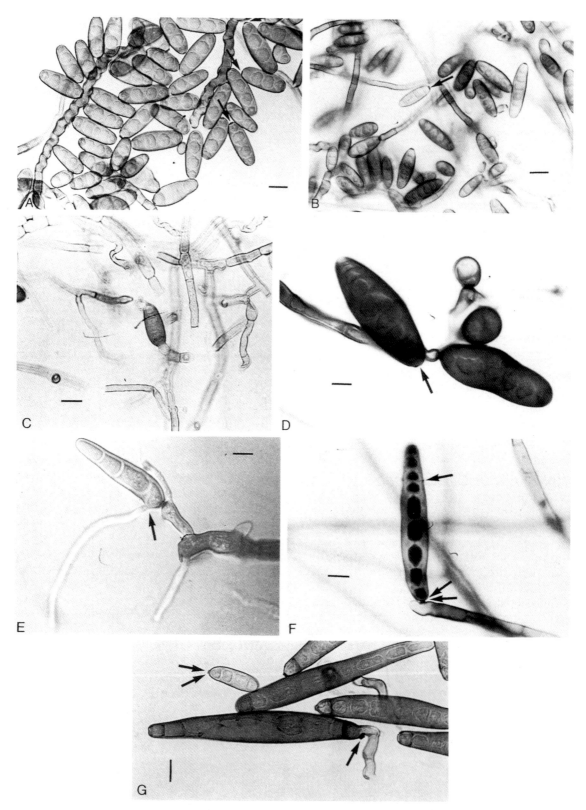

Figure 151. *A, Bipolaris spicifer* 2 condia with truncate hilum (*arrows*) produced from sympodial conidiosphore. Most conidia have three septa. 10 by 27 μm. *B, B. hawaiiensis* truncate hilum (*arrow*) and four to five septa; rarely three or six. 7 by 24 μm. *C, B. spicifera-*germinating at both ends. *D. Drechslera avenae* rounded basal end (*arrow*) without prominent hilum. *E, D. dictyoides.* Germ tube arising midway between hilum and wall of first septum (*arrow*), the germ tube is perpendicular to the axis of the conidium. *F. Exserohilum mcginnisii* basal cell with prominent hilum (*double arrow*) arising from elongating (sympodial) condiophore. This species has warty projections on conidial wall (*single arrow*). 13 by 83 μm. *G, E. rostratum* germ tube arising along the axis of conidium adjacent to prominent hilum (*arrow*). The growth of the mycelium is now bent. Note dark septum above hilum in basal cell. The size of the conidia is very variable in this species. Short conidia (*double arrow*) are 16 by 60 μm, and long conidia are 16 by 160 to 260 μm. The bar equals 10 μm in each. (Courtesty of M. McGinnis.)

Some of the reports on cases in the literature were previously under the genera *Helminthosporium* and *Drechslera.* Currently three species of *Bipolaris,* one species of *Drechslera,* and three species of *Exserohilum* have been reported in human cases.

Bipolaris, Drechslera, Exserohilum, and *Helminthosporium* spp. all grow rapidly, producing woolly, gray to black colonies. The conidiophores of *Bipolaris, Drechslera,* and *Exserohilum* spp. are sympodia and geniculates in contrast to *Helminthosporium* spp. which are straight and stop after the formation of the terminal conidium. The conidial characteristics are important in differentiation of the above genera. Table 9 has the characteristics of the conidia useful for differentiation of the three genera. The three pathogenic species of *Bipolaris, Drechslera,* and *Exserohilum* grow well between 37° and 40°C.

B. spicifera (Bain.) Subram. 1964. Conidia are straight, cylindrical to oblong, rounded at both ends with a protruding truncate hilum, and the conidial distosepta are usually 3, occasionally 2 or 4, with a finely roughened wall. See Figure 151a..

B. hawaiiensis (Ellis) Uchida et Aragaki, 1975. Conidia straight, elliptical to oblong, rounded at both ends, protruding truncate hilum, and the conidial distosepta are usually 4 to 5, occasionally 3 or 6, with a finely roughened wall. See Figure 151b.

B. Australiensis. Like *B. hawaiiensis* except usually 3 conidial distosepta, occasionally 4 or 5.

5. *Cladosporium* spp. Some species of *Cladosporium* are etiologic agents in subcutaneous phaeohyphomycosis as well as cutaneous, eye and nail infections. For more information on the colony and microscopic characteristics of the genus see the section on Common Contaminant Fungi, page 18.

Species of *Cladosporium* found in cases of phaeohyphomycosis are: *C. trichoides* and *C. bantianum,* causes of cerebral abscesses and subcutaneous abscesses; and *C. devriesii* as an etiologic agent of subcutaneous phaeohyphomycosis. *C. cladosporioides,* a common saprophyte has been isolated from an immunosuppressed patient with pulmonary intracavitary fungus ball.

C. bantianum (Sacc) Borelli, 1960 (Synonym: *Xyhlohyphya emmonsii* Padhye et al, 1988). Colonies are black with a velvety surface in Sabouraud agar. On malt extract or potato dextrose agar the colonies grow faster and are a dark-olive gray. The fungus is resistant to cycloheximide

but does not liquify gelatin. *C. bantianum* grows at temperatures between 14° and 30°C.

Microscopically, the brown conidia are smooth-walled, 3.5 to 6.0 by 7 to 17 μm in size, and oblong to ellipsoidal in shape with chains mostly unbranched, 5 to 20 in number.

C. trichoides Emmons, 1952 (Synonym: *Xylohypha bantiana* (Sacc.) McGinnis et al, 1986. The fungus is resistant to cycloheximide and grows well on Sabouraud glucose agar, but more rapidly on potato dextrose or malt extract agar. The colony is olive gray to brown or greenish-black with a velvety surface and blackish reverse side. The optimum temperature is 37° C, but the fungus will grow at 42°C, in contrast to *C. bantianum* which grows at temperatures of between 14° and 30°C.

Microscopically, long, usually unbranched chains of conidia are produced on poorly developed conidiophores at the tip or side of the hyphae. Conidia are pale brown, 2 to 4 μm wide and 3.8 to 18 μm long, one-celled, and ellipsoidal to oblong with a truncate base. The conidia chains tend to break up less than the saprophytic species. *Cladosporium carrionii* produces a similar colony to *C. trichoides* but has shorter conidia and grows slightly or not at all at 37°C.

C. devriesii Padhye et Ajello, 1984. Colonies are similar to other species of *Cladosporium.* The conidia are smooth-walled and resemble *C. carrionii* in conidial characteristics, but lack a *Phialophora* anamorph in culture and produce hyphae in place of sclerotic cells in tissue. *C. devriesii* can be separated from *C. trichoides* by no colonial growth above 37°C and from *C. bantianum* by having smaller conidia and numerous branches of conidial chains.

6. *Chaetomium* Kunze ex Fr. Three species have been reported in human cases of phaeohyphomycosis including a case of subcutaneous abscess, in an acute lymphocytic leukemia, and a cerebral infection in a renal transplant. Species of the genus are saprophytic on cellulose substrates. The three species are *C. funicolum, C. cochliodes,* and *C. globosum.* See the contaminant section, Chapter 2, for mycological characteristics of the genus (page 23).

7. *Curvularia* Boedijn. Currently 4 species and one variety have been causative agents of opportunistic infections, including paranasal sinusitis, endocarditis, mycetoma, eye infections, and pulmonary phaeohyphomycosis. In tissue the hyphae are hyaline to brown. The members of the genus are commonly found in the environment. *Curvularia* colonies are rapidly growing, woolly, and gray, grayish-brown, or black on agar media. (Figure 152 A. *Curvularia,* also see Chapter 2, page 19)

The conidiophores are simple or branched, septate, symmetrical, and geniculate. The conidia are two to several-celled, mostly curved, dark with pale ends and a dark hilum. See the contaminant section, Chapter 2, for illustrations (page 19). Reference should be made to Ellis (1971, 1976) if species need to be identified.

C. geniculata. The conidia are curved, ordinarily with four septa, 18 to 37 by 8 to 14 µm in size. Some cells are medium to dark brown.

C. lunata. The conidia are curved or almost straight, with three septa, 20 to 32 by 9 to 15 µm. The second cell in the conidium is usually darker.

C. pallescens. This species occurs more frequently in the tropics. The conidia are 17 to 32 by 7 to 12 µm in size, usually straight and all the cells are light to pale brown.

C. senegalensis. This species has been reported in mycotic keratitis and in an allergic sinusitis case. This species is similar to *C. lunata*, except conidia are usually with four septa instead of three septa.

8. *Dactylaria* Sacc. *D. gallopava* has been isolated from a subcutaneous abscess, and cases of dissemination to the brain in leukemia or lymphoma patients.

D. gallopava produces rapidly growing colonies reddish to brown-violet in color on Sabouraud glucose agar at 35° to 40°C. At 30°C the rate of growth is slower (Figure 153a, b).

Microscopically, conidia develop on cylindrical denticles (1 to 3 µm), grouped at the apex of conidiogenous cells. The conidia are 6 to 17 by 22.5 to 4.5 µm in size, light brown,-clavate, ovoid or clavate, frequently constricted as a central septum. The conidia resemble *Scolecobasidium constrictum*.

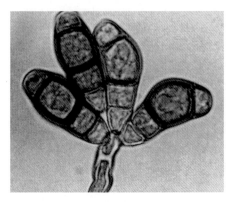

Figure 152. *Curvularia* sp.

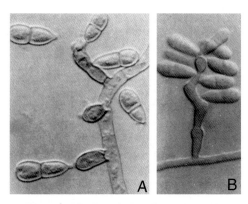

Figure 153. *Dactylaria gallopava,* a and b

9. *Exophiala* Carmichael, 1966. Species of *Exophiala* are commonly the etiologic agent of various cutaneous and subcutaneous phaeohyphomycosis. The nomenclature of species of *Exophiala* has been confusing with a number of synonyms for previous genera and species.

E. dermatitidis (Kano) De Hoogt, 1977 (synonyms: *Phialophora dermatitidis* (Kano) Emmons, 1963; *Wangiella dermatitidis* (Kano) McGinnis, 1977). This species has been isolated from cutaneous, subcutaneous, and systemic cases of phaeohyphomycosis.

The colony is near black in color, moist and slimy at first, then becomes velvety like *Cladosporium* spp. Most strains of the species grow well at 40°C. *E. dermatitidis* is differentiated from other *Exophiala* by growth at 40°C, a short conidiogenous tip and decomposition of tyrosine.

Microscopically, the yeast-like cells with buds predominate in the slimy colony. In the transition from slimy to velvety colonies the *Cladosporium*-like conidiophores may develop and then disappear in older colonies. Later conidiophores may form a chain of oblong cells or a straight hyphal branch with conidia accumulating near the mouth of the conidiogenous cells (Figures 154A, B). The conidiogenous cells may have connellidations.

E. jeanselmei (Langeron) McGinnis and Padhye, 1977 (Synonym: *Phaeoannellomyces elegans* McGinnis et Schell, 1987). This species is frequently isolated from mycetoma and the cyst form of subcutaneous phaeohyphomycosis.

Young colonies on Sabouraud glucose agar are black and slimy with many yeast-like cells (Figure 155), then gradually become velvety after hyphal formation, along with loss of slimy appearance.

Microscopically brown hyphae produce branched or unbranched conidiophores laterally or on the apex (Figures 155, 156, 157A, B). The conidiogenous cells are brown,

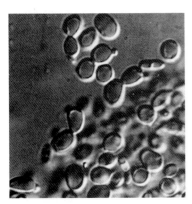

Figure 155. *E. jeanselmei*, yeast-like
cells with annellides

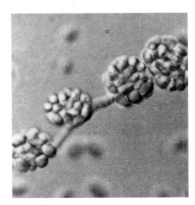

Figure 156. *E. jeanselmei*,
hyphae and conidia

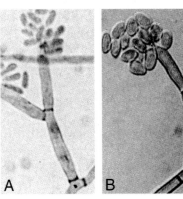

Figure 157. *E. jeanselmei*
a. Branched conidiasphore
b. Unbranched conidiophore

cylindrical annellides which arise near a septum or at the tip of the conidiophore. The conidia are one-celled, 0.75 to 3.0 by 1.0 to 6.0 μm in size, subglobose, cylindrical to elliptical, smooth-walled, hyaline, and aggregated in masses that readily move down the conidiophore or along the side of the hyphae.

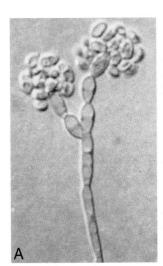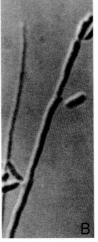

Figure 154. *Exophiala dermatitidis*
A. Conidiophore, conidia
B. Straight hyphal branch, conidia

E. moniliae De Hoog, 1977. This organism has been isolated from cases of subcutaneous phaeohyphomycosis.

The colony develops very slowly, dark olive to black in color. The surface texture varies from smooth, yeast-like to velvety.

Microscopically, dark, budding cells, subglobose to ellipsoidal, 4.4 to 7.4 by 33.3 to 6.7 μm in size. The germinating cells give rise to short, torulose, or smooth hyphae.

Conidiogenous cells are annellides with a swollen base and with long, neck-like extensions, with or without annellations. Conidia are hyaline, one-celled, thin-walled, ellipsoidal or cylindrical to curved in shape, 2.3 to 3.9 by 1.6 to 2.2 μm in size. Basal scars are inconspicuous. Both *E. dermatitidis* and *E. moniliae* decompose tyrosine and grow at 40°C. *E. moniliae* produces longer tips of conidiogenous cells than *E. dermatitidis*.

E. spinifera (Nielsen et Conant) McGinnis, 1977. This species has been isolated from cases of subcutaneous phaeohyphomycosis. This fungus occurs in organic wastes, debris and in enriched soil.

Young colonies are dark, moist, and yeast-like on Sabouraud glucose agar, they later become raised. The optimum temperature is 30°C.

Microscopically, young colonies budding cells, and chains of yeast-like cells are characteristic. Later more hyphae are formed. Conidiogenous cells, annellides, are either terminal or integrated with annellations. Hyaline conidia are single-celled, elliptical to oval, smooth-walled. The conidia aggregate at the tip of conidiogenous cells and tend to slide down along the side of the conidiophores.

10. *Exserohilum* Leonard et Suggs 1974. Infections due to *Exserohilum* have increased recently. Three species, *E. rostratum, E. longirostratum,* and *E. mcginnisii* have been isolated from human cases.

E. rostratum (Drechsler) Leonard et Suggs 1974 (synonym: *Drechslera rostrata* Richardson et Fraser, 1968). This fungus has been isolated from subcutaneous tissues, sinus, nasal polyp and aortic embolus. This genus has three species that may cause phaeohyphomycosis,

E. longirostratum, E. mcginnisii, and *E. rostratum.* See Table 9, page 119 concerning the separation of the three genera, *Bipolaris, Drechslera* and *Exserohilum.*

Microscopically, *Exserohilum rostratum* conidia are ellipsoidal to fusiform in shape with prominent protrusion from the truncate hilum. Mature conidia have thick, dark septa above the hilum on the end cells, while the other septa are not dark in color. The large multicelled conidia develop from sympodial conidiophores (see Figures 158, 159)

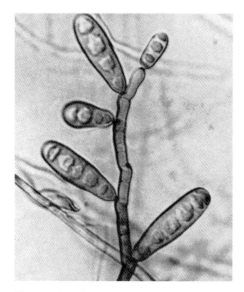

Figure 158. *E. rostratum.* Clavate, young conidia with no dark septa at the end cells

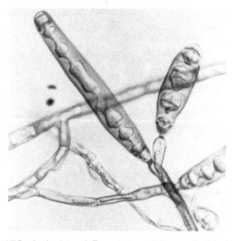

Figure 159. An isolate of *E. rostratum.* A long cylindrical conidium with a dark septum at the end cells

11. *Fonsecaea* Negroni, 1936. The two species of *Fonsecaea, F. pedrosoi* and *F. compacta* usually cause chromoblastomycosis. In two cases *F. pedrosoi* has been reported in a renal transplant patient and from a brain abscess. The cultural and microscopic characteristics are described under Chromoblastomycosis, page 106 in chapter 6.

12. *Phaeoannellomyces. P. werneckii* (Horta) McGinnis et Schell, 1985, is currently considered a synonym of *Exophiala werneckii* (Horta) von Arx, 1970.

13. *Phaeococcomyces.* Considered a synonym of *Wangiella.*

14. *Phialophora* Medlar, 1915. There are five etiologic agents in this genus, *P. verrucosa* is a causative agent of chromoblastomycosis and a phaeomycotic cyst. Three species, *P. bubakii, P. repens,* and *P. richardsiae* are causative agents of subcutaneous phaeohyphomycosis. *P. parasitica* has been reported in both subcutaneous phaeohyphomycosis and in disseminated infection.

P. bubakii has been isolated from a subcutaneous abscess of the forearm in a renal allograft case in Brazil.

P. parasitica. Colonies on Sabouraud glucose agar are white to light brown and glabrous, later becoming velvety, with furrows radiating from the center. Later the colony becomes grayish-brown in the center with cream colored edges.

Microscopically the conidiogenous cells developed from hyaline hyphae are short or long, flask-shaped phialides with funnel-shaped collarettes. Later the phialides become dark-brown toward the base usually with rough walls and proliferation (Figure 160a and Figure b). The latter proliferation is different from *P. repens.* The conidia in mature cultures are elliptical to ovoid, 2 to 8 by 1 to 4 μm in size.

P. repens develops a light to dark-brown colony with tufts of hyphae on Sabouraud agar.

Microscopically, phialides are developed singly or in groups, up to 15 μm long tapering from 2 to 4 μm across the base to 1 to 1.5 μm at the apex. The collarette is short and indistinct. The phialoconidia are hyaline, cylindrical or curved, 1.3 to 2.8 by 2.5 to 8 μm in size, in slimy droplets at the tip of the phialides.

P. richardsiae. Colonies are rapid in growth at 30°C. The color is olive-brown to grayish-brown with concentric bands. The brown pigment may diffuse in older colonies. The surface of colony is woolly and ropy. The hyaline hyphae darken to brown in a few days.

Microscopically, heavy sporulation occurs in this species on various media. The phialides vary in morphology and size being produced from the hyphae as tapering, lateral branches, 1 to 3 μm wide at the base and 2 to 30 μm in length with a narrow tip. The phialide tips are simple or produce a flaring, saucer-shaped collar up to 4 μm in diameter. See Figure 161a and Figure b. Two types of conidial development occur, one is nearly colorless, thin-walled, elliptical, 1 to 2 by 12 to 4 μm in size, and the other is spherical, 12.4 to 3 μm in size and brown in color. The second type of conidia are produced by phialides with flaring, saucer-shaped collarettes. These two types of conidia separate this species from *P. verrucosa*.

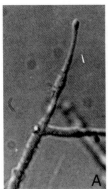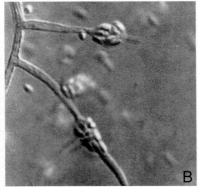

A B

Figure 160. *Phialophora parasitica*
a. A roughened, branched phialide
with conidium at the tip (X650)
b. Precurrently proliferating phialides (X650)

P. verrucosa usually is one of the etiologic agents of chromoblastomycosis. Two cases of subcutaneous infection have been reported, with short hyphae and sclerotic cells in the granuloma. Reference should be made to chromoblastomycosis on page 108, chapter 6 for colony and microscopic characteristics.

15. *Rhinocladiella*. The species, *R. aquaspersa* is a rare causative agent of chromoblastomycosis and phaeohyphomycosis.

16. *Scedosporium*. *Scedosporium apiospermum* (formerly known as *Monosporium apiospermum)* is the asexual state of *Pseudallescheria boydii* (previously known as *Petriellidium boydii* and *Allescheria boydii)*. This fungus may be the cause of mycetoma and also phaeohyphomycosis in the brain and lungs. The colony and microscopic characteristics are described under Mycetoma in chapter 6, page 105.

17. *Scytalidium*. Two species, *S. hyalinum* (a synanamorph of *Hendersonula toruloidea)* and *S. lignicola*. One case of a subcutaneous cyst was caused by *S. hyalinum*, and other was a subcutaneous phaeohyphomycosis caused by *S. lignicola*. The genus usually produced dark brown arthroconidia, but *S. hyalinum* has hyaline conidia.

18. *Wangiella*. This genus is currently considered a synonym of Exophiala (page 122).

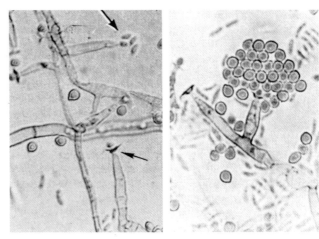

Figure 161. *Phialophora richardsiae,*
Two phialides with two types of phialoconidia

The following are occasional Dematiaceous causative agents.

Nigrospora sphaerica has been reported as the causative agent of an ulcerated lesion on the nose.

Oidiodendron cerealis was isolated from a patient with neurodermitis nuchae.

Phoma. Three species, *P. eupyrena*, *P. hibernica*, and *P. minutella* have been reported as causative agents of phaeohyphomycosis.

Note: There have been a number of dematiaceous fungi reported that may become more frequent in occurrence in the future.

Selected References

Adam RD, Paquin ML. 1986. Phaeohyphomycosis caused by the fungal genera *Bipolaris* and *Exserohilum*. Medicine 65:203

Ajello L. 1975. Phaeohyphomycosis: definition and etiology. Pan. Am. Health. Org. Sci. Publ. 304:126

Ajello L. 1981. The gamut of human infections caused by dematiaceous fungi. Jpn. J. Med. Mycol. 22:1

Ajello L. et al. 1980. *Drechslera rostrata* as an agent of phaeohyphomycosis. Mycologia 72:1094

Alcorn JL. 1983. Generic concepts in *Drechslera, Bipolaris,* and *Exoserohillum*. Mycotaxon 17:1

Anzinlt BJA. 1990. Subcutaneous phaeohyphomycosis due to *Exophiala jeanselmei* in an immunosuppressed patient: case report. N. A. Med. J. 103:321

Anandi V. et al. 1989. Cerebral phaeohyphomycosis caused by *Chaetomium globosum* in a renal transplant recipient. J. Clin. Microbiol. 27:2226

Baker JG, et al. 1987. First report of a subcutaneous phaeohyphomycosis of the foot cause by *Phoma milnutella.* J. Clin. Microbiol. 25:2395

Barnett JL, Hunter BB. 1987. Illustrated genera of imperfect fungi. 4th ed. Macmillan Publishing Co. New York, NY

Barron GL. 1968. The genera of Hyphomycetes from soil. The Williams & Wilkins Co., Baltimore, MD

Barale T, Fumey MH, Reboux G, Mallea M. 1990. Septicemie a *Chaetomium* sp. lors d'une autogreffe de moelle pour leucose aigue lymphoblastique. Bull de Societe Francaise Mycologie Medicale 10:43

Bartynski JM, McCaffrey TV, Frigas E. 1990. Allergic fungal sinusitis secondary to dematiaceous fungi *Curvularia lunata* and *Alternaria.* Otolaryngology - Head and Neck Surgery 103:32.

Benoldi D, Alinovi A, Polonelli L, Conti S, Gerloni M, Ajello L, Padhye AA, Hoog GS de. 1991. J. Med. Vet. Mycology 29(1):9

Bievre C de. 1991. Les *Alternaria* pathogenes pour l'homme: mycologie epidemiologique. J. Mycologie Med. 1:50

Blomquist K, Salonen A. 1969. *Oidiodendron cerealis* isolated from neurodermaṭitis nuchae. Dermatologica 139:1158

Body BA. et al. 1987. *Alternaria* species infection in a patient with acute lymphocytic leukemia. Pediatr. Infect. Dis. J. 6:418

Borges MC. et al. 1991. Pulmonary phaeohyphomycosis due to *Xylohypha bantiana.* Arch. Pathol. Lab. Meld. 115:627

Burges GE, Walls CT, and Maize JC. 1987. Subcutaneous phaeohyphomycosis caused by *Exeserohilum rostratum* in an immunocompetent host. Arch. Dermatol. 123:1346

Carmichael JW, et al. 1980. Genera of Hyphomycetes. University of Alberta Press. Edmonton, Canada. p. 210

Elewski BE, Greer DL. 1991. *Hendersonula toruloidea* and *hyalinum.* Arch. Dermatol. 127:1041

Ellis MB. 1971. Dematiaceous Hyphomycetes. Commonwealth Mycological Institute. Kew, England

Ellis MB. 1976. More Dematiaceous Hyphomycetes. Commonwealth Mycological Institute. Kew, England

Fader RC, McGinnis MR. 1988. Infections caused by dematiaceous fungi: chromoblastomycosis and phaeohyphomycosis. Infect. Dis. Clin. N. Am. 2:925

Friedman AD, et al. 1981. Fatal recurrent *Curvularia* brain abscess. J. Pediatr. 99:413

Kaczmarski EB. et al. 1986. Systemic infection with *Aureobasidium pullulans* in a leukemic patient. J. Infect. 13:239

Kendrick WB. (ed). 1971. Taxonomy of Fungi Imperfecti. University of Toronto Press. Toronto

Killingsworth SM, Wetmore SLJ. 1990. *Curvularia/ Drechslera* sinusitis. Laryngoscope 100:(1):932

Kwon-Chung KJ, Bennett JE. 1992. *Medical Mycology.* p. 866. Lea & Febiger, Philadelphia

Kwon-Chung KJ, Droller DD. 1984. Infection of the ole-

cranon bursa by *Anthopsis deltoidea.* J. Clin. Microbiol. 20:271

Kwon-Chung KJ, Wickes BL, Plaskowitz J. 1989. Taxonomic clarification of *Cladosporium trichoides* Emmons and its subsequent synonyms. J. Med. Vet. Mycol. 27:413

Lampert RP, et al. 1977. Pulmonary and cerebral mycetoma caused by *Curvularia pallescens.* J. Pediatr. 91:603

Loveless MO, et al. 1981. Mixed invasive infection with *Alternaria* species and *Curvularia* species. Am. J. Clin. Pathol. 76:491

MacMillan RH, et al. 1987. Allergic fungal sinusitis due to *Curvularia lunata.* Hum. Pathol. 18:960

McGinnis MR. 1980. Laboratory handbook of medical mycology. Academic Press, Inc. New York

McGinnis MR, Rinaldi MC, Winn RE. 1986. Emerging agents of phaeohyphomycosis: pathogenic species of *Bipolaris* and *Exserohilum.* J. Clin. Milcrobiol. 24:250

McGinnis MR, Borelli RD, Padhye AA, Ajello, L. 1986. Reclassification of *Cladosporium bantianum* in the genus *Xylohypha.* J. Clin. Microbiol. 23:1148

Moneymaker CS, et al, 1986. Primary cutaneous phaeohyphomycosis due to *Exserohilum rostratum* (*Drechslera rostrata*) in a child with leukemia. Pediatr. Infect. Dis. J. 5:380

Padhye AA, et al, 1986. *Phialophora bubakii*: isolamento de abscesso subcutaneo em transplatado renal. Rev. Inst. Med. Trop. Sao Paulo 21:106

Pasarell L, McGinnis MR, Standard PG, 1990. Differentiation of medically important isolates of *Bipolaris* and *Exserohilum* with exoantigens. J. Clin. Microbiol 128:1655

Salkin, IF, McGinnis, MR, Dykstra MJ, Rinaldi MG, 1988. *Scedosporium inflatum,* an emerging pathogen. J. Clin. Microbiol. 26:498

Rippon, JW, 1988. Medical Mycology. 3rd ed. WB Saunders, Philadelphia, pp. 297–324,

Rippon JW, et al, 1985. "Golden tongue" syndrome caused by *Ramichloridium schulzeri.* Arch. Dermatol. 121:892

Salkin JF, Martinez JA, Kenna ME, 1986. Opportunistic infection of the spleen caused by *Aureobasidium pullulans.* J. Clin. Microbiol. 23:828

Schnadig VJ, et al, 1986. *Phialophora verrucosa* induced subcutaneous phaeophyphomycosis, fine needle aspiration findings. Acta Cytol. 30: 425

Terreni AA, et al, 1990. Disseminated *Dactylaria gallopava* infection in a diabetic patient with chronic lymphocytic leukemia of the T-cell type. Am. J. Clin. Pathol. 94:104

Ventin M, Ramirez C, and Garau J, 1987. *Exophiala dermatitidis* de Hoog from a valvular aortal prothesis. Mycopathologia 99:45

Zaharopoulos, P, et al, 1988. Multiseptate bodies in systemic phaeohyphomycosis diagnosed by fine needle aspiration cytology. Acta Cytol. 32:885.

Chapter 7

TRUE SYSTEMIC MYCOSES

INTRODUCTION TO SYSTEMIC MYCOSES

The systemic diseases caused by fungi are separated into two very distinct groups. These two groups have important differences in host resistance and virulence. The first group includes diseases caused by the true pathogenic fungi: *Histoplasma, Coccidioides, Blastomyces,* and *Paracoccidioides*. These fungi are virulent and the host has normal defense mechanisms. The second group of fungi that remain mycelial or yeast forms in the immunocompromised or other forms of debilitation in the host include the etiologic agents of opportunistic infections: agents of hyalohyphomycosis (*Aspergillus, Fusarium*, etc.), *Candida, Cryptococcus*, and other yeasts, *Pseudallescheria*, agents of zygomycoses and miscellaneous fungi. The opportunistic infections with dark hyphae include agents of phaeohyphomycosis which are included with the subcutaneous group of fungi. All of these fungi in the second group are normal saprophytes that invade the immunocompromised or other form of debilitated host and remain in one form, yeast or mycelial. Table 12 (Table 14-1 Rippon) compares the true pathogenic fungus infections with the opportunistic fungus infections.

Table 12. The Systemic Mycoses

	True Pathogenic Fungus Infections	Opportunistic Fungus Infections
Diseases	Histoplasmosis	Aspergillosis
	Blastomycosis*	Candidiasis
	Paracoccidioidomycosis	Zygomycosis
	Coccidioidomycosis	Cryptococcosis
Host	Normal	Abrogated
Portal of entry	Primary infection polmonary	Various
Prognosis	99% of cases resolve spontaneously	Recovery depends on severity of impairment of host defenses
Immunity	Resolution imparts strong specific immunity	No specific resistance to reinfection
Host response	Tuberculoid granuloma; also mixed	Depends on degree of impairment—necrosis to pyogenic to granulomatous
Morphology in tissue	All agents show dimorphism to a tissue form	No change in morphology†
Distribution	Geographically restricted	Ubiquitous

*These diseases have significant exceptions to the usual patterns.
† *Candida* spp. are found as mixed yeasts and mycelial elements in tissue as well as in culture.

Through permission of J. W. Rippon, Textbook of Medical
Mycology, 3rd Ed, Philadelphia, W. B. Saunders Co, p. 374.

These mycoses will be covered in Chapter 7, Systemic Mycoses - True Pathogenic Fungi; Chapter 8 Opportunistic Infections - Yeasts; and Chapter 9 Opportunistic Infections - Mycelial Fungi.

TRUE PATHOGENIC FUNGI

The systemic mycoses due to the true pathogenic fungi may involve all of the internal organs of the body and in some stages the skin. Some of these mycoses involve bone as well as subcutaneous tissue. In many cases the systemic mycoses may be asymptomatic and can be recognized only by immunologic procedures, while other cases may have mild symptoms and be self-limited. In the progressive form of the disease symptoms are pronounced, internal organs may be damaged, and death may occur if the disease does not respond to chemotherapy.

Many of the fungi causing the systemic mycoses produce a different form in tissue or at 37°C in contrast to the mycelial form in culture at 24°C. These fungi are referred to as diphasic or dimorphic organisms. Fungi causing blastomycosis (North American blastomycosis), paracoccidioidomycosis (South American blastomycosis), coccidioidomycosis, and histoplasmosis are dimorphic. Sporotrichosis and chromoblastomycosis in the subcutaneous section (Chapter 6) also are dimorphic. Sporotrichosis changes from the mycelial form at 25°C to the yeast cells at 37°C or in tissue. Chromoblastomycosis remains mycelial at 25°C or higher but changes to sclerotic cells in tissue, or in special liquid culture.

Identification of these fungi depends upon several laboratory procedures. These include: (1) direct examination or staining of smears, (2) culture at 24°C and in some cases for the yeast form at 37°C, and (3) the use of serologic methods. The primary serologic tests include complement fixation (CF), immunodiffusion (ID), and latex agglutination (LA), for detection of antibodies in the serum. These serologic tests are available at the Fungus Immunology Section of the Center for Disease Control in Atlanta, through state health laboratories, or from commercial companies as test kits. Table 7 (see Chapter 6) illustrates possible genera and species of the etiolgic agents from clinical specimens from some of the subcutaneous and deep mycoses. More information is under the name of the disease and the corresponding genera of the etiologic agents.

Table 13. The Dimorphic Deep Mycoses

Disease, Fungus	Mycelial Form (25°)	Parasitic Form (37°C)
Blastomycosis *Blastomyces dermatitidis*	Colonies white to tan glabrous to velvety, septate hyphae,microconidia, globose or pyriform	Yeast with broad-based buds, 8-20 μm
Coccidioidomycosis *Coccidioides immitis*	Colonies white to buff, membranous to cottony septate hyphae, fragment into arthroconidia	Spherules,10-80 μm with endospores
Histoplasmosis *Histoplasma capsulatum*	Colonies white or buff, septate hyphae,tuberculate macroconidia and small oval microconidia	Small, single budding yeasts, l-5 μm (5-12 μm in var. *duboisii*)
Paracoccidioidomycosis *Paracoccidioides brasiliensis*	Similar to *B.dermatitidis*	Multiple budding yeasts, 20-60 μm

BLASTOMYCOSIS

(North American blastomycosis, Gilchrist's disease, Chicago disease)

Definition

This disease is a chronic verrucose, granulomatous, and suppurative mycotic infection that may occur in three clinical forms: cutaneous, pulmonary, and systemic (Figures 162 and 163). Symptoms may be similar to those of tuberculosis. Infection may occur in the pulmonary form or dissemination may occur to the skin, osseous system, central nervous system, urogenital system, and other organs.

Cutaneous blastomycosis is a rare form of the disease. The infection may involve any organ of the body except the intestinal tract.

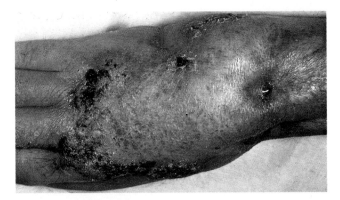

Figure 162. *Blastomycosis,* Hand and wrist

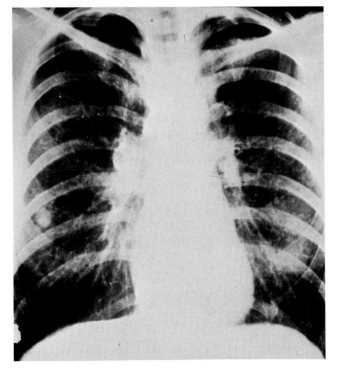

Figure 163. Pulmonary blastomycosis
Blastomyces dermatitidis, X-ray film

Etiologic Agent

Blastomyces dermatitidis Gilchrist and Stokes, 1898. The perfect state (or teleomorph state): *Ajellomyces dermatitidis* McDonough and Lewis, 1968.

Occurrence

Humans: Blastomycosis is found chiefly in North America, the highest incidence being south of the Ohio River and east of the Mississippi River. Other areas of disease concentration are North Carolina and the west side of Lake Michigan. A few cases have been reported in Mexico, Central America, northern South America, Tunisia, Israel, Lebanon, Saudi Arabia, Poland, India, and Africa.

Animals: Numerous cases of blastomycosis in dogs have been reported in North America. Cases in horses, a sea lion, and cats have also been reported.

Soil: The fungus has been recovered from soil samples and the bark of some trees, but the ecologic niche of *Blastomyces dermatitidis* has not been firmly established.

Laboratory Procedures

Specimen collection: *B. dermatitidis* can be isolated most easily from multiple minute abscesses in skin lesions. Scrapings, small pieces of tissue, sputum, or pus from the edge of the skin lesion should be collected. Pus from subcutaneous abscesses should be aspirated with a sterile syringe and needle, and sputum, urine, and spinal fluid should be submitted in suspected systemic cases. In case of bone infection, material should be collected from this area for examination in the laboratory.

Direct examination: Pus from human cases should be placed as a drop on a slide (using sterile technique) and pressed down with a coverglass. If there are no budding cells in the pus, this organism may resemble other fungi causing systemic mycoses. If opaque material is present, 10% KOH or Calcafluor white should be put on a slide with a coverglass. Biopsied material should be used for histopathology studies and culture. To keep infected pus material for future demonstrations, the pus may be mixed with lactophenol on a slide, a coverglass added, and the slide sealed with nail polish.

Microscopically, pus, sputum, or tissue shows large, spherical, thick-walled, yeastlike cells, 8 to 15 µm in diameter (rarely up to 30 µm) in direct mounts. Some walls in the cells may be sufficiently thick to look like a double contour or ring. Note the broad based buds on yeast cells which also form in culture at 37°C (Figure 167). The persistent attachment of bud to the mother cell is characteristic in *Blastomycosis.*

Culture: In order to isolate the fungus, the infected material should be cultured on blood agar, or brain-heart infusion agar at 37°C and on Sabouraud glucose agar or BHIA with chloramphenicol and/or Smith's (yeast extract phosphate) agar at 24°C. Keep four weeks before considering the culture negative.

Colonies: Colonies at 37°C on blood agar or brain-heart infusion agar develop slowly and are cream to tan in color, soft, wrinkled, and waxy in appearance (Figure 166). Conversion from the mycelial form usually takes four to five days. The surface of the medium should be moist.

Colonies at room temperature when first cultured on Sabouraud glucose agar may show a yeastlike growth in early stages of development. Later, coremia or hyphal projections may develop on the surface as the so-called "prickly stage," and finally the entire surface becomes downy or fluffy white (Figure 164). Older cultures become tan to brown in color. Try converting the mycelial form to the yeast form.

Microscopically, a slide mount from colonies grown at 37°C shows large, round, single budding, thick-walled cells similar to those in tissue, as well as short mycelial fragments. Check the size of these budding cells and the width of bud attachment to the parent yeast cell (Figure 167).

Slide cultures or mounts from colonies grown at room temperature should show numerous round to pyriform, one-celled conidia, 2 to 10 μm in diameter, attached directly on the hyphae or on short conidiophores. Older cultures have many chlamydoconidia, up to 18 μm in diameter, with thickened walls (Figure 165). If only grown at room temperature the organism must be converted to the yeast form at 37°C. BHIA is one of the media that may be used. The hyphal form of this organism will resemble *Chrysosporium* species.

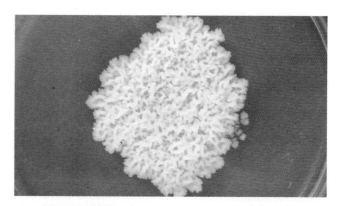

Figure 166. *Blastomyces dermatitidis,* colony 37°C

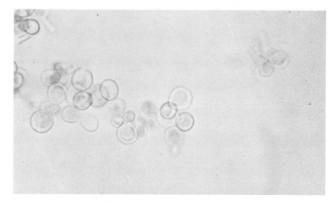

Figure 167. *Blastomyces dermatitidis,*
yeast cells 37°C X1000

Perfect state (Teleomorph state): *Ajellomyces dermatitidis* McDonough and Lewis, 1968. Yeast extract agar containing a suspension of pulverized bone meal (15 g/liter) is used as a medium in a modified block method (McDonough and Lewis, 1968) for study of the perfect state. The gymnothecia are tan in color, 200 to 300 μm in diameter, and develop thick-walled, closely coiled spiral hyphae that radiate out from a center in the gymnothecium. The spirals form on lateral hyphae, which branch to develop clusters of ascogenous hyphae in addition to branched hyphae with constrictions at the cross walls. Asci with eight smooth, spherical, hyaline or light tan ascospores, 1.5 to 2.0 μm in diameter. This fungus is heterothallic.

Histopathologic studies: Prepared stained slides are made from biopsy specimens taken from skin lesions or from internal areas in disseminated blastomycosis. The tissue reaction is usually a granulomatous and suppurative reaction. The granulomatous type giant cells are usually present, and the fungus cells usually are located in the necrotic areas and at times in the giant cells.

In the suppurative type, lesions have a polymorphonuclear exudate with many fungus cells scattered around the tissue

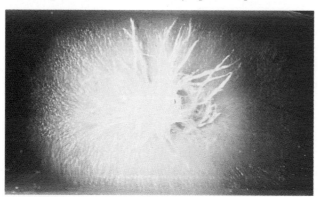

Figure 164. *Blastomyces dermatitidis,* colony 24°C

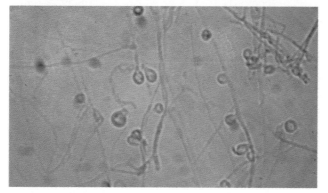

Figure 165. *Blastomyces dermatitidis,* conidia 24°C X800

or localized in abscesses. Skin lesions may be a mixture of granulomatous and suppurative types.

The fungus cells, which are about the same size as cells in the yeast form at 37°C, vary from 8 to 15 μm in diameter with double-contoured thick walls and usually single budding forms when reproducing (Figures 168 and 169). Each cell is multinucleate. The organism is readily stained with PAS, Gomori methenamine silver nitrate stain, or Gridley stain. H and E stain is satisfactory for *B. dermatitidis* in tissue.

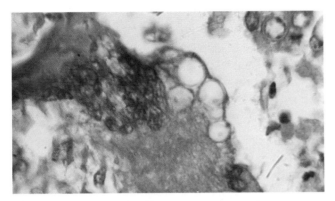

Figure 168. Blastomycosis, budding yeast cells in tissue X1200

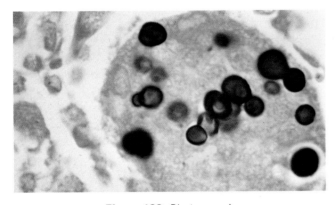

Figure 169. Blastomycosis, yeast cells in tissue X1200

Animal inoculation: Guinea pigs, rats, mice, or young male hamsters as well as monkeys and dogs may be inoculated intraperitoneally with infected material from lesions or with saline suspensions, 1 ml of a 1:200 suspension of the yeast form. Infection should reach a peak in about 21 days, and the animals may die. Intravenous injection of 0.1 ml of the suspension in mice may produce a rapidly fatal disease.

After autopsy, examine for nodules on the mesentery, omentum, and peritoneal surface. In addition the spleen, liver, and lung may have nodules that contain the yeastlike budding cells.

Direct slide mounts of pieces of smashed nodules in lactophenol, with the coverglass pressed down to spread the material out, should show the typical thick-walled budding cells. Stained slides may be made from sections of the infected materials. Slides with crushed material from these lesions mounted in lactophenol may be sealed with nail polish for future reference.

Serology and Immunology: Currently, due to the improvement in the diagnosis of blastomycosis with the availability of the purified antigen of *Blastomyces dermatitidis* (Turner and Kaufman, 1986), the EIA (Enzyme-linked immunosorbent assay) and ID tests are useful in serodiagnosis of blastomycosis. The CF test is not as sensitive as the EIA and the ID tests. The serologic tests for blastomycosis should be utilized when a patient has a respiratory infection that develops gradually with fever, weight loss, cough and purulent sputum, when skin lesions are present. These tests are also useful in patients with suspected blastomycotic meningitis.

The ID test for blastomycosis using a yeast form culture filtrate containing the A antigen results in a specific test. A positive test is the basis for immediate treatment of the patient. The EIA test is more sensitive than the ID but may occasionally be nonspecific. The EIA titers of 1:32 or greater are indicative of active blastomycosis. By using both the EIA and ID tests at the same time, the sensitivity is 85% and the specificity is 98%. Cultures should be done for additional confirmation especially if the serologic test is negative.

The A antigen from the yeast form culture filtrates is stable for several months at 4°C in phosphate buffer and has been used in all available tests. Sensitivity does vary according to patient population and the test format, ranging from 57 to 62% for the CF test, 52 to 79% for the ID test, and 80 to 100% for the EIA test. The EIA test may show some cross-reactions with sera from cases of histoplasmosis.

Excellent coverage of detailed procedures on the serodiagnosis of fungal diseases are covered by Kaufman and Reiss (1992). Although diagnosis by histologic or culture studies are very useful, more time is required and occasionally the results are negative.

Fungal reagents for use in ID tests are available from numerous commercial sources. Currently Immuno-Mycologics sells kits for immunoidentification of *B. dermatitidis*. Tests for exoantigens are useful whenever a white to tan fungus is isolated from any suspected case of blastomycosis especially if cultures are nonsporulating or are difficult to convert.

DNA Probe. The commercially available acridinium ester-labeled chemiluminescent DNA probe (Gen-Probe, BD probe. San Diego, CA) is available for *B. dermatitidis*. In a recent report on 306 isolates of various yeasts and other fungi with the BD probe, Stockman et al (1993) found a sensitivity of 91% and a specificity of 100% for *B. dermatitidis*. In a repeat testing of discrepant values, the sensitivity increased to 100%. This probe test is extremely useful because of ease and rapidity of identification of this dimorphic pathogen from a primary culture medium. The commercial kits from the manufacturer provide the methods for sample preparation and hybridization utilizing the fungal culture isolated from the patient. For more information see Laboratory procedures, page 45, DNA Probes. The probe is more reliable than the commercial exoantigen tests (Sandin, etc.).

Special nutritional requirements: The yeast phase requires 37°C for growth. No special nutrients are essential, unless biotin is absent. Less than 0.1 mg per 1,000 ml of medium is needed. Organic nitrogen, such as serine or hydroxyproline, increases the growth of the organism. The vitamin and nitrogen requirements are similar to the mycelial form.

Questions

1. Name other pathogenic fungi in tissue that may resemble budding cells or cells without buds.

2. Explain the differences in the ID, EIA, and CF tests. What is the exoantigen test?

Selected References

Baker RD. 1939. The effect of mouse passage on cultural characteristics and virulence for mice of organisms causing blastomycosis. Am. J. Trop. Med. 19:547

Bakerspigel A, Kane J, Schaus D. 1986. Isolation of *Blastomyces dermatitidis* from an earthen floor in southwestern Ontario. 1986. Canada J. Clin. Microbiol. 24:890

Beneke ES, Wilson RW, Rogers AL. 1969. Extracellular enzymes of *Blastomyces dermatitidis*. Mycopathologia 39:325

Busey JF. 1977. North American blastomycosis. Ariz. Med. 34:392

Campbell CC, Binkley GE. 1953. Serologic diagnosis with respect to histoplasmosis, coccidioidomycosis, and blastomycosis and the problem of cross reactions. J. Lab. Clin. Med. 42:896

Carman WF, et al. 1989. Blastomycosis in Africa. Mycopathologia 107:25

Chernisse EI, Waisbren BA. 1956. North American blastomycosis: A clinical study of forty cases. Ann. Intern. Med. 44:105

Chick EW, Sutliff WD, Rabich JH, et al. 1956. Epidemiological aspects of cases of blastomycosis admitted to Memphis, Tennessee hospitals during the period of 1922-1954. A review of 86 cases. Am. J. Med. Sci. 231:253

Conant NF, Howell A Jr. 1942. The similarity of the fungi causing South American blastomycosis (paracoccidioidal granuloma) and North American blastomycosis (Gilchrist's disease). J. Invest. Dermatol. 5:353

Conti Diaz IA, Smith CD, et al. 1970. Comparison of infection of laboratory animals with *Blastomyces dermatitidis* using different routes of inoculation. Sabouraudia 7:279

Crowe, H. M., Levitz, S. M, Sugar, A. M. 1987. Rapid method for the production of *Blastomyces dermatitidis* protoplasts. Exp. Mycol. 11:159

Denton JF, Di Salvo AF. 1964. Isolation of *Blastomyces dermatitidis* from natural sites at Augusta, Georgia. Am. J. Trop. Med. Hyg. 13:716

Denton JF, Di Salvo AF, Hirsch ML. 1967. Laboratory-acquired North American blastomycosis. JAMA 199:935

Denuys GA, Newman MA, Standard PA. 1983. Evaluation of a commercial exoantigen test system for the rapid identification of systemic fungal pathogens. Am. J. Clin. Pathol. 79:379

Emmons CW, Murray IG, Lurie HI, et al. 1964. North American blastomycosis: Two autochthonous cases from Africa. Sabouraudia Africa. Sabouraudia 3:30

Fraser VJ, Keath EJ, Powderly WG. 1991. Two cases of blastomycosis from a common source: Use of DNA restriction analysis to identify strains. J. Infect. Dis. 163:1378

Furcolow ML, Balows A, Menges RW, et al. 1966. Blastomycosis. An important medical problem in the central United States. JAMA 198:529

Garrison RG, Lane JW, et al. 1970. Ultrastructural changes during the yeastlike to mycelial phase conversion of *Blastomyces dermatitidis* and *Histoplasma capsulatum*. J. Bacteriol. 101:628

Gilardi GL. 1965. Nutrition of systemic and subcutaneous pathogenic fungi. Bact. Rev. 29:406

Gilchrist TC. 1896. Case of blastomycetic dermatitis in man. Johns Hopkins Hosp. Rep. 1:269

Guidry DJ, Bujard AJ. 1964. Comparison of the pathogenicity of the yeast and mycelial phases of *Blastomyces dermatitidis*. Am. J. Trop. Med. Hyg. 13:319

Kane J. Conversion of *Blastomyces dermatitidis* to the yeast form at 37°C and 26°C. J. Clin. Microbiol. 20:594

Kaufman L, Reiss E. 1992. *Serodiagnosis of fungal diseases. In* Rose NR, Friedman H (eds). Manual of Clinical Immunology. Am. Soc. Microbiol. 2nd ed. Washington, DC.

Kaufman L. et al. 1983. Detection of two *Blastomyces dermatitidis* serotypes by exoantigen analysis. J. Clin. Microbiol. 18:110

Klein BS, et al. 1986. Comparison of the enzyme immunoassay, immunodiffusion, and complement fixation tests in detecting antibody in human serum to the A antigen of *Blastomyces dermatitidis*. Am. Rev. Respir. Dis. 133:144

Kwon-Chung KJ. 1971. Genetic analysis on the incompatibility system of *Ajellomyces dermatitidis*. Sabouraudia 9:231

Lambert RS, George RB. 1987. Evaluation of enzyme immunoassay as a rapid screening test for histoplasmosis and blastomycosis. Am. Rev. Respir. Dis. 136:316

Lancaster MV, Sprouse RF. 1976. Isolation of a purified skin test antigen from *Blastomyces dermatitidis* yeast-phase cell wall. Infect. Immunol. 14:623

Lo CY, Notenboom RH. 1990. A new enzyme immunoassay specific for blastomycosis. Am. Rev. Respir. Dis. 141:84.

McDonough ES, Ajello L, Ausherman RJ, et al. 1961. Human pathogenic fungi recovered from soil in an area endemic for N. American blastomycosis. Am. J. Hyg. 73:75

McDonough ES, Chan DM, McNamara W. 1977. Dual infection by "+" and "-" mating types of *Ajellomyces* (*Blastomyces*) *dermatitidis*. Am. J. Epidemiol. 106:76

McDonough ES, Lewis AL. 1968. The ascigerous stage of *Blastomyces dermatitidis*. Mycologia 60:76

Medoff G, Painter A, Kobayashi G. 1987. Mycelial-to-yeast phase transitions of the dimorphic fungi *Blastomyces dermatitidis* and *Paracoccidioides brasiliensis*. J. Bacteriol. 169:4055

Pappas PG, Pottage JC, Powderly WG, Fraser VJ, Stratton CW, McKenzie S, Tapper MS, Chmel HJ, Bonerbrake FC, Blum R, Shafer RW, King C, Dismukes WE. 1992. Blastomycosis in patients with the acquired immunodeficiency syndrome. Ann. Inter. Med. 116 (10):847

Robbins ES. 1954. North American blastomycosis in the dog. J. Am. Vet. Med. Assoc. 125:391

Sandin RL, Hal GS, Longworth DL, Washington JA. 1993. Unpredictability of commercially available exoantigen culture confirmation tests in confirming the identity of five *Blastomyces dermatitidis* isolates. Am. J. Clin. Pathol. 99:542

Sarosi GA, Davies SF, Philips JR. 1986. Self-limited blastomycosis: a report of 39 cases. Semin. Respir. Infect. 11:40

Sekhon AS, Standard PG. 1986. Reliability of exoantigens for differentiating *Blastomyces dermatitidis* and *Histoplasma capsulatum* from *Chrysosporium* and *Geomyces* species. Diagn. Microbiol. Infect. Dis. 4:215

Smith CD, Brandsberg JW, Selby LA, et al. 1966. A comparison of the relative susceptibilities of laboratory animals to infection with the mycelial phase of *Blastomyces dermatitidis*. Sabouraudia 5:126

Stockman L, Clark KA, Hunt JM, Roberts GD. 1993. Evaluation of commercially available acridinium ester-labeled chemiluminescent DNA probes for culture identification of *Blastomyces dermatitidis*, *Coccidioides immitis*, *Cryptococcus neoformans* and *Histoplasma capsulatum*. J. Clin. Microbiol. 31(4): 845

Weeks RJ. 1964. A rapid, simplified medium for converting the mycelial phase of *Blastomyces dermatitidis* to the yeast phase. Mycopathologia 22:153

Witorsch P, Utz JP. 1965. North American blastomycosis. A study of 40 patients. Medicine (Baltimore) 47:169

PARACOCCIDIOIDOMYCOSIS

*(Paracoccidioidal granuloma,
South American blastomycosis)*

Definition

This disease is a chronic, progressive, granulomatous infection of the skin (Figure 170), mucous membranes, lymph nodes, gastrointestinal tract, and internal organs. Most infections are initiated as primary pulmonary lesions that are usually inapparent, and then disseminate to form ulcerative granulomas. In the early stages of infection symptoms resemble those of blastomycosis and coccidioidomycosis. The predominant form of the disease is on the face, especially around the mouth or nose.

Etiologic Agent

Paracoccidioides brasiliensis (Splendore) Almeida, 1930. (Synonym: *Blastomyces brasiliensis* Conant and Howell, 1941.)

Occurrence

Humans: Although most common in Brazil, especially in the state of Sao Paulo, the disease has been reported in all of South America except Chile, Nicaragua, and the areas of French Guiana, Guyana, Belize, the Caribbean islands and Suriname. It is also in Central America and Mexico. Recent observations show that primary infections are almost always pulmonary. The organism may be introduced into humans by the use of twigs or vegetation for cleaning of the teeth.

Animals: The fungus was isolated from the intestines of bats and from armadillos.

Soil: Reportedly isolated from soils of endemic areas in South and Central America, and cultured in the laboratories on moist soil, dust, dung, coffee leaves, and vegetation from woods.

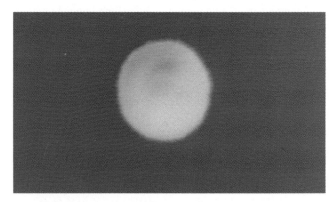

Figure 171. *Paracoccidioides brasiliensis*, colony 24°C

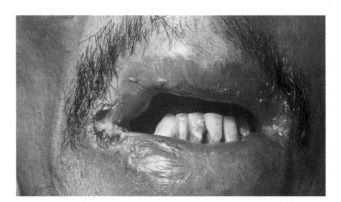

Figure 170. *Paracoccidioidomycosis, mouth*

Laboratory Procedures

Specimen collection: Material from biopsy of lesions, pus from lesions, sputum, or other body fluids would be the most likely material for laboratory diagnosis. Lymph nodes are a good source of the organism.

Direct examination: Pus, sputum, or other types of specimens should be placed on a slide with a coverglass for examination microscopically for multiple budding cells. If opaque material is present, 10% KOH or Calcafluor white should be put on a slide with the pus or sputum.

Microscopically, *P. brasiliensis* appears as single and multiple budding, thick-walled cells 10 to 60 μm in size, with double refractile walls. The presence of multiple buds with narrow-necks, is diagnostic (Figure 172b).

Culture: The infected material should be cultured for the mycelial form on Sabouraud glucose agar or preferably yeast extract agar (Restrepo and Correa, 1973) with antibacterial antibiotics and cycloheximide at 25° to 30°C. The colonies develop slowly with a white to light tan color and varied surface textures from glabrous and wrinkled to velvety to floccose on the surface (Figure 171).

At 37°C, up to three weeks are required for primary isolates to appear on sealed blood agar media. Smooth to cerebriform, waxy, cream to tan, yeastlike colonies develop on the surface. Mycelial cultures that are thought to be *P. brasiliensis* should be transferred to an enriched medium, such as brain-heart infusion agar or blood-glucose-cysteine agar, and incubated at 37°C, keeping the surface of the medium moist. Transformation to the tissue form will confirm identification (Figure 172a).

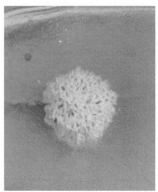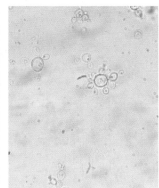

Figure 172. *Paracoccidioides brasiliensis*
a. *Colony 37°C*   b. *Multiple budding yeast cells 37°C X800*

Microscopically, slide mounts from colonies grown at 37°C show single and multiple budding cells similar to the tissue form. The multiple budding cells, 6 to 30 μm in diameter, have buds 1 to 5 μm in diameter with narrow base to mother cell.

At room temperature, the fungus grows slowly on Sabouraud glucose agar with poor sporulation on this medium. The use of water agar or yeast extract agar on a slide culture will produce racquet hyphae and arthroconidia. Recently isolated cultures from clinical material may produce pyriform to oval conidia on the sides of the hyphae.

Histopathologic studies: Stained slides may have either granulomatous or suppurative tissue reactions similar to those seen in North American blastomycosis. The budding cells may be in the giant cells in the abscesses or scattered in the granulomatous tissue. The budding cell is around 12 to 20 μm with buds varying from 2 to 5 μm in diameter. Some cells may not be in the multiple budding stage or may not have any buds present. Multiple peripheral budding with narrow base to mother cell must be present for specific diagnosis (Figure 173). Satisfactory stains are PAS, Gridley, and Gomori methenamine-silver stains.

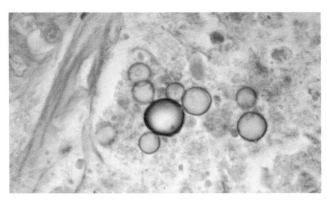

Figure 173. *Paracoccidioides brasiliensis,*
yeast cells in tissue X1200

Animal inoculation: It is usually not necessary to inoculate animals for the identification of clinical materials. The disease may be produced by inoculating infected material or a saline suspension of the yeast form intratesticularly into the guinea pig. After two to three weeks orchitis develops and draining sinuses should appear. Pus should be removed for examination on slide mounts. Some strains may produce granulomas or nodular bodies in the mesentery area of mice after about four to six weeks by intraperitoneal injection of a saline suspension of the organism. The granules may be smashed into thin pieces, or frozen sections may be made and placed on a slide containing lactophenol or other mounting media. Observations are made with a coverglass under the microscope for characteristic budding structures. The frozen sections should be stained.

Try reisolating the fungus in culture from the infected animal. This will fulfill Koch's postulates.

Serology: Complement fixation (CF) and immunodiffusion (ID) tests are useful in the diagnosis of paracoccidioidomycosis as well as in following the course of the disease through chemotherapy. By using both tests for serodiagnosis of this disease, over 95% accuracy can be obtained. The CF test detects antibodies in 80 to 96% of the cases, but is technically difficult to do without experience. Titers of 1:8 or greater are considered presumptive evidence of the disease. A decline in titer usually indicates effective therapy, while a clinical relapse is associated with an increase in humoral antibodies. A fluctuating high titer indicates a poor prognosis (Kaufman and Reiss, 1992)

The ID test is around 80 to 95% accurate. The sera of patients may contain one to three precipitins to *P. brasiliensis*. The ID test is very useful for the diagnosis of progressive pulmonary and disseminated paracoccidioidomycosis (Kaufman and Reiss, 1986). Band 1 is located near the antigen well and is usually found in up to 98%

of seroactive cases and is considered to be sensitive and a specific means of serodiagnosis (Restrepo and Moncada, 1974). Bands 2 and 3 nearer the serum well are usually present.

Delayed hypersensitivity reactions in skin tests have been used in South America (Lacaz, 1956) to evaluate the immune state of the patient. Skin test reactivity plus a negative immunodiffusion test indicates a subclinical or mild, self-limiting infection. A dilution of 1:100 for the skin test antigen, paracoccidioidin, is considered specific (Mackinnon, 1970). The antigen developed by Restrepo and Moncada (1970) is very specific, with rare cross-reactions with cases of histoplasmosis. Surveys using the skin test by Greer et al (1971) and Restrepo and Espinal (1968) have shown that the disease is widespread, most cases being self-limiting.

DNA probe. The first species-specific probe to *P. brasiliensis* was produced by Jigueroa, et al, 1990. Commercially produced kits may become available in the near future.

LOBOMYCOSIS

(Keloidal blastomycosis, Lobo's disease)

This disease is discussed in the section on Subcutaneous Mycoses, page 113.

Selected References (paracoccidioidomycosis)

Benard GF, et al. 1990. Paracoccidioidomycosis in a patient with HIV infection: immunological study. Trans. Royal Soc. Trop. Med. and Hygiene 84(1):151

Blumer SO, Jalbert M, and Kaufman L. 1984. Raid and reliable method for production of a specific *Paracoccidioides brasiliensis* immunodiffusion test antigen. J. Clin. Microbiol. 19:404

Brummer E. et al. 1988. Production of *Paracoccidioides brasiliensis*: the influence of *in vitro* passage and storage. Mycopathologia 109:13

Camargo ZP de, et al. 1988. Production of *Paracoccidioides brasiliensis* exoantigens for immunodiffusion tests. J. Clin. Microbiol. 26:2147

Cano LE, and Restrepo A. 1987. Predictive value of serologic tests in the diagnosis and follow-up of patients with paracoccidioidomycosis. Rev. Inst. Med. Trop. Sao Paulo 29:276

Conant NF, Howell A Jr. 1942. The similarity of the fungi causing South American blastomycosis (paracoccidioidal granuloma) and North American blastomycosis (Gilchrist's disease). J. Invest. Dermatol. 5:353

Ferreira MS, et al. 1990. Isolation and characterization of a *Paracoccidioides brasiliensis* strain from a dog food probably contaminated with soil in Uberlandia, Brazil. J. Vet. Med. Mycol. 28:253

Figueroa JI, et al. 1990. Preparation of species-specific murine monoclonal antibodies against the yeast phase of *Paracoccidioides brasiliensis*. J. Clin. Microbiol. 28(8):1766

Furtado JS, DeBrito T, Freymuller E. 1967. The structure and reproduction of *Paracoccidioides brasiliensis* in human tissue. Sabouraudia 5:226

Greer DL, D'Costa de Estrade D. 1971. Dermal reactions to paracoccidioidin among family members of patients with paracoccidioidomycosis. Panamerican Health Organization Sci. Publ. 254, Washington, DC.

Greer DL, Restrepo MA. 1977. La epidemiologia de la paracoccidioidomycosis. Bull. Oficina Sanitaria Panam. 82:428

Grose E, Tamsitt FR. 1965. *Paracoccidioides brasiliensis* recovered from the intestinal tract of three bats (*Artibeus Ilituratus*) in Columbia, S. A. Sabouraudia 4:124

Johnson WD, Lang CM. 1977. Paracoccidioidomycosis (South American blastomycosis) in a squirrel monkey (*Saimiri sciureus*). Vet. Pathol. 14:368

Kaufman L, and Reiss E. 1992. Serodiagnosis of fungal diseases. Chapter 78 pp. 506-528. *In* N. R. Rose, H. Friedman, and J. L. Fahey (ed.). *Manual of clinical laboratory immunology*. 4th ed. American Society for Microbiology, Washington, D. C.

Lacaz CS. 1956. South American blastomycosis. Ann. Fac. Med. Univ. Sao Paulo 29:1

Negroni P. 1966. El *Paracoccidioides brasiliensis* vive saprofiticamente en el suelo argentino. Prensa med. argent. 53:2381

Restrepo MA, Correa I. 1973. Comparison of two culture media for primary isolation of *Paracoccidioides brasiliensis* from sputum. Sabouraudia 10:260

Restrepo MA, and Moncada LH. 1974. Characterization of the precipitin bands detected in the immunodiffusion test for paracoccidioidomycosis. Appl. Microbiol. 28:138.

Restrepo A, Restrepo M, de Restrepo F, et al. 1978. Immune responses in paracoccidioidomycosis. A controlled study of 16 patients before and after treatment. Sabouraudia 16:151

San-Blas G, San-Blas F. 1977. *Paracoccidioides brasiliensis*. Cell wall structure and virulence. A review. Mycopathologia 62:77

Salfelder KJ, Schwarz J, Johnson CE. 1968. Experimental cutaneous South American blastomycosis in hamsters. Arch. Dermatol. 97:69

COCCIDIOIDOMYCOSIS

(Coccidioidal granuloma, Valley fever, San Joaquin fever)

Definition

Coccidioidomycosis occurs as a primary infection, which is an acute self-limiting respiratory or rarely a cutaneous disease, and as a chronic infection, known as progressive coccidioidomycosis (coccidioidal granuloma), a pulmonary condition or as a systemic disease, which may be fatal, involving the cutaneous tissues, subcutaneous tissues, pulmonary, visceral organs, and bony tissue and meninges (Figures 174, 175). The disease is usually acquired through inhalation of spores.

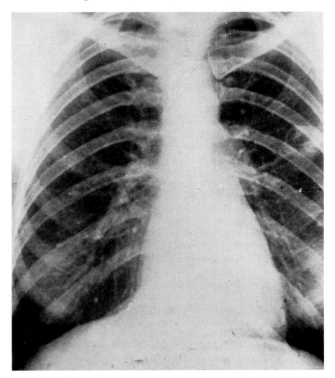

Figure 174. Pulmonary coccidioidomycosis X-ray showing eggshell cavity

Etiologic Agent

Coccidioides immitis Rixford and Gilchrist, 1896.

Occurrence

The fungus has been isolated from soil and air in endemic areas on numerous occasions.

Humans: Coccidioidomycosis is endemic to the arid southwestern United States. Other areas where the disease has been reported are northern Mexico, Honduras, Guatemala, Venezuela, Bolivia, Columbia, Paraguay, and Argentina. Thus the disease is a new world disease.

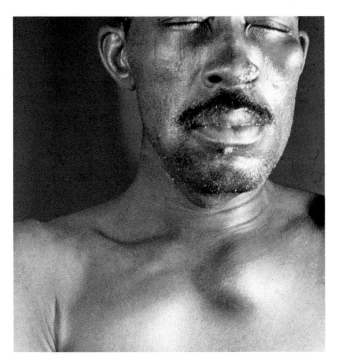

Figure 175. Coccidioidomycosis *Coccidioides immitis*

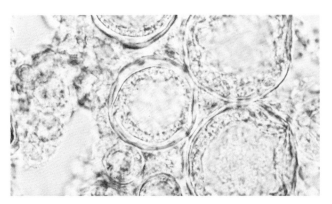

Figure 176. Coccidioidomycosis,
Young spherules X1200

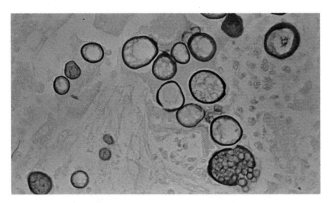

Figure 177. Coccidioidomycosis,
Spherules in lymph node X600

Animals: A number of cases have been reported in cattle, while occasional cases have occurred in dogs, sheep, horses, swine, primates, and various wild animals including the cottontail rabbit, Townsend mole, European rabbit, mountain gorilla, American monkey, and desert rodents.

Laboratory Procedures

Specimen collection: Sputum, gastric contents, spinal fluid, pus from subcutaneous abscesses, or exudates from cutaneous lesions or tissue biopsy should be collected in sterile containers for laboratory examination.

Direct examination: Sputum, gastric contents, spinal fluid exudate, or pus should be examined directly as a wet mount on a slide with a coverglass. The addition of 10% KOH is desirable if some of the material needs clearing. If a wet mount without KOH is sealed with petrolatum and allowed to remain for three to eight hours, the spherules with endospores will develop hyphae. Due to the hazards involved in handling of cultures of *C. immitis,* the clinical laboratory must have a biosafety level of 3 for culture studies.

Microscopically, round, double refractile, thick-walled spherules 20 to 80 µm in diameter with many small endospores 2 to 5 µm in diameter, should be found in the infected material. The spherules are much smaller that the large sporangia (up to 300 µm in diameter) of *Rhinosporidium seeberi.* Immature spherules of *C. immitis* are smaller and may have a central vacuole (Figures 176 and 177). In experimentally infected mice the spherule may reach 200 µm.

Culture: Infected material should be isolated at room temperature or 37°C and cultivated in a well-stoppered bottle or test tube slant containing Sabouraud glucose agar, or blood agar with or without chloramphenicol and cycloheximide. For better sporulation a modified cornmeal or a glucose-yeast extract agar or yeast extract phosphate medium is useful. Due to the hazards of handling the cultures, a laminar flow hood should be used for subcultures of the fungus. Cultures may be killed by covering the colonies in the tubes or bottles with 1.0% formaldehyde, or with lactophenol.

Colonies: The colony develops moderately fast in three to five days as a moist, membranous gray to steel-gray culture, and later develops abundant aerial mycelium, white in color. Older colonies of some strains become browner in color (Figure 178). Because of the infectious hazard from arthroconidia, it is better not to use Petri dishes for culture of *C. immitis.* Some surface areas become glabrous as the aerial mycelium becomes flattened. The diagnostic arthrospores develop in about 10 to 14 days. Some strains have extensive variation in the color, texture, and morphology of the colonies (Figure 179).

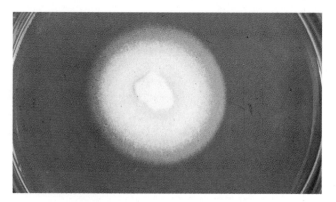

Figure 178. *Coccidioides immitis,* Colony

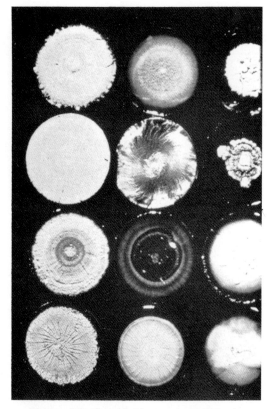

Figure 179. Coccidioidomycosis. Variation in
morphology, texture, and color in isolants of *Coccidioides immitis.*
(From Huppert, M., S. H. Sun, et al. Copyright 1967. Natural variability
in *Coccidioides immitis.*
In *Coccidioidomycosis.* Proceedings of Second Coccidioidomycosis
Symposium. Ajello, L. (ed.) Tucson, University of Arizona Press, p.
323, by permission)

Microscopically, slide mounts with lactophenol and cotton
blue, prepared from cultures containing saline or from
killed cultures, should show branching septate hyphae and
chains of thick-walled, barrel-shaped arthroconidia separated by clear spaces, the remnants of empty cells. Older culture mounts show numerous free arthroconidia that are in

the highly infectious stage (Figure 180). The arthroconidia
are 2.5 to 4 by 3 to 6 μm in size.

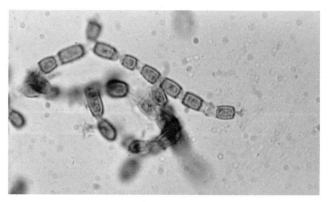

Figure 180. *Coccidioides immitis,* Arthroconidia X800

The spherules can be produced in the laboratory using
Converse liquid medium (Sun et al 1976) inoculated with
a large number of arthroconidia, and incubated at 37-40°C
with a mixture of 10% CO_2 to 90% air. To differentiate
other similar fungi Sun, et al (1976) used Brosbe's modified
Converse liquid medium with agar on a slide culture to
convert arthroconidia into spherules in 3 to 5 days to distinguish *C. immitis* from other similar fungi. This type of
slide culture must be done in a safety hood (Biosafety hood
level of 3).

NOTE: Special precaution should be exercised in transfer
of cultures that contain the highly infectious arthroconidia.
Transfers should be done only in a safety hood. A saline
solution poured into and flooding the surface of the tube
near a flame under the hood should help prevent contamination of the laboratory worker. A syringe may be used to
insert the saline without removing the cotton plug. The
arthroconidia are killed readily in four minutes at 60°C
(Roessler, et al, 1946), or by injecting lactophenol into the
test tube.

Histopathology: The lesions in coccidioidomycosis resemble those of several other infections, especially the tubercu-
lous lesions. If stained slides from a biopsy specimen are
made or are available for class study, look for the typical
spherules with or without endospores, the giant cells, and
the granulomatous or suppurative reaction.

The H and E stain may be adequate; however, special fungus
stains such as periodic acid-Schiff, Gomori methenamine-silver, or Gridley stain show more contrast.

Animal inoculation: Saline suspensions of viable arthroconidia from a virulent strain in cultures or from clinical

materials may be injected intraperitoneally or into the scrotum of the mouse. After seven to ten days the mice should be sacrificed and the peritoneum, liver, lungs, or spleen examined for lesions or nodules that contain the spherules. By smashing a piece of the nodule or lesion exudate on a slide containing lactophenol and adding a coverglass, the spherules should be visible if the mount is sufficiently thin. Look for different stages in spherule formation, including small young spherules, larger ones with vacuole formation, and mature ones with endospores. Other animals readily infected are rats, guinea pigs, dogs, and monkeys.

Stained sections of the infected material from the laboratory animal may be made for pathologic studies. Try isolating the fungus from the infected animal.

Laboratory animals are useful for immunologic studies related to possible vaccine production that would be suitable for active immunization against this disease.

Serology: Much of the information concerning the serology of the disease has been reported by Smith, et al (1948, 1950, and 1956), and later by Huppert, et al (1968), Levine, et al (1973), Pappagianis, et al (1967), and Kaufman (1976). An excellent coverage of serodiagnosis of fungal diseases has been published recently by Kaufman and Reiss (1992). The tube precipitin (TP) test, and the complement-fixation (CF) test are valuable for determining the diagnosis and prognosis of coccidioidomycosis. The latex particle agglutination (LPA) test, and the immunodiffusion (ID) test are also useful diagnostic techniques. The coccidioidin skin test is of limited diagnostic value but is of considerable value in epidemiologic studies.

1. Coccidioidin for skin tests. Coccidioidin is a filtrate from the liquid culture of the organism used for skin tests (commercially available). Positive reaction in 24 to 36 hours to coccidioidin indicates past infection or present infection. Up to one month may be required before a positive reaction occurs after exposure to the spores, or two to three days after the symptoms appear. Normally the ability to show a positive reaction lasts for years except in the final stages of a disseminated case. Three to five percent of chronic cavitary cases have produced negative skin tests, but this does not indicate poor prognosis. False positives may occur from cross reactions with histoplasmosis. Coccidioidin skin tests do not elicit a homologous humoral antibody response, as do histoplasmin skin tests (Wallraff et al, 1967).

2. Tube precipitin (TP) test. This test is useful to detect infection before the rise in the CF titer can be detected. The precipitin test can be done seven days after symptoms develop. The titer reaches a maximum in 21 days and then drops gradually. Three dilutions of coccidioidin, constant amounts of serum, and a control are used to perform tube precipitin tests for coccidioidomycosis. Precipitinogens are not affected by heat at 60°C for 30 minutes but the CF antigens are destroyed. The TP test is probably the most specific, but duration of precipitins is short, approximately six months from onset of symptoms.

3. Complement fixation (CF) test. This is one of the most useful tests for diagnosis of progressive coccidioidomycosis. Spherulin appears less sensitive than coccidioidin for the complement fixation test (Huppert et al, 1977). The CF antibodies appear later than precipitins. In primary coccidioidomycosis, the CF antibody titer is low until recovery begins, then the titer drops. In progressive types, the titer goes up rapidly and remains high until the patient improves. Generally if the patient shows progressive development of the disease, the titer remains high or rises until the patient is near death.

For the preparation of the antigen (coccidioidin) for both precipitin and complement-fixation tests, reference may be made to Kaufman and Reiss (1992).

4. Immunodiffusion (ID) test (available commercially). This test is performed using agar gels and matrices, patient's serum, coccidioidin, and positive reference anti-C. *immitis* antiserum which will produce a specific F precipitin band with homologous antigen. The antisera and antigen diffuse toward each other. If the F precipitin band is continuous or identical for the patients serum and the reference antiserum, the test is positive. Two or more lines are seen in active disease and one line in stable chronic infection. A positive test indicates the patient may have or has had coccidioidomycosis. Results of this test correlate with those of the CF test (Palmer, et al (1977).

5. Latex particle agglutination (LPA) test (available commercially). This test is performed by placing latex particles sensitized with coccidioidin in heat at 60°C for 30 minutes and adding inactivated sera (patient's and reference serum) to tubes in proper arrangements. These are rotated at 180 rpm for four minutes and observed for agglutination (Huppert et al, 1968). A positive reaction should be confirmed by TP or CF test (Chick et al, 1973). At the present time a combination of CF and TP tests (over 90% positive) or LPA and ID tests have comparable results (Kaufman, 1976). The LPA and ID tests can be used in laboratories not equipped to do the CF and TP tests.

DNA Probe. The commercially developed acridinium ester-labeled chemiluminescent DNA probe (Gen-Probe,

CI probe, San Diego, CA) is available for *C. immitis*. The sensitivity and specificity of the probe was determined by probing cultures of *C. immitis* (target) and nontarget fungi. For *C. immitis* the sensitivity and specificity are 99.2 and 100% respectively. This probe test is most useful for easy and rapid, accurate identification of this fungus from a primary culture medium. The commercial kit from the manufacturer provides the methods for sample preparation and hybridization, utilizing the fungal culture isolated from the patient. See Laboratory procedures for more information, DNA Probe (page 45).

Questions

1. Diagram the life history of *Coccidioides immitis*, including both forms.

2. In what way does *Rhinosporidium seeberi* resemble *C. immitis*? Any differences?

3. What are similarities and differences microscopically between *C. immitis* and *Geotrichum* spp.?

4. Explain the significance of changes in the precipitin and complement fixation tests during different stages in primary and progressive coccidioidomycosis.

5. What are the similarities and differences in macroscopic and microscopic characteristics in culture and in tissue for *Geotrichum* spp., *Blastomyces dermatitidis*, and *C. immitis*?

6. What are the advantages or disadvantages of serological methods, culture, and DNA probe for the determination of a fungus disease in a patient?

Selected References

Baker EE, Mrak EM, Smith CE. 1943. The morphology, taxonomy and distribution of *Coccidioides immitis*. Rixford and Gilchrist, Farlowia 1:199

Beaman L, Pappagianis D, Benjamin E. 1977. Significance of T cells in resistance to experimental murine coccidioidomycosis. Infect. Immunol. 17:580

Bennett HD, Milder JW, Baker LA. 1954. Coccidioidomycosis, possible fomite transmission. J. Lab. Clin. Med. 43:633

Breslau AM, Kubota MY. 1964. Continuous in vitro cultivation of spherules of *Coccidioides immitis*. J. Bacteriol. 87:468

Campins H. 1950. Coccidioidomycosis: Un nuevo problema de salud publica en Venezuela. Rev. San Caracas 15:1

Carmichael JW, Kendrick WB. 1980. Genera of Hyphomycetes. Edmonton, Canada, University of Alberta Press

Chick EW, Baum GL, Furcolow ML, et al. 1973. The use of skin tests and serologic tests in histoplasmosis, coccidioidomycosis, and blastomycosis. Am. Rev. Respir. Dis. 180:156

Clemons KV, Leathers CR. and Lee KW. 1985. Systemic *Coccidioides immitis* infection in nude and beige mice. Infect. Immun. 47:814

Emmons CW. 1942. Isolation of *Coccidioides* from soil and rodents. Public Health Rep. 57:109

Emmons CW. 1967. Fungi which resemble *Coccidioides immitis*. *In* Coccidioidomycosis. Edited by L. Ajello. Proceedings of Second Coccidioidomycosis Symposium. University of Arizona Press, Tucson. pp. 333

Florek KK, and Rogers AL. 1978. Viability of lactophenol exposed endospores and spherules of *Coccidioides immitis*. Abstr Ann. Meet. Amer. Soc. Microbiology, Las Vegas, NV

Galgiani JN, Ampel NM. 1990. Coccidioidomycosis in human immunodeficiency virus-infected patients. J. Inf. Dis. 162:1165

Galgiani JN, Grace GM, and Lundergan LL. 1991. New serologic tests for early detection of coccidioidomycosis. J. Infect. Dis. 163:671

Huppert M, Peterson ET, Sun SH, et al. 1968. Evaluation of a latex particle agglutination test for coccidioidomycosis. Am. J. Clin. Pathol. 49:96

Huppert M, Sun SH, Rice EH. 1978. Specificity of exoantigens for identifying cultures of *Coccidioides immitis*. J. Clin. Microbiol. 8:346

Johnson JE, Perry JE, Fekety FR, et al. 1964. Laboratory acquired coccidioidomycosis. A report of 210 cases. Ann. Intern. Med. 60:941

Johnson JE, Jeffery B, Huppert M. 1984. Evaluation of five commercially available immunodiffusion kits for detection of *Coccidioides immitis* and *Histoplasma capsulatum* antibodies. J. Clin. Microbiol. 20(3):530

Kaufman L, Reiss E. 1992. Serodiagnosis of fungal diseases. *In* Rose NR, Friedman H (eds). Manual of Clinical Immunology. Am. Soc. Microbiol., Washington, DC, Ch 78

Maddy KT. 1954. Coccidioidomycosis of cattle in the southwestern United States. J. Am. Vet. Med. Assoc. 124:456

Negroni P, Negroni R. 1963. Estudios sobre el *Coccidioides immitis*. XV. Su ecologia en la Argentina. Bol. Acad. Na. Med. [Rio de Janeiro] 41:493

Pappagianis D, and Zimmer BL. 1990. Serology of coccidioidomycosis. Clin. Microbiol. Rev. 3:247

Rixford E, Gilchrist TC. 1896. Two cases of protozoan (coccidioidal) infection of the skin and other organs. Bull. Johns Hopkins Hosp. 1:209

Rutala PJ, Smith JW. 1978. Coccidioidomycosis in potentially compromised hosts: The effect of immunosuppressive therapy in dissemination. Am. J. Med. Sci. 275:283

Sinski JT, Smith FX, Lowe EP. 1968. Survival of dry *Coccidioides immitis* at 4 C for five years. Mycologia 60:444

Smith CE, Saito MI, Simons SA. 1956. Pattern of 39,500 serological tests in coccidioidomycosis. JAMA 160:546

Swatek FE. 1970. Ecology of *Coccidioides immitis*. Mycopathologia 40:3

Stockman L, Clark KA, Hunt JM, Roberts GD. 1993. Evaluation of commercially available acridinium ester-labeled chemiluminescent DNA probes for culture identification of *Blastomyces dermatitidis*, *Coccidioides immitis*, *Cryptococcus neoformans*, and *Histoplasma capsulatum*. J. Clin. Microbiol. 311:845

Sarosi G, et al. 1988. Clinical usefulness of skin testing in histoplasmosis, coccidioidomycosis, and blastomycosis. Am. Rev. Respir. Dis. 138:1081

Sun SH, Huppert M, Vukovich KR. 1976. Rapid in vitro conversion and identification of *Coccidioides immitis*. J. Clin. Microbiol. 3:186

HISTOPLASMOSIS

(Darling's disease, reticuloendotheliosis)

Definition

Histoplasmosis, a disease involving primarily the reticuloendothelial system, probably results in widespread dissemination even in mild or inapparent cases. The skin and almost every tissue or organ in the body may be involved. The infection is initiated after inhalation of the fungus spores. About 95% of infections are inapparent, subclinical, or benign. These primary forms may be diagnosed by x-ray detection of areas of pulmonary calcification or by a positive histoplasmin skin test. The remaining 5% become either a chronic progressive lung infection, a chronic cutaneous or systemic disease, or a rapidly fatal systemic infection (Figure 181, and Figure 182). The progressive forms of histoplasmosis may cause emaciation, leukopenia, anemia, and ulceration in the nasal region, intestines, and lungs. The liver, spleen, and lymph nodes usually enlarge. In endemic areas a high percentage of AIDS patients are becoming infected or reinfected with *Histoplasma capsulatum*.

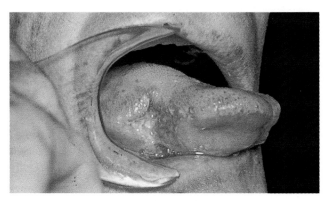

Figure 181. Histoplasmosis, *Histoplasma capsulatum,* tongue

Etiologic Agent

Histoplasma capsulatum Darling, 1906. Perfect (teleomorph) state: *Ajellomyces capsulatus* (Kwong-Chung) McGinnis et Katz, 1979 (Synonym: *Emmonsiella capsulata* Kwon-Chung, 1973). There are three varieties: *H. capsulatum* var. *capsulatum*, *H. capsulatum* var. *duboisii*, and *H., capsulatum* var. *farciminosum*.

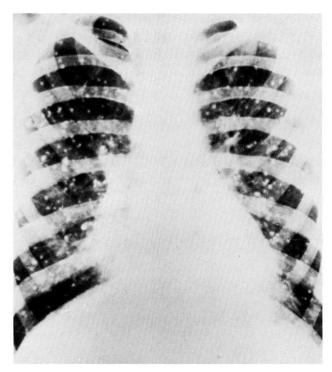

Figure 182. Pulmonary histoplasmosis, *Histoplasma capsulatum,* X-ray film

Occurrence

Histoplasmosis, especially in the primary or benign form, is known to be very common. Skin tests show that up to 90% of the population in the Mississippi Valley are or have been infected. Based on skin tests in 48 states in the

United States approximately 40 million people have been infected. The chronic forms of the disease require antimycotic therapy.

The organism has been isolated from soils, especially around chicken houses, bat guano, and areas used by starlings and occasionally pigeons. The spores are inhaled during the saprophytic stage in the soil by humans and animals for the usual route of infection.

Humans: The disease is somewhat restricted to the central Mississippi Valley, the Ohio Valley, and along the Appalachian Mountains in the United States. It has been reported in over 60 countries throughout the world in temperate and tropical climates. An African form, *H. capsulatum* var. *duboisii* is found in subcutaneous lesions and cranial bones (more information on page 144). *H. capsulatum* var *capsulatum* is also found in Africa.

Animals: The fungus has been isolated from dogs, cats, rats, mice, raccoons, opossums, skunks, foxes, and woodchucks in the United States. Histoplasmosis has also been found in cows, horses, bats, and African monkeys and baboons. Positive histoplasmin tests have been reported in cattle, horses, sheep, swine, and chickens. Epizootic lymphangitis of horses and mules is endemic in Asia, Europe, and Africa, caused by *H. capsulatum* var. *farcinimosum*.

Laboratory Procedures

Specimen collection: Specimens from peripheral blood, bone marrow, lymph nodes, sputum, bronchial wash, urine, biopsy, or cutaneous or mucosal lesions should be smeared for staining and for placing directly on agar media.

Sputum should be collected in all cases in sterile containers. One ml or more taken early in the morning after the patient has rinsed out his mouth and then placed in a 0.2-mg/ml chloramphenicol solution. This should be repeated to determine if a diagnosis of pulmonary histoplasmosis can be established. Gastric lavage should be done early in the morning before the patient is fed. The containers with the material should be refrigerated temporarily or cultured immediately.

Spinal fluid is taken only if meningeal or cerebral areas are involved and is spun down to obtain the sediment for use in culture studies.

Direct examination: KOH mounts are not useful. Peripheral blood, buffy coat and sediment from centrifuged blood, sputum, material from biopsy or stenal puncture, or bone marrow should be spread on a micro-

scope slide, fixed with methanol for ten minutes, then stained with Giemsa stain, PAS, or the Wright method. Other stains may be used, such as Gomori methenamine-silver. Overstaining will emphasize the yeast cells. These cells are found primarily in the macrophages or the monocytes or outside broken cells.

Microscopically, under immersion oil, the fungus should appear as small, round or oval, yeastlike cells, 2 to 5 µm in diameter, within the phagocytic cells, mononuclear and macrophage cells, or occasionally the polymorphonuclear cells (Figure 183). Look for these structures in the freshly prepared slides or in the demonstrations for class study. At times, cells of *Histoplasma* are found free in the tissue (Figure 184). Giemsa stain shows the cell wall as light blue, with a clear space between the wall and the dark-blue protoplasm. Dark oval to crescent-shaped chromatin material appears in the protoplasm. The wall is violet-red to pink with pale colored protoplasm filling the cell if PAS stain is used. Buds are usually detached from the parent cell during staining. When present, they occur at the small end of the mother cell.

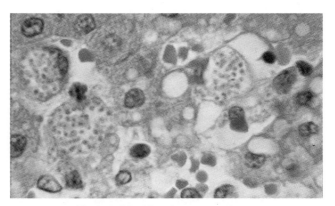

Figure 183. *Histoplasma capsulatum,* Liver, mononuclear cells, hematoxylin-eosin X1000

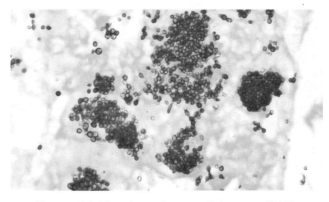

Figure 184. Histoplasmosis, extracellular yeasts X1000

Culture: Infected material such as sputum, pus, bone marrow, centrifuged gastric washings, or lysis-centrifugation to concentrate blood for inoculating immediately on several media: brain-heart infusion agar with blood, yeast extract phosphate agar, or SABHI agar with or without chloramphenicol or penicillin and streptomycin, and incubated at 25° to 30°C. If the infected specimen is contaminated, yeast extract phosphate agar is the best choice. The tissue form may be isolated on glucose-cysteine-blood agar or BHI agar plus 10% blood at 37°C; however this is not as productive as incubation at 25° to 30°C for the hyphal form. Cultures should be retained for at least four weeks in taped plates or plastic bags with moisture.

At 37°C the yeast growth appears in a few days as a granular to rough, or smooth cream-colored, round, convex colony turning tan in a couple of weeks. Brain-heart infusion agar slants, BHIA plus 1% cysteine, Francis cysteine blood agar, Sabhi blood agar, and Salvin synthetic medium are satisfactory to maintain or convert the mycelial form to the yeast form. Surface moisture is an important factor in the conversion, in addition to temperature, medium, and sealed tubes (Figure 186).

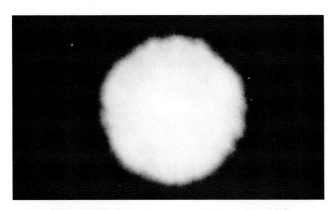

Figure 185. *Histoplasma capsulatum,* colony 24°C

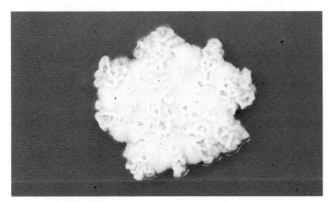

Figure 186. *Histoplasma capsulatum,* colony 37°C

At room temperature on brain-heart infusion medium or Emmons' modified Sabouraud glucose agar or other media, two types of colonies may appear from infected

material from patients or from soil. The albino type "A" consists of white, coarse aerial hyphae, while the Brown type "B" consists of flat colonies with light-tan to dark-brown color in seven days (Berliner, 1968). The white type may become buff color with age. The tan to brown colonies produce an abundance of macroconidia at first but become white upon repeated transfers, and is reversible. Both types may occur in the same patient. Potato dextrose agar or modified cornmeal agar is a good sporulation medium. (For colony appearance see Figure 185.)

Microscopically, slide mounts of the yeast form show oval or round, small (2 to 3 by 3 to 4 µm) single cells with buds at the narrow end of the parent cell (Figure 187). Slide cultures or mounts from colonies grown at 25°C should show septate hyphae with small (2 to 5 µm), smooth or spiny-walled, round or pyriform conidia borne on short lateral hyphae or sessile on the side of the hyphae. Large (8 to 14 µm), round to pyriform, tuberculate macroconidia, also known as chlamydoconidia, are also produced (diagnostic). See Figure 188. The tubercles are 1 to 8 µm in length. The "A" type produces smooth or at times tuberculate macroconidia, while the "B" type has masses of tuberculate macroconidia. The saprophytic species of the genus *Sepedonium* produces tuberculate spores somewhat like *H. capsulatum* but no microconidia. Species of three other genera may be confused with *Histoplasma capsulatum*. *Histoplasma capsulatum* usually has macroconidia and can be converted to the yeast form. The species of the other genera do not have the macroconidia and *Chrysosporium* and *Renispora* species cannot be converted to a yeast form. The use of exoantigens is an excellent test for *H. capsulatum*.

NOTE: The yeast form if an original isolate should be cultured at room temperature to verify conversion to the mycelial phase and the formation of tuberculate macroconidia (chlamydoconidia). Conversion of mycelium to yeast form aids in identification.

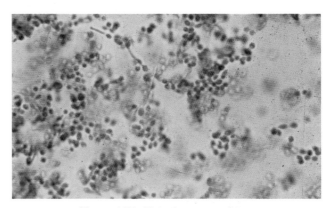

Figure 187. *Histoplasma capsulatum,* yeast cells 37°C X1200

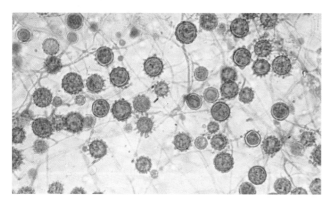

Figure 188. *Histoplasma capsulatum,* Macroconidia and microconidia 24°C X400

Perfect state (teleomorph): *Ajellomyces capsulatus* (Kwon-Chung, 1973) McGinnis et Katz, 1979. *(Synonym: Emmonsiella capsulata* Kwon-Chung, 1973), is heterothallic, producing ascocarps characteristic of the Ascomycota. The buff-colored gymnothecia are globose, later becoming irregularly star-shaped with age as the coils grow beyond the peridia. The gymnothecia differ from those in *Ajellomyces dermatitidis* by the highly branched hyphae arising from the coils, irregularly curved, and the lack of constrictions at the cross walls or the cells. The club-shaped asci contain eight globose, smooth-walled (spiny with electron microscopy), hyaline ascospores, 1.5 µm in diameter.

Histopathology: Stained sections of biopsy material should be examined, especially when the organism is not readily found in blood smears. If stained slides are available, study the pathologic changes. Sections through lesions usually show the organisms developing intracellularly in macrophages, and occasionally in giant cells, as the yeast form, 2 to 5 µm in diameter, surrounded by a "capsule" which is unstained space between the cell wall and the shrunken protoplasm of the host cell (Figure 179). H and E, Gridley, periodic acid-Schiff, or Gomori methenamine-silver nitrate stain may be used. The organisms resemble *Leishmania donovani* in size and shape but lack the central nuclear material and the blepharoplast in the stained preparations. *Toxoplasma* is smaller and is not found in histiocytes nor will it stain with fungal stains. *Torulopsis glabrata* and *Candida albicans* need to be differentiated in tissue.

Animal inoculation: Mice, guinea pigs, and dogs are susceptible to the yeast form or to spores of the filamentous phase. Mice are best to use for laboratory studies since they are the most sensitive laboratory animals for isolation of *Histoplasma* from contaminated soil and air samples or from pathologic material.

For sputum add 1 ml of a stock solution containing 7 mg of penicillin and 10 mg of streptomycin per 5 ml (or 0.1 mg of chloramphenicol for each 5 ml of sputum), before injecting intraperitoneally into mice. A pure culture of the yeast form may be used by injecting 1.0 ml or more of a suspension intraperitoneally into mice for laboratory or class study.

Sacrifice the mice at the end of three or more weeks and use the liver and spleen for smears and for culture. Hold cultures for one month before considering them negative. The intracerebral injection of mice as recommended by Howell (1947), with at least 20,000 or more yeast cells should kill the animals in seven to ten days. This may be used as a more rapid method for study of the tissue form or the organism in class. After autopsy, look for enlarged liver, spleen, and lymph nodes in the animal. Care in handling mice or other laboratory animals should be practiced at all times, as feces of mice have been shown to contain the fungus in the yeast form.

a. Prepare blood smears from these organs and stain with Giemsa or periodic acid-Schiff stain. If sections are made of the organs, use the stains mentioned under Histopathology. Look for the small, oval to round cells in the mononuclear blood cells using the oil immersion lens.

b. Try isolating the organism from the animal at 37°C and at room temperature. Soil samples that may contain spores of the organism are combined with saline in the ratio of 1 to 5, antibiotics are added, the mixture is shaken well, and after one hour 1 ml of the supernatant is inoculated intraperitoneally into mice. One month later the mice are sacrificed, and the spleen and liver are cultured on BHI or blood agar (without antibiotics) at 37°C and on BHI agar with antibiotics in sealed tubes. For further reference see Emmons (1961).

Serology: Histoplasmin skin sensitivity test has been used to indicate present or past infection and for epidemiologic studies. This test should not be done prior to taking serum for other tests. The complement fixation (CF), immunodiffusion (ID), and latex agglutination (LA) tests are aids in the clinical diagnosis of the disease and are of prognostic value.

1. Histoplasmin: This is a filtrate from a broth culture of *H. capsulatum* grown in asparagine broth (see page 39) in the same way as for *C. immitis.* The undiluted filtrate or stock may be stored in the refrigerator for a couple of years with dilutions made up with a reference standard. Positive reactions will occur in one to two months after infection.

Sensitivity in individuals continues indefinitely. A positive skin reaction in one to two-year old children indicates an active infection is likely, while in older individuals this may indicate past infection. A negative reaction to the skin test may indicate no infection or anergy and grave prognosis. The histoplasmin test has little value in diagnosis and may interfere with the CF tests for coccidioidomycosis and histoplasmosis. This antigen and the yeast form antigen may be purchased from Baxter Scientific Products, Immuno-Mycologics, M.A. Bioproducts, and Meridian Diagnostics.

2. Complement-fixation test: Since the sensitivity of the yeast form antigens is usually greater than that of histoplasmin antigen, the yeast form antigen should be used in the diagnostic laboratory and supplemented with the histoplasmin for the CF test. The CF titer develops gradually within a few weeks or months after infection. If the patient develops the disseminated form of the disease, a titer of 1:8 or greater is presumptive while titers above 1:32 are strong evidence for the disease. In the progressive form of the disease, the titer usually remains high. If a patient improves, the titer gradually falls. Terminal cases may show a rapid drop in the titer prior to death. Cross-reactions may occur in sera from patients with other fungus infections, including blastomycosis and coccidioidomycosis. This test should be performed by well-trained individuals as the CF tests are rather complex and expensive. Over 90% of cases with positive cultures may be positive with the CF test if serum samples are collected at 2 to 3 week intervals.

3. Immunodiffusion test: This test is useful in screening for or as an adjunct in the serologic diagnosis of histoplasmosis. Concentrated histoplasmin and antisera from the patient diffuse from the wells in the agar to form two significant bands of diagnostic value (Heiner, 1958). The H band close to the serum well is usually from active or progressive cases of histoplasmosis. This H band usually disappears after recovery, but may be present for up to two years. The M band, near the antigen well, indicates active or past infection, or a recent histoplasmin skin test. The M band may indicate early infection if no recent skin test has been given and if it appears before the H band. The M band can be present without an H band (for more detailed information see Kaufman and Reiss, 1992). Serum from nearly 70% of patients with proven histoplasmosis contains M precipitins while only 10% of the sera may contain both the H and M precipitins.

4. Latex agglutination test: Serum is mixed with histoplasmin-coated latex particles (available from Immuno-Mycologics). This test may be positive before the CF test and is useful when the serum is anticomplementary.

False-positives or false-reactions and cross-reactions may be ruled out if other serologic tests are run. Some individuals consider a titer of 1:16 or greater as significant while others recommend titers of 1:32 as good evidence for an active or very recent disease.

Special nutritional requirements: The yeast phase requires biotin, thiamine, thioctic acid, and sulfhydryl compounds (cysteine) in addition to glucose and inorganic salts in the basal medium for growth factors. The mycelial form utilizes inorganic ammonium as the best nitrogen source and has no other special requirements.

DNA Probe. The acridinium ester-labeled chemiluminescent DNA probe is commercially available (Gen-Probe, HC probe, San Diego, CA) for *H. capsulatum*. In a recent report on 86 target and 164 nontarget fungi tested, Stockman, et al (1993) found a sensitivity of 100% and a specificity of 100%. This probe test is very useful due to ease and rapidity of identification of this dimorphic pathogen from a primary culture medium. The commercial kits provide the methods for sample preparation and hybridization utilizing the fungal culture isolated from the patient. See Laboratory procedures (page 45) for additional information. Currently the cost is a factor for the laboratories.

AFRICAN HISTOPLASMOSIS

A different type of histoplasmosis occurs in Africa caused by a large form of the fungus. Over 127 cases have been reported as of 1983. The granulomatous tissue has giant cells with oval to round, thick-walled budding cells, 7 to 20 μm in diameter. This is primarily a cutaneous, subcutaneous, and osseous tissue infection. The thick-walled budding cells resemble those of *B. dermatitidis* in size, but each cell is uninucleate except at the time of budding, and the isthmus between mother cell and bud is usually narrow. The mycelial form is similar to *H. capsulatum* var. *capsulatum* in culture. At 37°C after conversion to the yeast form, the *H. capsulatum* var. *duboisii* yeast cells develop as small *H. capsulatum* var. *capsulatum* type yeast cells and later the large, thick-walled cells (12 to 15 μm) are produced. This organism is considered to be *Histoplasma capsulatum* var. *duboisii* (Vanbr.) Ciferri, 1960.

Histoplasmosis farciminosum (Epizootic Lymphangitis): Epizootic lymphangitis is an infection of horses and mules caused by *H. capsulatum* var *farciminosum*. The disease is widespread in Scandinavia, Russia, Europe, Africa, India and Southern Asia. The disease commonly involves subcutaneous and ulcerated lesion of the skin, the front and hind legs, neck, and areas rubbed by the harness. The budding yeast cells in tissue are 3 to 5 by 2.5 to 3.5 μm in size. The fungus is isolated and identified on similar media as the *H. capsulatum* var. *histoplasmum*. The fungus should be grown on soil extract agar, producing a slow-growing, gray-brown, dry, folded colony. At 37°C the fungus, which is more difficult in some strains to convert, develops white to brownish yeast like colony.

Questions

1.   Are there any other pathogenic fungi that attack the reticuloendothelial system?

2.   Differentiate leishmaniasis and toxoplasmosis from histoplasmosis in stained sections of tissue on slides.

3.   Compare the similarities and differences between *Histoplasma capsulatum* and *Sepedonium* spp. in culture and microscopically.

4.   What cross-reactions may occur with histoplasmin?

Selected References

Ajello L. 1971. Coccidioidomycosis and histoplasmosis: A review of their epidemiology and geographic distribution. Mycopathologia 45:221

Ajello L, Runyon LC. 1953. Infection of mice with single spores of *Histoplasma capsulatum*. J. Bacteriol. 66:34

Ankobiah, W. A., et al. 1990. Disseminated histoplasmosis in AIDS. N. Y. State J. Med. 90:234

Berliner MD. 1968. Primary subcultures of *Histoplasma capsulatum*. I. Macro and micro-morphology of the mycelial phase. Sabouraudia 6:111

Blumer S, Kaufman L. 1968. Variation in enzymatic activities among strains of *Histoplasma capsulatum* and *Histoplasma duboisii*. Sabouraudia 6:203

Campbell CC, Binkley GE. 1953. Serologic diagnosis with respect to histoplasmosis, coccidioidomycosis, and blastomycosis and the problem of cross reactions. J. Lab. Clin. Med. 42:896

Conant NF. 1941. A cultural study of the life cycle of *Histoplasma capsulatum* Darling (1906). J. Bacteriol. 41:563

Darling STA. 1906. A protozoan general infection producing pseudotubercles in the lungs and focal necroses in the liver, spleen and lymph nodes. JAMA 46: 1283

Dismakes WE, Royai SA, Tynes BS. 1978. Disseminated histoplasmosis in corticosteroid-treated patients. Report of five cases. JAMA 240: 1495

DiSalvo AF, Corbett DS. 1976. Apparent false positive

histoplasmin latex agglutination tests in patients with tuberculosis. J. Clin. Microbiol. 3:306

Duncan JT. 1958. Tropical African histoplasmosis. Trans. R. Soc. Med. Trop. 52:468

Emmons CW. 1949. Isolation of *Histoplasma capsulatum* from soil, Pub. Health Rep. 641:892

Emmons CW. 1958. Association of bats with histoplasmosis. Pub. Health Rep. 73:590

Ehrhard HB, Pine L. 1972. Factors influencing the production of H and M antigens by *Histoplasma capsulatum*: effect of physical factors and composition of medium. Appl. Microbiol. 23:250

Furcolow ML, Schubert J, Tosh FE, et al. 1962. Serologic evidence of histoplasmosis in sanatoriums in the U.S. JAMA 180:109

Gabal MA, Hassan FK, Siad AA, and Karim KA. 1983. Study of equine histoplasmosis farciminosi and characterization of *Histoplasma farciminosum*. Sabouraudia. 21:121

Garrison RG, Boyd SK. 1978. Electron microscopy of yeastlike cell development from the microconidium of *Histoplasma capsulatum*. J. Bacteriol. 133:345

Gilardi GL. 1965. Nutrition of systemic and subcutaneous pathogenic fungi. Bact. Rev. 29:406

Gonzales, Ochoa A. 1959. Histoplasmosis primaria pulmonar aguda en la republica Mexicana. Rev. Inst. Salubr. Enferm. Trop. (Mex) 19:341

Goodman NL, Sprouse RF, Larsh HW. 1968. Histoplasmin potency as affected by culture age. Sabouraudia 6:273

Grayston JT, Altman PL, Cozad CC. 1956. Experimental histoplasmosis in mice. Pub. Health Monogr. 39:99

Gugnani HC, Egere JU, Larsh H. 1991. Skin sensitivity to capsulatum and duboisii histoplasmin in Nigeria. J. Trop. Med. Hyg. 94:24

Heiner DC. 1958. Diagnosis of histoplasmosis using precipitin reactions in agar gel. Pediatrics 22:616

Howard DH. 1965. Intracellular growth of *Histoplasma capsulatum*. J. Bacteriol. 89:518

Johnson JE, Goodman NL. 1985. Variation in complement fixation test results with three Histoplasma capsulatum yeast phase antigens. J. Clin. Microbiol. 22:1066

Kaufman L, Reiss E. 1992. Serodiagnosis of fungal diseases. *In* Rose N.R., Friedman H (eds). Manual of Clinical Immunology. Am. Soc. Microbiol., Washington D.C. Ch 78

Kaufman L, Standard P. 1987. Specific and rapid identification of medically important fungi by exoantigen detection. Ann. Rev. Microbiol. 41:209

Kwon-Chung KJ. 1973. Studies on *Emmonsiella capsulata*. Heterothallism and development of the ascocarp. Mycologia 65:109

Kwon-Chung KJ. 1974. Perfect state (*Emmonsiella capsula-*

ta) of the fungus causing large-form African histoplasmosis. Mycologia 67:980

Larsh HW, Hinton A, Furcolow ML. 1953. Laboratory studies of *Histoplasma capsulatum*. III. Efficiency of the flotation method in isolation of *Histoplasma capsulatum* from soil. J. Lab. Clin. Med. 41:478

Lopez JF, Grocott RG. 1968. Demonstration of *Histoplasma capsulatum* in peripheral blood by the use of methenamine-silver nitrate stain (Grocott's). Am J. Clin. Pathol. 50:692

McGinnis MR, Katz B. 1979. *Ajellomyces* and its synonym *Emmonsiella*. Mycotoxin 8:157

McVeigh I, Morton K. 1965. Nutritional studies of *Histoplasma capsulatum*. Mycopathologia 25:294

Menges RW, Furcolow ML, Hinton A. 1954. The role of animals in the epidemiology of histoplasmosis. Am. J. Hyg. 59:113

Mok WY, Buckley HR, Campbell CC. 1977. Characterization of antigens from type A and B yeast cells of *Histoplasma capsulatum*. Infect. Immunol. 16:461

Murray JF, Howard DH. 1964. Laboratory acquired histoplasmosis. Am. Rev. Respir. Dis. 89:631

Nethercott JR, et al. 1978. Histoplasmosis due to *Histoplasma capsulatum* var *duboisii* in a Canadian immigrant. Arch. Dermatol. 114:595

Nightingale SD, et al. 1990. Disseminated histoplasmosis in patients with AIDS. South. Med. J. 83(6):624

Peeters P, et al. 1987. Disseminated African histoplasmosis in a white heterosexual male patient with the acquired immunodeficiency syndrome. Mykosen 30:449

Pine L. 1970. Growth of *Histoplasma capsulatum*. VI. Maintenance of the mycelial phase. Appl. Microbiol. 19:413

Pine L. 1977. *Histoplasma* antigens: Their production, purification and uses. Contrib. Microbiol. Immunol. 3:138

Rowley DA, Huber M. 1955. Pathogenesis of experimental histoplasmosis in mice. I. Measurement of infecting dosages of the yeast phases of *Histoplasma capsulatum*. J. Infect. Dis. 96:174

Salvin SB. 1949. Cysteine and related compounds in the growth of the yeastlike phase of *Histoplasma capsulatum*. J. Infect. Dis. 84:275

Smith CD, Furcolow ML. 1964. Efficiency of three techniques for isolation *Histoplasma capsulatum* from soil, including a new flotation method. J. Lab. Clin. Med. 64:342

Spitzer ED, et al. 1990. Temperature-sensitive variants of *Histoplasma capsulatum* isolated from patients with acquired immunodeficiency syndrome. J. Infect. Dis. 162:258

Stockman L, Clark KA, Hung JM, Roberts GD. 1993. Evaluation of commercially available acridinium ester-labeled *Blastomyces dermatitidis*, *Coccidioides immitis*, *Cryptococcus neoformans* and *Histoplasma capsulatum*. J. Clin. Microbiol. 311(4):845

Strauss RE, Kiigman AM. 1951. The use of gastric mucin to lower resistance of laboratory animals to systemic fungus infections. J. Infect. Dis. 88: 151

Vanbreuseghem R. 1964. L'histopiasmose africaine ou histoplasmose causee par *Histoplasma duboisii* Vanbreuseghem 1952. Bull. Acad. Roy. Med. Beig., 7th Ser. 4:543

Weeks RJ, Padhye AA, and Ajello L. 1985. *Histoplasma capsulatum* variety *farciminosum*: a new combination for *Histoplasma farciminosum*. Mycologia 77:964

Wheat LJ, Kohler RB, Tewari RP. 1986. Diagnosis of disseminated histoplasmosis by detection of *Histoplasma capsulatum* antigen in serum and urine specimens. N. Engl. J. Med. 314:82

Wheat LJ, et al. 1983. Immunoglobulin M and G histoplasma antibody response in histoplasmosis. Am. Rev. Respir. Dis. 128:65

Chapter 8

OPPORTUNISTIC INFECTIONS—YEASTS

YEASTS OF MEDICAL IMPORTANCE

The number of yeast infections in humans reported in the literature has greatly increased in recent times. Yeasts most commonly isolated from human sources are *Candida albicans*, other species of *Candida*, and *Cryptococcus neoformans; Torulopsis glabrata, Geotrichum candidum*, and *Trichosporon* spp. as well as other yeasts or yeastlike fungi may be implicated at times. This significant increase is mainly due to clinical alteration of the patient's defenses as in AIDS patients, the use of corticosteroids and immuno-suppressive agents, anticancer agents, or broad-spectrum antibacterial agents, by long-term intravenous therapy or inadequate catheter care and by some alteration of the host's physiology. In these situations almost all yeasts are potential pathogens by some alteration of the host's physiology.

Yeast infections are among the most common fungus infections in humans. Their form ranges from localized cutaneous or mucocutaneous lesions to fungemia or disseminated systemic mycoses.

Yeasts are ubiquitous organisms. They are found in almost all types of organic substrates. *Candida albicans*, the most frequent yeast pathogen, is a normal colonizer of the gastrointestinal tract (20% to 40%) and the female urogenital area. Due to the frequent association of yeasts with both our internal and external environments, their incidence in clinical specimens and as pathogenic agents is relatively high.

Yeasts isolated routinely from sputum, vaginal discharge, urine, and fecal specimens are significant for *Candida* species if buds and pseudohyphae are present to indicate a pathogenic condition. In urine, the isolation of more than 10,000 cells in 1 ml is significant for identification. The presence of *C. neoformans* in urine is significant.

Yeasts under normal environmental conditions are mostly spherical to oval, 2.5 to 6 µm in diameter, unicellular, budding, or fission organisms. They produce glabrous, moist, creamy, mucoid, or membranous colonies. Under reduced oxygen, in an increased CO_2 atmosphere or in tissues, many yeasts may produce hyphae and/or pseudohyphae. The pseudohyphae result from elongation of blastoconidia that remain in chains.

Yeasts are separated into three groups according to the method of sexual reproduction: (1) Blastomycetes (Deuteromycota or Fungi Imperfecti), with no usual sexual reproduction in laboratory cultures, and illustrated by the majority of species of *Candida*, and *Torulopsis*, (2) Hemiascomycetes (Ascomycota) which produce ascospores as a result of sexual reproduction and are exemplified by the genera *Saccharomyces, Pichia*, and *Hansenula* and (3) Heterobasidiomycetes (Blastomycota) with formation of basidiospores as a result of sexual reproduction and illustrated by the genera *Filobasidiella*, and *Leucosporidium*.

Identification of medically important yeasts is based on both morphologic and physiologic characteristics. The morphologic characteristics may include such structures as: capsules, germ tubes, chlamydoconidia, arthroconidia, blastoconidia, pseudohyphae, hyphae, ascospores, and basidiospores. The physiologic characteristics may include: assimilation and fermentation of carbohydrates, production of urease, assimilation of nitrate, caffeic acid reaction, temperature tolerance, and cycloheximide resistance. On the following page there is a flow chart (Table 14) using these characteristics as a basis for separation of some of the medically important yeasts. Reference should be made to J. Lodder, *The Yeasts, A Taxonomic Study* (North Holland Publishing Co., Amsterdam, 1970) for more information on yeasts.

Table 14. Flow Diagram, Yeasts

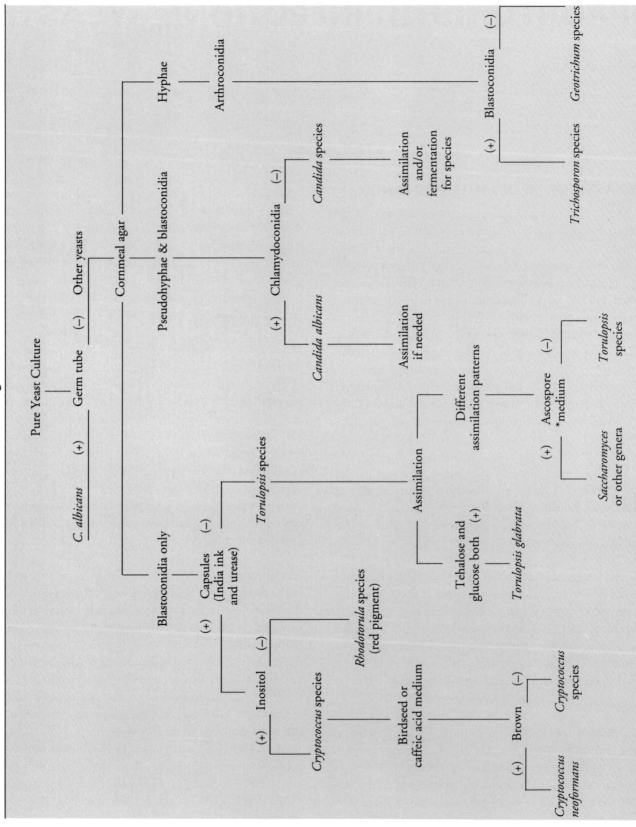

*Ascospores will not, at times, develop on ascospore or other media under routine laboratory conditions.

CANDIDIASIS

(Candidosis Moniliasis, thrush, mycotic vulvovaginitis, *Candida* paronychia, *Candida* endocarditis)

Definition

Candidiasis is a disease with varied manifestations. The acute or chronic infection may show lesions in the mouth (Figure 189), pharynx, vagina (Figure 191), skin, nails (Figure 190), bronchopulmonary system, intestines, or perianal area (Figure 192), and occasionally may manifest as endocarditis, meningitis, fungemia, or infections of other organs,

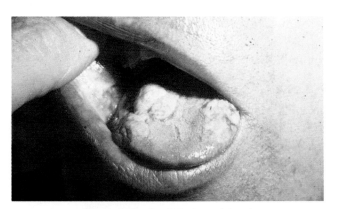

Figure 189. Candidiasis, oral thrush

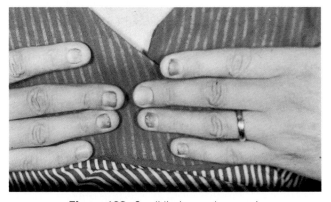

Figure 190. Candidiasis, onychomycosis

Etiologic Agents

Candida albicans (Robin) Berkhout, 1923, is usually the pathogenic species in the genus. Some synonyms are: *Oidium albicans* Robin, 1853; *Monilia albicans* Zopf, 1890; and *Endomyces albicans,* Vuillemin, 1898; *Candida stellatoidea* Jones et Martin, l938.

A part of the normal human flora and may become an opportunistic disease.

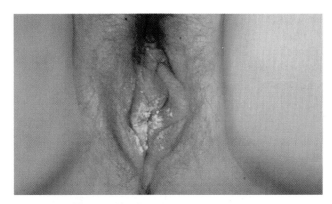

Figure 191. Candidiasis, diabetic patient

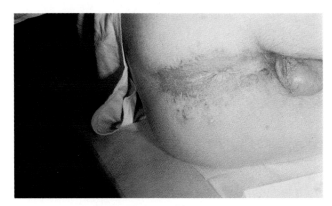

Figure 192. Perianal candidiasis,
result of long-term antibiotic treatment

Other species of the genus *Candida* are occasionally pathogenic:

C. guilliermondii (Castellani) Langeron and Guerra, 1938 (synonym: *Endomyces guilliermondii* Castellani, 1912). Perfect state: *Pichia guilliermondi.* This organism is occasionally associated with human infections.

C. kefyr (Beijerinck) van Uden et Buckley 1970. (synonym: *C. pseudotropicalis* (Castellani) Basgal, 1931; *Endomyces pseudotropicalis* Castellani, 1911; *Monilia pseudotropicalis* Castellani and Chalmers, 1913; *M. mortifera* Martin, Jones, Yao, and Lee, 1937). Perfect state: *Kluyveromyces fragilis.* This yeast may cause various clinical forms of candidiasis. It is frequently isolated from nails.

C. krusei (Castellani) Berkhout, 1923 (synonym: *Saccharomyces krusei* Castellani, 1910; *Monilia krusei* Castellani and Chalmers, 1913). Perfect state: *Pichia kudriavezii.* This species is frequently found colonizing gastrointestinal, respiratory, and urinary tracts of patients undergoing therapy with fluconzole; also associated with some forms of infant diarrhea.

C. lusitaniae van Uden et do Carmo-Sousa, 1959. (synonymy *C. parapsilosis* (Ashf.) Langeron et Talice var *obtusa*

Dietrichson 1954; *Candida obtusa* (Dietrichson) van Uden et do Carmo-Sousa ex van Udeen et Buckley, 1970). Perfect state: *Clavispora lusitaniae*. This species is mostly associated with blood, urine, and the respiratory tract, and is resistant to amphotericin B.

C. parapsilosis (Ashford) Camargo, 1934 (synonym: *Monilia parapsilosis* Ashford, 1928; *M. parakrusei* Castellani and Chalmers, 1934; *C. brumpti* Langeron and Guerra, 1935). Frequently involved in cases of endocarditis,fungemia, and in nail disease.

C. stellatoidea Jones and Martin, 1938, a synonym of *C. albicans*.

C. tropicalis (Castellani) Berkhout, 1923 (synonym: *Monilia candida* Hansen, 1888; *Oidium tropicalis* Castellani,1910; *Mycotorula dimorpha* Redaelli and Ciferri, 1935; *M. trimorpha* Redaelli and Ciferri, 1935). This species is a major pathogen causing disseminated infections in immunocompromised patients.

C. viswanathii Sandhu et Randhawa 1962. Rarely isolated from human cases. Isolates of *C., tropicalis* that do not ferment sucrose are phenotypically similar to *C. viswanathii*.

Occurrence

Pathogenic species of *Candida* may be isolated from various body sites as a normal saprophyte, ranging from 2 to 69% in the oral cavity (Odds,1988), Cohen et al (1968) in the study of the gastrointestinal tract found the prevalence of yeast at 35% in the oropharynx, 50% in the jejunum, 60% in the ileum, and 70% in the colon. Most studies report under 30% yeasts in the vagina of normal women. The most prevalent species (Odds, 1988) in the gastrointestinal tract are: *C. albicans* (51%), followed by *Torulopsis glabrata* (9.l%), *C. parapsilosis* (5.4%), *C. krusei* (2.9%), and *C. tropicalis* (2.3%). Infants aged 1 week to 18 months have a higher carriage (46.3%) than neonates up to 1 week old (17.3%). Under certain conditions these organisms may change to pathogens. The organism has been isolated from soil probably contaminated with feces of humans or animals, and from fruits.

Humans: Candidiasis is a relatively common mycosis of worldwide distribution. It occurs at all ages and in both sexes. Certain predisposing factors favor the development of the disease: malnutrition, diabetes, pregnancy, antibiotic therapy, iatrogenic immunosuppression, intravenous catheters, cytoreductive chemotherapy, hematologic malignant diseases, neutropenia, burns, and intravenous drug abuse, and use of corticosteroids.

Animals: The disease has been reported in chickens, turkeys, ducks, geese, pigeons, pheasants, ruffed grouse, quail, guinea-fowl, dogs, cattle, pigs, colts, lambs, monkeys, hedgehogs, guinea pigs, horses, dolphins, and rodents. The total includes 58 or more animal species (Odds, 1988).

Laboratory Procedures

Specimen collection: Collection of infected material for examination will vary considerably depending upon the type of clinical symptoms. Skin or nail scrapings; mucous patches from the mouth, vagina, or anus; sputum, blood, or cerebrospinal fluid should be collected for laboratory study in sterile containers, as smears on slides, or cultured directly. Only freshly collected material is reliable for diagnostic purposes, as the organism multiplies rapidly.

Candida spp. may be normal flora in some of the above areas and may appear as budding cells in direct examination. The material should be examined as soon as possible to avoid multiplication of numbers while standing.

Direct examination: Skin and nail scrapings, and other clinical specimens should be mounted in 10% KOH in the usual manner, with a coverglass, and heated gently. The wet mount is rapid and useful for detecting the yeasts. The use of calcofluor white stain in a wet mount gives a better contrast with a fluorescence microscope. Sputum or mucous material should be on a slide and stained by Gram's method, Wright's, or Giemsa stain. The material may also be mounted in lactophenol cotton blue. (When doing the Gram stain of infected material, or from material provided in the laboratory, try making smears from scrapings from the mouth, especially from around the base of an exposed tooth, to see if any yeast cells are present.)

Microscopically, species of *Candida* appear on the stained slides or direct mounts both as budding cells and as fragments of pseudohyphae. In a patient with candidiasis the pseudohyphae or hyphae predominate. The small, oval, thin-walled budding cells and the pseudophypae are about 2 to 6 μm in diameter (Figure 193). Figure 194 shows pseudohyphae in an acridine orange stain. Since nonpathogenic yeasts may look similar to pathogenic yeasts, special methods of culturing are necessary for identification.

Stool, spinal fluid, bronchial washings, or urine after centrifugation or passage through a membrane filter should be examined in the same manner as sputum.

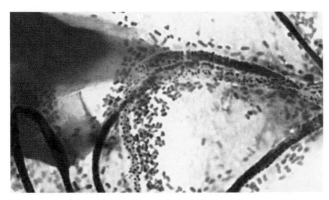

Figure 193. Candidiasis, smear showing pseudohyphae

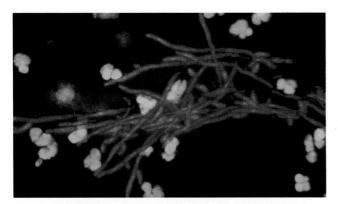

Figure 194. Candidiasis, pseudohyphae,
acridine orange X450

ial antibiotics and incubated at 30°C. The biphasic brain heart infusion medium may be used although not as effective as the Isolator method. The biphasic bottles should be vented.

Colonies: Colonies of *C. albicans* on Sabouraud glucose agar appear in three or four days as cream-colored, smooth, glistening, and have a yeasty odor (Figure 195). Older colonies (1 month) are cream colored, waxy or soft, smooth or wrinkled, and may have submerged hyphal growth resembling feathers deep in the agar resembling fringes.

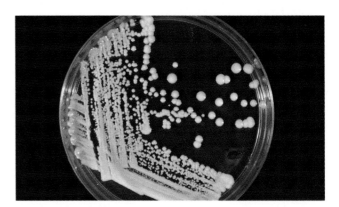

Figure 195. *Candida* spp., colonies

Culture: Only freshly collected infected material, including scrapings, swabs, sputum, and pus should be cultured on a variety of media. The addition of penicillin and streptomycin or chloramphenicol to Sabouraud glucose agar is desirable to reduce contamination in the cultures. *Candida krusei, C. tropicalis,* and *C. parapsilosis* are inhibited by cycloheximide. The cultures usually grow at room temperature or 37°C. On media containing larger amounts of fermentable carbohydrates, the organism grows primarily as a budding yeast. Without fermentable carbohydrates, and with less aerobic conditions, along with the addition of nitrogen to the medium, pseudohyphae, blastoconidia, and in some cases, chlamydoconidia develop. Blood agar is useful for isolation of yeasts in clinical material.

The isolation of species of *Candida* from peritoneum, joint aspirates, cerebrospinal fluid, bone marrow, or biopsies should be considered as significant in debilitated patients. Urine cultures may be useful in cases of disseminated candidiasis caused by *C. tropicalis*. The presence of numerous yeast cells in urine (10^4/ml or more) is significant. For recovery of *Candida* species from blood, a 10 ml lysis centrifugation system (Isolator) is useful. The sediment after centrifugation of the isolator tubes should be streaked on slants or plates of Sabouraud glucose agar with antibacter-

Microscopically, a slide mount from Sabouraud glucose agar will show oval, budding cells 2.5 to 4 by 6 μm in size and some pseudomycelium if taken from submerged growth. The pseudomycelium consists of elongate, undetached cells with clusters of blastoconidia at constrictions.

Production of chlamydoconidia in chlamydospore agars is usually sufficient for identification of *C. albicans*. If none are present, carbohydrate fermentations and especially assimilations are useful for species determination. The very rapid germ tube method is another useful procedure for identification of *C. albicans*. In sputum the presence of numerous pseudohyphae of *Candida* species is usually significant.

1. ***Chlamydoconidial* formation.** Cornmeal agar (including freshly prepared cornmeal agar) plus 0.5% to 1% Tween 80, zein agar, rice infusion agar, cream of rice agar, or other types of media are used for the production of chlamydoconidia by *C. albicans*. All inoculated media for chlamydoconidia should be incubated at 24°C.

If a yeastlike colony has developed on Sabouraud glucose agar, streak a little of the colony into the cornmeal or other similar media. Add a flamed coverglass over the streak. The other species of *Candida* may also be streaked on the same agar for comparison. An identified *C. albicans* should be streaked into the agar for comparison with the unknown. The streak may be made against the bottom of a petri dish as a furrow in the agar. Incubate at 24°C for two or three days. Growth can be checked from the bottom under a microscope.

Under the low-power objective, examine the streak on the bottom of the plate or the coverglass on the agar in the petri dish and look for branching mycelium or pseudohyphae with clusters of blastoconidia along the sides and the thick-walled round chlamydoconidia terminating the hyphae. *C. albicans* produces the characteristic chlamydoconidia (Figure 196). These are 8 to 12 μm in diameter. Occasionally *C. tropicalis* produce chlamydoconidia.

2. **Germ tube method.** The production of filaments or germ tubes by a low concentration of cells of *C. albicans* in 0.5 ml of human, rabbit, guinea pig, fetal calf or sheep serum, albumin, 1% peptone, or commercially available germ-tube media gives a rapid presumptive identification within two or three hours with a control at 37°C (Taschdjian, Burchall, and Kozinn, 1960). Make a slide mount at the end of two or three hours and examine for germ tube formation. The isolates are most likely to be *C. albicans* if germ tubes form. A germ tube without constrictions at septa is about one-half the width and three to four times the length of the mother cell from which it develops (Figure 197). Some strains of *C. albicans* on rare occasions will not form germ tubes.

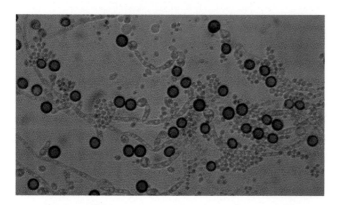

Figure 196. *Candida albicans,* chlamydoconidia X450

On TOC medium (Tween 80, oxgall, caffeic acid) *C. albicans* will develop germ tubes in three hours at 37°C and chlamydoconidia in 18 to 24 hours at 28°C.

A number of factors may prevent the formation of germ tubes, including too high a concentration of the yeast cells, temperatures above 41°C or below 31°C, and heat coagulated serum.

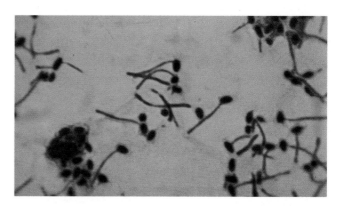

Figure 197. *Candida albicans,* germ tubes X600

Carbohydrate fermentation and assimilation tests: If chlamydoconidia are lacking or no germ tubes are produced, it is necessary to determine a specific pattern of carbohydrate fermentation and assimilation (see Table 15) to determine the species of *C. albicans, C. guilliermondii, C. kefyr (pseudotropicalis), C. krusei, C. lusitaniae, C. parapsilosis, C. tropicalis,* and *C. viswanathii.*

1. **Carbohydrate fermentation.** Fermentation reactions are less dependable than carbohydrate assimilations and the only reliable result of fermentation is the formation of gas. All carbohydrates fermented will also be assimilated, but not all assimilated carbohydrates will be fermented.

For each organism to be checked, set up six tubes, each containing a solution of one of the following 1% sugars: glucose, sucrose, lactose, maltose, galactose, and trehalose with a Durham tube in each or sealed with wax or vaseline. For inoculation, a suspension is prepared equivalent to a McFarland Standard #4-7 using sterile distilled water and the yeast to be tested. Add 0.2 ml of the suspension to each tube. Incubate at 37°C for 48 hours. Gas is necessary for a positive reaction and is usually accompanied by a color change. Commercial kits are available.

2. **Carbohydrate assimilation** (auxanographic technique). For each organism to be tested prepare plates according to the directions given on page 39. The inoculum suspension used for fermentation may be used to inoculate the assimilation media by streaking with a swab or making a suspension before solidification of the medium in a pour plate. Disks are added which have been impregnated with 20% solutions of the following carbohydrates: glucose, maltose, sucrose, lactose, galactose, trehalose, inositol, melibiose, celibiose, raffinose, dulcitol, and xylose.

Incubate at 24° to 30°C for 24 to 72 hours. Growth around the disk indicates the utilization of the carbohydrate contained in the disk (positive test). Quality control

Table 15. Physiologic Characteristics of *Candida* spp. and Other Yeasts

Organism	Surface Growth on Sabouraud Broth	Sugar Assimilation																			Sugar Fermentation					
		Glucose	Maltose	Sucrose	Lactose	Galactose	Melibiose	Cellobiose	Inositol	Xylose	Raffinose	Trehalose	Glycerol	D-Ribose	L-Rhamnose	Melezitose	Erythritol	Ribitol	D-Mannitol	Methyl α-D-glucoside	Glucose	Maltose	Sucrose	Lactose	Galactose	Trehalose
C. albicans	0	+	+	+	0	+	0	0	0	+	0	+	v	v	v	v	0	v	+	v	+	+	+	0	+	+
C. guilliermondi	0	+	+	+	0	+	+	+	0	+	+	+	+	+	v	v	v	v	+	±	+	0	+	0	+	+
C. Kefyr (pseudo-tropicalis)	0	+	0	+	+	+	0	+	0	+*	+	0	v	0	0	0	0	0	v	0	+	0	+	+	+	+
C. krusei	+ (film)	+	0	0	0	0	0	0	0	0	0	0	+	0	0	0	0	0	0	0	+	0	0	0	0	0
C. lusitaniae	0	+	+	+	0	+	0	+	0	+	0	+	+	+	v	+	0	+	+	+	+	+	+	0	0	0
C. parapsilosis	0	+	+	+	0	+	0	0	0	+	0	+	+	v	v	+	0	+	+	v	+	0	0	0	+	+
C. tropicalis	+ (film)	+	+	+	0	+	0	v	0	+	+	−	v	v	0	+	0	v	+	±	+	+	+	0	+	+
C. viswanathii	0	+	+	+	0	+	0	+	0	0	0	+	+	0	0	v	0	0	+	+	0*	0	0	0	0	0
Saccharomyces cerevisiae	0	+	+*	v	0	+	+*	0	0	0	+	+*	v	0	0	v	0	0	0	v	+	0	+	0	+	+*
Geotrichum candidum	0	+	0	0	0	+	0	0	0	+	0	0	+	NA	NA	0	NA	0	0	0	0	0	0	0	0	0
Torulopsis glabrata	0	+	0	0	0	+	0	0	0	0	0	+	v	0	0	0	0	0	0	0	+	0	0	0	0	+
Trichosporon cutaneum	0	+	+*	v	+	+	+*	v	+*	+	+	+*	v	0	0	0	v	v	v	v	0	0	0	0	0	0

*Strain variation.   acid and gas; + = reaction; 0 = no reaction. v = variable

is important in these tests. A yeast with a known assimilation pattern should be used as a check.   See Table 15 for the fermentation and assimilation patterns.   There are several commercial identification kits available based on carbohydrate assimilation profiles.   These widely used systems are rapid and very accurate for identification of most of the medically important species.   The commercially available kits include API 20 C, the Abbott Quantum, the Vitek yeast identification system, and other systems are widely acceptable for use.   See Table 15 for sugar assimilations.

Colony and microscopic morphology of *Candida* species.

The following *Candida* species have a brief description of the colony and microscopic appearances. The microscopic appearance of some of the *Candida* species have a characteristic growth pattern microscopically on cornmeal agar.

Candida albicans (Robin) Berkhout, 1923.   In the nucleic acid studies of Stenderup and Bak (1969) there is a general agreement that *C. albicans* has two large serologic groups, A and B, with the former including *C. tropicalis*. Serotypes A and B are based on differences in the mannan structure (Hasenclever and Mitchell, 1961).

Colony morphology: The colony after three days on Sabouraud glucose agar is white to creamy, smooth, and after 30 days become creamy, glistening, waxy, soft, smooth to rough, and sometimes wrinkled.

Microscopic morphology: After three days the yeast cells are globose, short ovoid (5 to 7 µm) and sometimes elongate cells (4 to 6 by 6 to 10 µm).   On cornmeal (3 days), mycelium and pseudomycelium form with masses of blastoconidia (3 to 4 µm) at the internodes. Characteristic terminal, thick-walled chlamydoconidia usually form. A positive germ tube test is also characteristic of this species.

Candida guilliermondii (Castellani) Langeron et Guerra, 1938.

Colony morphology: The colony after three days on Sabouraud glucose agar is thin, flat, cream to pinkish and glossy.   After one month the colony is yellowish cream to pink, smooth or dull, glistening and wrinkled.

Microscopic morphology: After three days the cells are short ovoid or elongate (2 to 5 by 3 to 7 µm) along with small and cylindrical cells. On cornmeal (3 days), the very fine and short pseudomycelium with small cells which may bear ramified chains of small ovoid cells or stalactoid, verticillated blastoconidia.

Candida kefyr (Beijerinck) van Uden et Buckley, 1970

(Synonym: *Candida pseudotropicalis* (Cast.) Basgal, 1931).

Colony morphology: On Sabouraud glucose agar after three days, the colony is creamy, smooth and in one month cream to yellowish, with a rather dull, soft, smooth or a small amount of reticulations.

Microscopic morphology: A three day old colony usually has abundant pseudomycelium with very elongated cells that fall apart and remain parallel like a stream full of "logs".   On cornmeal, pseudomycelium may be abundant and fall apart in parallel masses.

Candida krusei (Castellani) Berkhout, 1923.

Colony morphology: A three day old colony on Sabouraud glucose agar is flat, dry, and dull. A month later the colony becomes greenish-yellow, soft, dull, smooth, or wrinkled with fringe of mycelium around the edges.

Microscopic morphology: In three days varied size cylindrical and a small number of ovoid cells (3 to 5 by 6 to 20 µm) develop.   On cornmeal agar after three days elongated cells are arranged like a tree or "crossed matchsticks". Blastoconidia are elongated, growing in verticillate branches from the mycelium.   Only a few blastoconidia may develop in some strains.

Candida lusitaniae van Uden et do Carma-Sousa, 1959.

Colony morphology: Colonies that develop in three days on Sabouraud glucose agar are white to cream in color, soft, glistening, and smooth.

Microscopic morphology: After three days the colony has yeast cells that are subglobose, ovoid, or elliptical, and 1.5 to 6.0 by 2.5 to 10 µm in size.   On cornmeal the colony develops elongated to oval cells.

Candida parapsilosis (Ashford) Langeron et Talice, 1932.

Colony morphology: A three-day-old culture on Sabouraud glucose agar has colonies similar to *Candida albicans*: soft, smooth, white, becoming cream to yellowish, glistening, and smooth or wrinkled in older colonies.

Microscopic morphology: Young colonies have short-ovoid to long-ovoid cells (2.5 to 4 by 2.5 to 9 µm).   On cornmeal agar in three days thin pseudomycelium is produced with branched chains of elongated cells with clusters of blastoconidia around the septa. Thick pseudomycelium and giant cells may occur.

Candida tropicalis (Castellani) Berkhout, 1923.

Colony morphology: Colonies are like *C. albicans*. Old colonies become hairy and tough.

Microscopic morphology: Three-day-old colonies contain globose-ovoid or short-ovoid cells (4 to 8 by 5 to 11 μm). On cornmeal agar in three days abundant pseudomycelium develops composed of elongate cells with extensive branching, and blastoconidia formed singly or in clusters along the mycelium. The pseudohyphae at times produce globose to pear-shaped cells resembling chlamydoconidia with thin walls.

Candida viswanathii Sandhu et Randhaw, 1959.

Colony morphology: Three-day-old cultures are cream-colored, soft, and glistening, becoming wrinkled and hairy on the surface in older cultures.

Microscopic morphology: Young colonies contain globose, ovoid to cylindric cells (2.5 to 7 by 4 to 12 μm). On cornmeal agar, long wavy mycelium has irregular branches at up to 90 degree with verticillately arranged chains of globose to ovoid blastoconidia.

Histopathology: The organisms are not likely to occur in biopsy material unless taken from the pulmonary region, the mucous membrane of the alimentary tract or bronchi, or from endocarditis and systemic cases. Hyphae, pseudohyphae 3 or 4 μm in diameter, and blastoconidia (buds) are usually present in tissue in place of oval to round budding cells. The organisms can be readily demonstrated in the Gridley, PAS, or Gomori methenamine-silver nitrate stains. H and E stain is satisfactory for demonstration of the organisms in tissue. The demonstration of the organism in tissue is sufficient to designate the genus *Candida* (Figure 198). Study sections containing granulomatous lesions or abscesses.

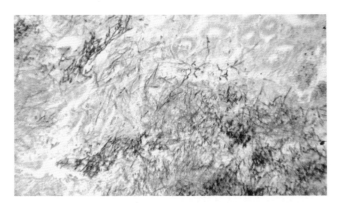

Figure 198. Candidiasis, pseudohyphae in kidney. Gomori methenamine-silver stain X200

Animal inoculation: *C. albicans* and *C. tropicalis* (both

may have germ tubes), and are pathogenic in mice and rabbits. Inject rabbits intravenously with 1 ml of a 1% saline suspension of the organism. In four or five days the animal should die with abscessed kidneys. For mice, 1 ml saline suspension of the fungus should be injected intraperitoneally or 0.2 ml suspension of 10^3 cells to 10^4 or 10^6 yeast cells should be injected intravenously. In seven to ten days examine the kidney for abscesses.

Prepare sections or smears of the kidney with white abscesses from the infected rabbit or from the infected mouse and stain by Gram's method. Look for Gram-positive, short, irregularly formed hyphae, pseudohyphae, and budding cells in the section or smear under the immersion oil lens.

NOTE: Animal inoculations are usually of little diagnostic value in determining the significance of the organism in a patient.

Serology: The serology of *Candida* species has been extensively studied.

The Latex agglutination (LA), immunodiffusion (ID), and the counterimmunoelectrophoresis (CIE) are useful for detecting antibodies to *Candida* species in sera from patients with candidemia, pneumonitis, endocarditis, intra-abdominal abscess, and indwelling urinary or intravenous catheters (Kaufman and Reiss, 1992). A negative test may indicate the exclusion of systemic candidiasis in the diagnosis. The detection of precipitins or a fourfold change or a titer of 8 or greater by LA is presumptive for systemic candidiasis. The ID, CIE, and LA tests have a sensitivity of around 80% for proven candidiasis cases in immunologically intact patients. The LA test is quantitative and has some prognostic value. The *decision to treat a patient should not* be based on serologic data only.

The antibody tests are of limited value for the diagnosis of systemic candidiasis in immunosuppressed patients, antigen test are more useful. The detection of about 2mg of serum mannan per ml by EIA and a titer of about 8 with the Cand-Tec test should be diagnostic for invasive candidiasis in neutropenic patients.

In the ID test, one to seven precipitates may form with *C. albicans* antigens and the antisera from a patient with candidiasis. The production of one or more lines constitutes a positive reaction. When serial serum specimens demonstrate conversion or an increase in the number of bands, systemic candidiasis is suspected.

Commercial kits available: API 20 C Yeast Identification System (API 20 C), Analytab Products Inc, Plainview, NY;

BBL Minitek system, Cockeysville, MD; Microdrop Yeast Identification System, Clinical Sciences, Inc., Whippany, NJ; Uni-Yeast Tek System, Flow Laboratories, Inc., McLean, VA.; Biomerieux Vitek System, Hazelwood, MO; Microscan Yeast, Baxter Microscan.

Serology kits: Cand-Tec, Ramco Laboratories, Inc., Houston, TX; Pastorex *Candida*, Sanofi Diagnostics, Pasteur; Candida Latex Test, Difco Laboratories, Detroit, MI.

A kit for detection of serum enolase antigen in patients with systemic candidiasis may show promise (Walsh, et al, 1991).

Media for detection of Fungemia: BACTEC high-blood-volume fungal medium (HBV-FM), BACTEC Plus 26 (BP26), Becton Dickinson Diagnostic Instrument Systems, Sparks, MD; and Isolator (IS) Centrifugation-Lysis Blood Culture System, Wampole Laboratories, Cranbury, NJ.

Summary: Yeasts isolated from most patients will be *Candida albicans*. Determination of this species by formation of germ tubes or chlamydoconidia is usually sufficient. Other possible pathogenic yeasts will require assimilation and/or fermentation tests for species determination.

Questions

1. Where does *Candida albicans* occur under normal conditions?

2. What conditions apparently enhance the development of candidiasis?

3. Compare *Candida* spp. with *Saccharomyces cerevisiae*. What are the similarities and differences between these two genera?

4. What are the similarities and differences between the pathogenic *Candida* species in disease development? Compare the locations of *Candida* infections in the normal and the immunocompromised hosts.

Selected References

Anderson A, Yardley J. 1972. Demonstration of candida in blood smears. N. Engl. J. Med. 286:108

Auger P, Joly J. 1977. Factors influencing germ tube production in *Candida albicans* directly from clinical specimens. Mycopathologia 61:151

Bak AL, Stenderup A. 1969. Deoxyribonucleic acid homology in yeasts. Genetic relatedness within the genus Candida. J. Gen. Microbiol. 59:21-30

Bille J, Edson RS, Roberts GD. 1986. Clinical evaluation of the lysis-centrifugation blood culture system for the detection of fungemia and comparison with a conventional biphasic broth blood culture system. J. Clin. Microbiol. 19:126-128

Buckley HR, Van Uden N. 1963. The identification of *Candida albicans* within two hours by use of an egg white slide preparation. Sabouraudia 2:205

Burrow ML, Stewart WW. 1960. *Candida albicans*. Experience with Pagano-Levin culture medium for its identification in clinical material. A report of 294 cultures. Harlem Hosp. Bull. An. Ser. 1:88

Businco L, et al. 1977. Disseminated arthritis and osteitis by *Candida albicans* in a two-month old infant receiving parenteral nutrition. Acta. Paediatr. Scand. 66:393-395

Cohen R, et al. 1968. Fungal flora of the normal human small and large intestine. N. Engl. J. Med. 279:340-344

Cooper BH, Johnson JB, Thaxton ES. 1978. Clinical evaluation of the Uni-Yeast-Tek system for rapid presumptive identification of medically important yeasts. J. Clin. Microbiol. 7:349

Dealler SF. 1991. *Candida albicans* colony identification in five minutes in a general microbiology laboratory. J. Clin. Microbiol. 29:1081

El-Zaatari, et al. 1990. Evaluation of the updated Vitek yeast identification database. J. Clin. Microbiol. 28(9):1938.

Faix RG. 1984. Systemic candida infections in infants in intensive care nurseries: high incidence of central nervous system involvement. J. Pediatr. 105:616-622

Fischer JB, Kane J. 1968. Production of chlamydospores by *Candida albicans* cultivated on dilute oxgall agar. Mycopath. Mycol. Appl. 35:223

Fox BC, et al. 1989. The use of DNA probe for epidemiological studies of candidiasis in immunocompromised hosts. J. Infect. Dis. 159:488-494

Giger D, et al. 1978. Experimental murine candidiasis: pathological and immune responses in T-lymphocyte-depleted mice. Infect. Immun. 21:729

Gordon MA, Elliott JC, Hawkins TW. 1967. Identification of *Candida albicans*, other *Candida* species, and *Torulopsis glabrata* by means of immunofluorescence. Sabouraudia 5:323

Guerra-Romero L, et al. 1987. Comparison of Du Pont Isolator and Roche Septi-Chek for detection of fungemia. J. Clin. Microbiol. 25(9):1623-1925

Hasenclever HF, Mitchell WO. 1961. Antigenic studies of *Candida*. I. Observation of two antigenic groups in *Candida albicans*. J. Bacteriol. 82:570-573

Holzschu DL, et al. 1979. Identification of *Candida lusitaniae* as an opportunistic yeast in humans. J. Clin, Microbiol. 10:202

Huppert M, Harper G, Sun S, et al. 1975. Rapid methods for identification of yeasts. J. Lab. Clin. Med. 2:21

Johnson DE, et al. 1984. Systemic candidiasis in very low birth-weight infants (<l,500 grams). Pediatrics 73:138

Kaji H, Asanuma Y, Ide H, et al. 1976. The auto-brewery syndrome - the repeated attacks of alcoholic intoxication due to the overgrowth of *Candida albicans* in the gastrointestinal tract. Materia Medica Poiona 8:429

Kaufman L, Reiss E. 1992. Serodiagnosis of fungal diseases. *In* Rose NR, Friedman H (eds). Manual of Clinical Immunology. Am. Soc. Microbiol., Washington, DC.

Kennedy MJ, Volz PA. 1985. Effect of various antibiotics on gastrointestinal colonization and dissemination by *Candida albicans*. J. Med. Vet. Mycol. 23:265-273

Herent P, et al. 1992. Retrospective valuation of two latex agglutination tests for detection of circulating antigens during invasive candidosis. J. Clin. Microbiol. 30:2158

Kwon-Chung KJ, Wickes BL, Whelan WL. 1987. Ploidy and DNA content of the yeast cells of *Candida stellatoidea*. Infect. Immun. 55:3207

Land GA, Vinton EC, Adcock GB, et al. 1975. Improved auxanographic method for yeast assimilations: A comparison with other approaches. J. Clin. Microbiol. 2:206

Land GA, et al. 1991. Evaluation of the Baxter-MicroScan 4-hour enzyme based yeast identification system. J. Clin. Microbiol. 29:718

Landau JW, Dabrowa N, Newcomer VD. 1965. The rapid formation in serum of filaments by *Candida albicans*. J. Invest. Dermatol. 44: 171

Lodder J (ed.). 1970. The Yeasts, A Taxonomic Study, 2nd ed. North Holland Publishing Co, Amsterdam. The Netherlands

Louria DB, Brayton RG, Finkei G. 1963. Studies on the pathogenesis of experimental *Candida albicans* infections in mice. Sabouraudia 2:271

MacDonald EM, Wegner MJ. 1962. A slide culture technique for the identification of *Candida albicans*. Tex. Rep. Biol. Med. 20:128

Mackenzie DW. 1962. Identification of *Candida albicans* by serum tube method. J. Clin. Pathol. 15:563

Marier R, Andrioie VT. 1978. Usefulness of serial antibody determinations in diagnosis of candidiasis as measured by discontinuous counterimmunoelectrophoresis using HS antigen. J. Clin. Microbiol. 8:15

Mason AB, Brandt ME, Buckley HR. 1989. Enolase activity associated with *C. albicans* cytoplasmic antigen. Yeast. 5:S231

Mason MM, Lasker BA, Riggsby WS. 1987. Molecular probe for identification of medically important *Candida* species and *Torulopsis glabrata*. J. Clin. Microbiol. 25(3):563

Montes LF, Patrick TA, Martin SA, et al. 1965. Ultrastructure of blastospores of *Candida albicans* after permanganate fixation. J. Invest. Dermatol. 45:227

Munoz P, et al. 1990. Impact of the BACTEC NR system in detecting *Candida* fungemia. J. Clin. Microbiol. 28:639

Murray PR. 1991. Comparison of the lysis-centrifugation and agitated biphasic blood culture systems for detection of fungemia. J. Clin. Microbiol. 229(1):96

Murray PR, Spizzo AW, Niles AC. 1991. Clinical comparison of the recoveries of bloodstream pathogens in SeptiChek brain heart infusion broth with saponin, Septi-Chek tryptic soy broth, and the Isolator lysis-centrifugation system. J. Clin. Microbiol. 29(5):901

Meyer SA, Payne RW, Yarrow D. 1993. *Candida* Berkhout. *In* The Yeasts: A Taxonomic Study, 4th Ed. Edited by C. P. Kurtzman and J. W. Fell. Elsevier Science Publishers, Amsterdam.

Myerowitz RL, Pazin GJ, Allen CM. 1977. Disseminated candidiasis: Changes in incidence, underlying diseases, and pathology. Am. J. Clin. Pathol. 68:29

Ness MJ, Vaughan WP, Woods GL. 1989. Candida antigen latex test for detection of invasive candidiasis in immunocompromised patients. J. Infect. Dis. 159:495

Nickerson WJ, Mankowski Z. 1953. A polysaccharide medium of known composition favoring chlamydospore formation in *Candida albicans*. J. Infect. Dis. 92:20

Odds FC. 1988. *Candida* and *Candidosis*. 2nd Ed. Bailliere Tindall, London.

Pagano J, Levin JD, Trejo W. 1958. Diagnostic medium for differentiation of species of *Candida*. Antibiot. Ann. 1957 8:137

Patriquin H, et al. 1980. Neonatal candidiasis: renal and pulmonary manifestations. AJR, 135:1205

Roberts GD, Horstmeier C, Hall M, et al. 1975. Recovery of yeast from vented blood culture bottles. J. Lab. Clin. Med. 2:18

Roberts GD, Wang HS, Hollick GE. 1976. Evaluation of the API 20C Microtube System for the identification of clinically important yeasts. J Lab Clin Med 3:302

Rogers AL, Beneke ES. 1964. Human pathogenic fungi recovered from Brazilian soil. Mycopathol Mycol. Appl. 22:15

Salvin SB, Cory JC, Berg MK. 1952. The enhancement of the virulence of *Candida albicans* in mice. J. Infect. Dis. 90:177

Sanchez ML, et al. 1992. Diagnosis of disseminated candidiasis in hospitalized patients using the Cand-Tec agglutination assay. Mycopath. 188(3):153

Schwartz DS, Larsh HW, Bartels PA. 1977. Enumerative

fluorescent vital staining of live and dead pathogenic yeast cells. Stain Tech. 52:203

Seeleger H. 1955. Ein neus Medium zur Pseudomycelbildung von *Candida albicans.* Zeitschr. für Hyg. 141:488

Sekhon AS, Padhye AA, Garg AK, Gowa AH. 1988. Evaluation of the "Yeast-IDENT for the identification of medically important yeasts. Mycoses 331(12):627

Shinoda T. Kaufman L, Padhye AA. 1981. Comparative evaluation of the Iatron serological *Candida* check kit and the API 20C kit for identification of medically important *Candida* species. J. Clin. Microbiol. 13:513

St.-Germain G, Beachesne D. 1991. Evaluation of the MicroScan Rapid Yeast Identification panel. J. Clin. Microbiol. 29(10):2296

Taschdjian CL, Burchail JJ, Kozinn PJ. 1960. Rapid identification of *Candida albicans* by filamentation of serum and serum substitutes. J. Dis. Child. 99:212

Walsh TJ, et al. 1991. Role of anticandida enolase antibody diagnosis of invasive candidiasis. *In* Proceedings of the InterScience Conference on Antimicrobial Agents and Chemotherapy. Chicago, Am. Soc. Microbiol. p. 178

Walsh TJ, et al. 1989. Clinical microbiological and experimental animal studies of *Candida lipolytica.* J. Clin. Microbiol. 27:927

Warren JW, Piatt R, Thomas RJ, et al. 1978. Antibiotic irrigation and catheter-associated urinary-tract infections. N. Engl. J. Med. 299:570

Whelan WL, Partridge RM, Magee PT. 1980. Heterozygosity and segregation in *Candida albicans.* Mol. Gen. Genet. 180:107

Wickerham LJ, Borton KA. 1948. Carbon assimilation tests for the classification of yeasts. J. Bacteriol. 56:363

Wilson ML, et al. 1993. Controlled comparison of the BACTEC High-Volume Fungal Medium, BACTEC Plus 26 Aerobic Blood Culture Bottle, and 10-Milliliter Isolator Blood Culture System for detection of fungemia and bacteremia. J. Clin. Microbiol. 31:865

TORULOPSOSIS

Definition.

Torulopsosis occurs primarily in debilitated persons including AIDS, usually as an opportunist, but on rare occasions in patients without underlying disease. Microabscesses are the usual pathologic symptom, with less frequent occurrence of small granulomas containing giant cells. The yeast has been found in cases of fungemia, pyelonephritis, septicemia, pulmonary infections, endocarditis, meningitis and hyperalimentation. Lesions are found most frequently in the lungs and kidney but fungemia may occur followed by dissemination and/or a septic shock due to a toxic reaction to the yeast. The organism may be seen in rare cases intracellularly within macrophages of the infected lung. In such locations the organism must be differentiated from *Histoplasma capsulatum. Torulopsis* has a broader isthmus between the bud and yeast cell and is culturally different (Figure 199). *T. glabrata* as a nosocomial agent may cause an endophthalmitis following ketoplasty after the use of organ cultured cornea.

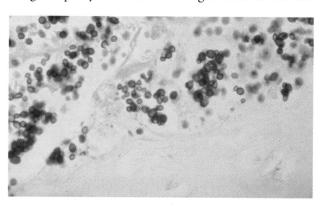

Figure 199. *Torulopsis glabrata* with a broad isthmus between the bud and the yeast cell

Etiologic Agents and Occurrence

Torulopsis glabrata (Anderson) Lodder et De Vries, 1938, and *Torulopsis haemulonii* van Uden et Kolpinski, 1962.

Laboratory Procedures

Specimen collection: Occurs as normal flora in the oral cavity, gastrointestinal tract, and urogenital area of humans and animals, as well as in the soil. Material for the laboratory includes urine, and occasionally blood, sputum, spinal fluid, and AIDS.

Examination of infected material: Stained smears or tissue sections show oval to spherical cells, 1 to 2 by 2 to 3 µm to 2 to 3 by 4 to 5 µm in size, no capsule, no hyphae, and no ascospores. Blastospores are connected by a broader isthmus than that in yeast cells of *H. capsulatum.* In urine, 10^4 yeast cells per milliliter or over is considered significant and is the probable cause of the infection.

Torulopsis glabrata:

Culture: Rapid growth on ordinary media. Sabouraud glucose agar, blood, or other media are suitable for culture. This organism is resistant to cycloheximide but media without this agent should also be used.

Colonies: Colonies of *T. glabrata* are pasty, smooth to glossy, white to cream in color at first, later becoming grayish-tan. The yeast cells are 2.5 to 4.5 by 4.6 µm.

Biochemical characteristics: *T. glabrata* forms acid and gas in glucose. Glucose and trehalose are assimilated. No other carbohydrates are assimilated. Inositol is assimilated by *Cryptococcus* spp. but not by *Torulopsis*. Urease is negative and KNO_3 is not assimilated.

T. haemulonii (van Uden et Kolipinski) Meyer et Yarrow 1978 has been reported from cases of fungemia (Marjolet, 1986).

Animal inoculation: In mice altered physiologically with alloxan, x-irradiation, or cortisone, infection can be produced by *T. glabrata*.

Questions

1. How is *Torulopsis glabrata* differentiated from *Cryptococcus neoformans* in culture?

2. How is *T. glabrata* differentiated from *H. capsulatum* in tissue or in the laboratory animal?

3. Separate the genera *Torulopsis, Candida, Trichosporon, Rhodotorula,* and *Geotrichum.*

Selected References

Ahearn DG, Jannach JR, et al. 1966. Speciation and densities of yeasts in human urine specimens. Sabouraudia 5:110

Courcol RJ, et al. 1992. BioArgos a fully automated blood culture system. J. Clin. Microbiol. 30:1995

Flynn P, et al. 1987. *Torulopsis glabrata* infection in immunocompromised children. S. Med. J. 80:237

Hickey WF, Sommerville LH, Schoen FJ. 1983. Disseminated *Candida glabrata:* report of a uniquely severe infection and a literature review. Am. J. Clin. Pathol. 80:724

Howard DH, Otto V. 1967. The intracellular behavior of *Torulopsis glabrata* Sabouraudia 5:235

Kremer M, Basset M, Koenig H. 1977. Frequence de *Torulopsis glabrata,* etude de la C.M.I. de certains antifungiques. Bull. Soc. Francaise Mycol. Med. 6:301

Jansson E. 1963. Yeasts isolated from urine specimens. Ann. Med. Intern. Fenn. 52:267

Lavarde VF, et al. 1984. Peritonite mycosique a *Torulopsis haemulonii.* Bull. Soc. Fr. Mycol. Med. 13:173

Larsen PA, Lindstrom RL, Doughman D. 1978. *Torulopsis glabrata* endophthalmitis after keratoplasty with an organcultured cornea. Arch. Ophthal. 96:1019

Marjolet M. 1986. *Torulopsis ernobii, Torulopsis haemulonii:* levures opportunistes chez l'immunodeprime? Bull. Soc. Fr. Mycol. Med. 15:143

Marks MI, O'Toole E. 1970. Laboratory identification of *Torulopsis glabrata* Typical appearance on routine bacteriological media. Appl. Microbiol. 19:184

Sekhon AS, et al. 1992. Evaluation of the Pro-Lab ID ring system for the identification of medically important yeasts. Mycopath , 119:11

Vaidivieso M, Luna M, Rodriguez GP, et al. 1976. Fungemia due to *Torulopsis glabrata* in the compromised host. Cancer 38:1750

Walter EB Jr, Gingras JL, McKinney RE Jr. 1990. Systemic *Torulopsis glabrata* infection in a neonate. Sout. Med. J. 83:837

Wickerham LJ. 1957. Apparent increase in frequency of infections involving *Torulopsis glabrata.* JAMA 165:47

Wildfeuer A. 1978. Experimenteile Sprosspiizinfektion des Gastrointestinaltraktes der Maus. Mykosen 21:157

CRYPTOCOCCOSIS

(European blastomycosis, torulosis, Buschke's disease)

Definition

Cryptococcosis is a subacute or chronic infection involving primarily the skin (Figure 202), skeleton, or other parts of the body. The organism enters by the respiratory tract, producing a primary pulmonary infection that is usually transitory, mild, and unrecognized. The chronic infections involve primarily the brain (Figure 201), meninges and at times the lungs (Figure 200). Infection is usually initiated by inhalation into the lungs. Cryptococcosis occurs in about 8% of AIDS patients in the United States (Kovacs, et al, 1985), and accounts for more than 50% of the total cases. Cryptococcosis is not *only* an opportunistic disease.

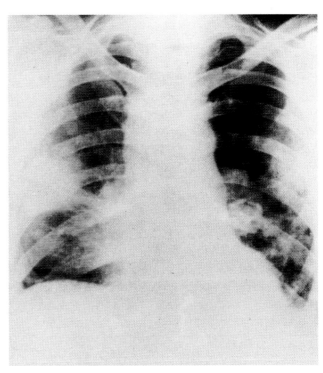

Figure 200. Pulmonary cryptococcosis, *Cryptococcus neoformans,* X-ray film

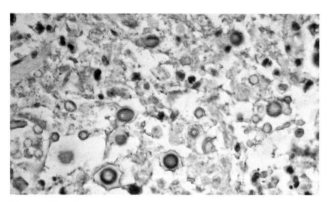

Figure 201. Cryptococcosis, brain tissue with capsules around yeast cells. Mayer's mucicarmine X600

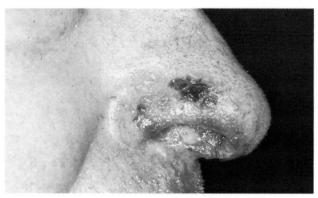

Figure 202. Cryptococcosis, *Cryptococcus neoformans*, skin lesion

Etiologic Agent

Cryptococcus neoformans has two varieties in the imperfect (anamorph) and perfect (teleomorph) states.

Cryptococcus neoformans (Sanfelice) Vuillemin var. *neoformans* 1901. Some synonyms: *Saccharomyces neoformans* Sanfelice, 1895; *Torula neoformans* Weis, 1902 *Torula histolytica* Stoddard and Culter, 1916; *Cryptococcus bacillisporus* Kwon-Chung, Bennett et al, 1978, and *Debaryomyces hominis* Todd and Herrman, 1936. Teleomorph *Filobasidiella neoformans* Kwon-Chung var. *neoformans,* 1975. Serotypes A and D.

Cryptococcus neoformans (Sanfelice) Viullemin var. *gattii* Vanbreuseghemm et Takashio in DeVroly et Gatti, 1989. Synonym: *C. neoformans* (Sanfelice) Vuillemin, 1901; *C. bacillispora* Kwon-Chung et Bennett, 1978. Teleomorph: *Filobasidiella neoformans* var. *bacillispora* Kwon-Chung, 1982. Serotypes B and C.

Occurrence

C. neoformans var. *neoformans* has been isolated as a saprophyte from soil, plants, fruits, milk, skin, feces of normal people, and pigeon dung. The only known source of *C. neoformans* var. *gattii* is on *Eucalyptus camaldulensis.*

Humans: The disease is worldwide in distribution.

Animals: The disease has been reported especially in dogs, cats, pigs, horses, foxes, ferrets, cows, cheetahs, monkeys, and sheep.

Laboratory Procedures

Specimen collection: Pus from skin lesions or subcutaneous tumorlike formations should be obtained by aspiration if possible. All material collected, including cerebrospinal fluid, sputum, urine, pus, or visceral organs from autopsies should be put in sterile containers for laboratory examination.

Direct examination: Place a loopful of pus, sputum, urine, or other body fluids in a drop of India ink (nigrosin) mix, cover with a coverglass, and examine for cells with capsules. Calcofluor white is also a useful technic. Even macerated biopsy tissue may be placed into India ink to observe for cells with capsules. Spinal fluid should be centrifuged and a part of the pellet or the sediment is placed on the slide with the drop of India ink, then a coverglass added. If the India ink is too dark, dilute to 50% with water. The right light intensity, usually low, is important for observing the cell and capsule in the slide under the microscope. The remainder of the pellet and the supernate should be used for isolation and for the latex agglutination test.

Microscopically, India ink mounts of the infected material should show round to oval thin-walled budding cells, ranging from 5 to 20 µm in diameter. The organisms are usually surrounded by wide refractile, polysaccharide, gelatinous capsules. Notice that the capsule may be more than twice as wide as the diameter of the cell (Figure 139). Buds develop at any point on the parent cell surface and are attached by a thin-walled, narrow pore. Occasionally more than one bud may develop at a time. All species of *Cryptococcus* may produce capsules except *C. luteolus.*

Culture: Sputum, spinal fluid, cisternal fluid, or urine may be cultured on Sabouraud glucose agar with antibacterial antibiotics. Capsule formation is enhanced in glucose medium in an atmosphere high in CO_2. Other excellent media for isolation are birdseed (niger seed) agar and caffeic acid agar which produce brown to black colonies (melanin pigments) within 5 days. Both media are useful for identification of *C. neoformans* at 37°C and for separation of other species of *Cryptococcus* which do not produce the specific brown pigment. Cycloheximide should not be used in the media as *C. neoformans* is inhibited.

The thistle (bird) seed agar was developed as a selective medium by Shields and Ajello (1966), for isolation of *C. neoformans* from heavily contaminated materials. This medium contains glucose, creatinine, chloramphenicol, diphenol, and an extract of thistle seed *Guizotia abyssinica.* (See page 40) Colonies of *Cryptococcus neoformans* assimilate creatinine and absorb the color from the seed extract, resulting in development of a brown-black color. Other species of *Cryptococcus* and *Candida* grow on this medium without the production of a brown color. L-dopa medium (see page 40) is also useful for checking brown-black color development.

Colonies: Colonies at room temperature or 37°C on Sabouraud glucose agar develop slowly and are mucoid, slimy, and cream to brown in color. Primary isolates at room temperature have small capsules, are wrinkled and granular in appearance and upon transfer become mucoid, and will run down a slant of medium (Figure 203). Colonies appear in a couple of days but mature in a couple of weeks.

Microscopically, India ink mounts of a portion of the colony will have thick-walled, ovoid to spherical budding cells up to 20 µm in diameter, with a gelatinous capsule surrounding the cells (Figure 204). The polysaccharide capsule varies in thickness, being up to twice the radius of the cell. In some primary isolates, capsules may not develop until the colony is transferred. No hyphae are present (except in rare cases).

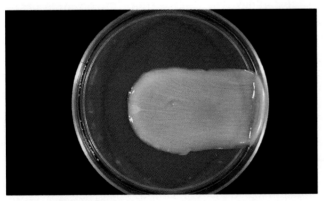

Figure 203. *Crptococcus neoformans,* colony

Perfect (Teleomorph) states: *Cryptococcus neoformans* has two perfect states: *Filobasdidiella neoformans* var *neoformans,* and *F. neoformans* var. *bacillispora.* When mating types a and *a* of serotype D of *F. neoformans* var *neoformans* are crossed on malt extract agar, V-8 juice or hay-infusion agar, conjugation occurs in submerged medium, and long hyphae develop with clamp connections and dolipore septa. Aerial hyphae and basidia are produced after about three weeks. The slender basidia are subglobose to flask-shaped at the apex and are nonseptate. Basidia pro-

duce sessile, slightly roughened or smooth, oval, pyriform, cylindrical to elliptical (1.8 to 3 by 2 to 5 µm) basidiospores by budding at four points on the apex. Basidiospores may form in chains. Crosses of A × D or A x A less readily produce the *Filobasidiella* state.

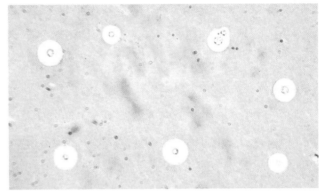

Figure 204. *Crptococcus neoformans* X400. Budding cells in India ink

The perfect state of *F. neoformans* var *bacillispora* is the same as for *F. neoformans* var *neoformans* except the basidiospores are rod-shaped (bacillary), 1 to 1.8 by 3 to 8 µm in size and smooth (Figure 205), when serologic strains B and C are crossed.

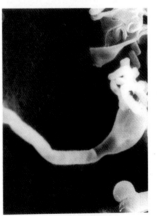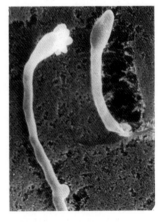

Figure 205. *F. neoformans var. bacillispora* Rod shaped basidiospores

In order to separate the two imperfect or perfect varieties of *Cryptococcus* or *Filobasidiella*, the colonies of *Cryptococcus* should be grown on Canavanine-glycine-bromthymol blue (CGB). No color changes occur on the CGB medium for *C. neoformans* var *neoformans*, while the medium changes to blue for *C. neoformans* var *gattii*.

Special tests for identification of species of Cryptococcus:

1   *Urease production.* All species of *Cryptococcus* are urease-positive, while other yeasts are urease-negative except *Trichosporon pullulans* and *Rhodotorula* spp. which are positive, with variable reactions in *T. cutaneum* and *Candida krusei.*

Table 16. Physiologic Characteristics of *Cryptococcus* Spp.*

	C. neoformans	C. albidus var. albidus	C. albidus var. diffluens	C. gastricus	C. laurentii	C. luteolus	C. terreus	C. unigatulatus
Growth at 37°C	+	0	0†	0	+	0	+	0
Nitrate assimilation	0	+	+	0	0	0	+	0
Urease test	+	+	+	+	+	+	+	+
Sugar assimilation								
Glucose	+	+	+	+	+	+	+	+
Maltose	+	+	+	+	+	+	+†	+
Sucrose	+	+	+	0†	+	+	0†	+
Lactose	0	+†	+	0	+	0	0†	0
Galactose	+†	0†	0†	+	+	+	+†	0†
Melibiose	0	0†	+†	0	+†	+	0	0
Cellobiose	+	+	+	+	+	+	+	0†
Inositol	+	+	+	+	+	+	+	+
Xylose	+	+	+	+	+	+	+	+
Raffinose	+	+	+	0	+	+	+	+
Trehalose	+	+†	+	+	+†	0†	0	+†
Melezitose	+	0†	0†	+	+	+	+	+†
Erythritol	0†	0†	0†	−	0†	+	0†	+
Ribitol	+	0†	0†	−	0†	0†	0†	−

*Fermentations are all negative for *Cryptococcus* spp.
†Variable reactions.
0 = negative, + = positive

Inoculate the surface of the urea agar (see page 44, media) with a loopful of a pure culture and incubate at 25° to 30°C for four days. A deep-red color throughout the medium indicates a positive reaction for urease.

2. *Rapid nitrate assimilation.* See page 42 for preparation of the medium. The tip of a swab containing medium is coated with yeasts by sweeping it over yeast colonies several times, and swirling against the bottom of the test tube to imbed the yeast cells into the swab. After incubation for 10 minutes at 45°C, the swab is inserted into a second tube containing two drops each of a-naphthylamine and sulfanilic acid (substitutes for these substances, see page 38). The swabs containing all nitrate positive yeasts turn a bright cherry red.

3. *Sugar assimilation.* Carbohydrate assimilation tests may be performed by one of the following methods: (1) auxanography (method on page 39) with several variations, as (a) inoculation of the medium by swabbing the surface of Wickerhams yeast nitrogen base or seeding the agar; (b) the addition of carbohydrates into wells, on impregnated disks, or as drops of concentrated solutions; and (c) the addition of pH indicators to the agar; (2) Wickerham and Burton (1948) broth technique; or (3) assimilation agar slant technique by Adams and Cooper (1974). Commercial kits are also available (API 20°C, Uniyeast Tek, BBl Minitek system, etc.). After inoc-

ulation, incubate at a temperature between 25° and 30°C for 24 to 72 hours or for 14 days if the tube method is used. Slants should be read every 24 hours.

The various physiologic tests are indicated in Table 16.

Histopathology: In tissue sections the organism can be demonstrated with hematoxylin and eosin stain. The most satisfactory stains for demonstrating the organisms are: periodic acid-Schiff (PAS) stain, Gomori methenamine-silver stain (GMS), Alcian blue stain, Gridley stain, or Mayer's mucicarmine stain. There is little tissue reaction around the capsules containing budding cells (Figure 201). Look for the budding cells in the various types of stained slides if available for study. See references for additional information on pathology of the disease.

Animal inoculation: *Cryptococcus neoformans* may be differentiated from other species by pathogenicity tests in mice. About 0.5 ml of infected material or a saline suspension of the culture should be injected intraperitoneally into the mouse. In two to four weeks, an autopsy of the intraperitoneally injected animal should show gelatinous masses in the visceral cavity, spleen involvement, and in more virulent strains, infection of the lung and brain. Pathogenicity for mice is correlated with capsular substance (Bulmer and Sans, 1967).

Make India ink preparations of the infected tissue or gelatinous mass and look for the typical budding cells with capsules. These mounts, not good after the ink dries, should be sterilized after use. Try to isolate the fungus from the lesions in the mouse or rat.

Intravenous route: Intravenous or intracerebral injection is a preferred route. An intravenous injection of 1×10^3 to 1×10^6 cells in the tail vein of a mouse is usually fatal after the mouse has 5×10^6 to 10^7 cells in a gram of brain tissue. The mouse usually develops lesions in the brain, lungs, and other organs. Death may occur in 10 to 14 days. Intravenous injection of rabbits produces an immediate fever response.

Intracerebral route: A suspension of a young culture (three to four days old), diluted 1:100 or containing about 100,000 cells per ml, is used for injection. Inoculate the mice intracerebrally with 0.02 to 0.04 ml of the suspension, using a 26-gauge needle. In one to two weeks the skull may become swollen, and at autopsy, the gelatinous material from the brain should show budding cells with capsules when put in a drop of India ink.

Serology: Recent works have developed diagnostically and prognostically useful tests. The following procedures for cryptococcal antibodies tests are: an indirect fluorescent antibody (IFA) technic, an enzyme immunoassay (EIA), and a tube agglutination (TA). Procedures for detecting cryptococcal antigens are: the latex agglutination (LA) test and the EIA test. The antibody tests are useful in the detection of either early or localized cryptococcosis and to determine prognosis, however the antigen tests are more specific. The EIA test takes several hours to run in contrast to several minutes for the LA test. The LA test is very specific and of diagnostic and prognostic value, thus is widely used (Kaufman, and Reiss, 1992).

The LA test has been successful in detecting cryptococcal antigens in the sera and in spinal fluid. This test is valuable in diagnosing active meningeal and nonmeningeal cryptococcosis, especially the former. The sensitivity of the LA test of approximately 92% from spinal fluids is greater than that of the India ink test for diagnosing cryptococcal meningitis. Sera from patients with severe rheumatoid arthritis may give a false-positive, otherwise incorrect tests are rare. In untreated patients a titer of 1:4 or lower is suggestive of cryptococcal infection. Higher titers of 8 or more indicates an active case of cryptococcosis. A further increase in the titer indicates progressive infection with a poor prognosis while a lowering of the titer indicates the patient is responding to chemotherapy and probable recovery. False positives have been reported in patients infected with *Trichosporon beigelii*.

1. Latex agglutination (LA) test (for antigens). The latex particles are coated with rabbit cryptococcal antiserum, which is the mixed with dilutions of serum or spinal fluid from a patient with suspected cryptococcosis. If the serum or spinal fluid has cryptococcal polysaccharide antigen, agglutination will occur. For details refer to Kaufman and Reiss (1992). Kits are available for this test: Crypto-LA (International Biological Laboratories, Rockville, MD); Immy (Immuno-Mycologics, Inc., Norman OK); Myco-Immune (Baxter-Microscan, W. Sacramento, CA), Enzyme immunoassay (Meridian Diagnostics, Inc., Cincinnati, OH); and Serodirect Eiken Cryptococcus (Eiken Chemical Co., Tokyo, Japan).

2. Indirect fluorescent antibody (IFA). This is a test for antibodies. The test involves antigens which are fixed to a slide and then covered with 1:16 dilution of heat-inactivated serum or spinal fluid. An antigen-antibody complex will form if antibodies are present in the fluids. These complexes are detected by the addition of fluorescein-labeled rabbit antihuman globulin that will react with the antibodies. For details see Palmer et al (1977). This test is of value for detecting early or localized cryptococcosis.

3. Tube agglutination (TA) test. This test is for *C. neoformans* antibodies. The test involves formalin-killed yeast cells in a concentration of 15×10^6, and heat inactivated serum set up in serial twofold dilutions. This is mixed and incubated at 37°C for two hours, and for 72 hours at 4°C. The highest dilution that has any agglutination is the titer. Positive and negative controls must be used. For details refer to Palmer, et al (1977). The TA test may be of prognostic value when the antigen titer declines, indicating effective chemotherapy.

DNA Probe. The commercially developed acridinium ester-labeled chemiluminescent DNA probe (Gen-Probe, CN probe, San Diego, CA) is available for *C. neoformans*. The sensitivity and specificity of the probe was determined by probing 100 isolates of *C. neoformans* (target) and 230 nontarget fungi. All 230 nontarget fungi were negative while 97 of the *C. neoformans* isolates were positive and after a retest the 3 remaining isolates were positive. This probe test is most useful for easy and rapid, accurate identification of this encapsulated yeast from a primary culture. The commercial kit from the manufacturer provides the methods for sample preparation and hybridization. See Laboratory procedures for more information on DNA Probes, page 45.

Important characteristics for identification: The organism produces capsules, buds, grows at 37°C, does not assimilate nitrates, is urease-positive, and produces a brown pigment in media containing either creatinine or caffeic acid. A closely related genus, *Rhodotorula*, may be distinguished from *Cryptococcus* by the usual carotenoid pigments and the inability to utilize inositol.

Questions

1. How does cryptococcosis differ from blastomycosis in tissue?

2. What are diagnostic characteristics that may be used to differentiate the virulent *Cryptococcus* from the non-virulent cryptococci?

3. Differentiate *C. neoformans* from *Saccharomyces cerevisiae* and *Rhodotorula* spp.

Selected References

Adams ED, Cooper BH. 1974. Evaluation of a modified Wickerham medium for identifying medically important yeasts. Am. J. Med. Tech. 40:377

Ajello L. 1958. Occurrence of *Cryptococcus neoformans* in soil. Am. J. Hyg. 67:72

Bennett JE, Kwon Chung KJ, Howard D. 1977. Epidemiologic differences among serotypes of *Cryptococcus neoformans*. Am. J. Epidemiol. 105:582

Bennett, JE, Kwon Chung KJ, Theodore T. 1978. Biochemical differences between serotypes of *Cryptococcus neoformans*. Sabouraudia 16:167

Berlin L, Pincus JH. 1989. Cryptococcal meningitis: false-negative antigen test results and cultures in nonimmunosuppressed patients. Arch. Neurol. 46:1312

Bulmer GS, Sans MD. 1967. *Cryptococcus neoformans*. II. Phagocytosis by human leukocytes. J. Bacteriol. 94:1480

Clancy MN, et al. 1990. Isolation of *Cryptococcus neoformans* var. *gattii* from a patient with AIDS in southern California. J. Infect. Dis. 161:809

Denning DW, Stevens DA, Hamilton JR. 1990. Comparison of *Guizotia abyssinica* seed extract (bird seed) agar with conventional media for selective identification of *Cryptococcus neoformans* in patients with acquired immunodeficiency syndrome. J. Clin. Microbiol. 23:2565

Denton JF, Di Saivo AF. 1968. The prevalence of *Cryptococcus neoformans* in various natural habitats. Sabouraudia 6:213

Ellis D, Pfeiffer TJ. 1990. Natural habitat of *Cryptococcus neoformans* var *gattii*. J. Clin. Microbiol. 28:1642

Emmons CW. 1955. Saprophytic sources of *Cryptococcus neoformans* associated with the pigeon(*Columbia livia*). Am. J. Hyg. 62:227

Fleming WH III, Hopkins JM, Land GA. 1977. New culture medium for the presumptive identification of *Candida albicans* and *Cryptococcus neoformans*. J. Clin. Microbiol. 5:236

Hamilton JR, et al. 1991. Performance of *Cryptococcus* antigen latex agglutination kits on serum and cerebrospinal fluid specimens of AIDS patients before and after pronase treatment. J. Clin. Microbiol. 29:333

Heelan J, Corpus L, Kessimian N. 1991. False-positive reactions in the latex agglutination test for *Cryptococcus neoformans* antigen. J. Clin. Microbiol. 29:1260

Hopfer RL, Blank E. 1975. Caffeic acid-containing medium for identification of *Cryptococcus neoformans*. J. Clin. Microbiol. 2:115

Huahua T, Rudy J, Kunin CM. 1991. Effect of hydrogen peroxide on growth of *Candida*, *Cryptococcus*, and other yeasts in simulated blood culture bottles. J. Clin. Microbiol. 29:328

Kao CJ, Schwarz J. 1957. The isolation of *Cryptococcus neoformans* from pigeon nests, with remarks on the identification of virulent cryptococci. Am. J. Clin. Pathol. 27:652

Kaufman L, Reiss E. 1992. Serodiagnosis of fungal diseases. *In* Rose NR, Friedman H (eds). *Manual of Clinical Immunology*. Am Soc Microbiol, 4th ed. Washington, DC Chap 78

Kaufman L, Cowart G, Blumer S, et al. 1974. Evaluation of a commercial latex agglutination test kit for cryptococcal antigen. Appl. Microbiol. 27:620

Khardori N, Butt F, Rolston KVI. 1988. Pulmonary cryptococcosis in AIDS. Chest. 93:1319

Kwon-Chung KJ. 1976. A new species of *Filobasidiella*, the sexual state of *Cryptococcus neoformans* B and C serotypes. Mycologia 68:942

Kwon-Chung KJ. 1976. Morphogenesis of *Filobasidiella neoformans*, the sexual state of *Cryptococcus neoformans*. Mycologia 68:821

Kwon-Chung KJ, Polacheck I, Benett JE. 1982. Improved diagnostic medium for separation of *Cryptococcus neoformans* var. *neoformans* (serotype A and D) and *Cryptococcus neoformans* var. *gattii* (serotype B and C). J. Clin. Microbiol. 15:535

Leggiadro RJ, Barrett FF, Hughes WT. 1992. Extrapulmonary cryptococcosis in immunocompromised infants and children. Ped. Infect. Dis. J. 11(1):43

Mrak EM, Phaff HJ, Douglas HC. 1942. A sporulation stock medium for yeasts and other fungi. Science 96:432

Malabonga VM, Basti J, Kamholz SL. 1991. Utility of Bronchoscopic sampling techniques for cryptococcal disease in AIDS. Chest. 99:370

Muchmore HG, Felton FG, Scott EN. 1978. Rapid presumptive identification of *Cryptococcus neoformans*. J. Clin. Microbiol. 8:166

Neilson JB, Fromtling RA, Bulmer GS. 1977. *Cryptococcus neoformans*. Size range of infectious particles from aerosolized soil. Infect. Immunol. 17:634

Pfeiffer T, Ellis D. 1991. Environmental isolation of *Cryptococcus neoformans gatti* from California. J. Infect. Dis. 163:929

Polacheck I, Kwon-Chung KJ. 1988. Melanogenesis in *Cryptococcus neoformans*. J. Gen. Microbiol. 134:1037

Porges DY, Krueger JG. 1992. A novel use of the cryptococcal latex agglutination test for rapid presumptive diagnosis of cutaneous cryptococcosis. Arch. Derm. 128:461

Prevost E, Neweil R. 1978. Commercial cryptococcai latex kit: Clinical evaluation in a medical center hospital. J. Clin. Microbiol. 8:529

Rodrigues de Miranda, L. 1984. *Cryptococcus* Kutzing emend. Phaff et Spencer. In The Yeasts: A Taxonomic Study. 3rd ed. Edited by N.J.W. Kreger-van Rij. Amsterdam. Elsevier Sci. Publ. p. 845

Ruiz A, Bulmer GS. 1981. Particle size of airborne *Cryptococcus neoformans* in a tower. Appl. Environ. Microbiol. 41:1225

Salkin IF, Hurd NJ. 1982. New medium for differentiation of *Cryptococcus neoformans* serotype pairs. J. Clin. Microbiol. 15169

Seeliger HP. 1956. Use of a urease test for the screening and identification of cryptococci. J Bacteriol 72:127

Shadomy HJ, Utz JP. 1966. Preliminary studies on a hypha-forming mutant of *Cryptococcus neoformans*. Mycologia 58:383

Shields AB, Ajello L. 1966. Medium for selective isolation of *Cryptococcus neoformans*. Science 151:208

Staib R, Mishra SK, Abel T, et al. 1976. Growth of *Cryptococcus neoformans* on uric acid agar. Zentral Bakteriol Parasitenkunde, Infektionskrankheiten Hygiene, IA 236:374

Stockman L, Clark KA, Hunt JM, Roberts GD. 1993. Evaluation of commercially available Acridinium Ester-Labeled Chemiluminescent DNA Probes for culture identification of *Blastomyuces dermatitidis*, *Coccidioides immitis*, *Cryptococcus neoformans* and *Histoplasma capsulatum*. J. Clin. Microbiol. 31:845

Swatek FE, Wilson JW, Omieczynski DT. 1967. Direct plate isolation method for *Cryptococcus neoformans* from the soil. Mycopath. Mycol. Appl. 32:129

Vogel RA. 1966. The indirect fluorescent antibody test for the detection of antibody in human cryptococcal disease. J. Infect. Dis. 116:573

Wickerham LJ, Burton KA. 1948. Carbon assimilation tests for the classification of yeasts. J. Bacteriol. 56:363

Yao JD, et al. 1990. Disseminated cryptococcosis diagnosed on peripheral blood smear in a patient with acquired immunodeficiency syndrome. Am. J. Med. 89:100

Yasin MS, et al. 1988. Laboratory isolation of *Cryptococcus albicus* from two cases of meningitis. Trop. Biomed. 5:145

MISCELLANEOUS YEAST INFECTIONS

1. *Malassezia* species

Definition

Normally the cause of tinea versicolor, *Malassezia* spp may cause catheter acquired fungemia in adults and especially in neonates while receiving intravenous lipid treatments. These patients may develop small embolic lesions in the lungs or other organs. On occasions *M. furfur* has been involved in peritonitis during chronic ambulatory peritoneal dialysis, in nipple discharge, or in sinusitis. In humans the infectious process of *M. pachydermatis* resembles that of *M. furfur*. The yeasts have been recovered from urine, cerebrospinal fluid, eye or ear discharges, trachial aspirate, blood, and vaginal swabs.

Etiologic agents

Malassezia furfur (Robin) Baillon, 1889 and *M. pachydermatis* Weidman 1925.

Laboratory Procedures

See chapter 4, page 54 on procedures for examination of clinical material, culture, and microscopic characteristics of *M. furfur* and *M. pachydermatis*. Most routine culture media are not adequate to detect the causative agent unless the surface of the Sabouraud glucose agar with chloramphenicol and cycloheximide is covered with a thin layer of sterile olive oil after inocation with specimens. Incubation should be at 37°C for 7 to 14 days. In contrast to *M. furfur*, *M. pachydermatis* grows readily on Sabouraud glucose agar without oil in 8 to 10 days, varying in shape and size. The cells are globose-to ellipsoidal, with the small cells measuring 2.5 to 4.8 by 2.5 to 5 μm, and the large cells measure 3.8 to 6 by 4.8 to 7 μm.

2. *Trichosporonosis*

Definition

In addition to being the causative agent of white piedra in the hair shaft, *Trichosporon beigelii* may colonize or cause disseminated infections in immunosuppressed patients. *Trichosporon* infections have been more frequently associated with leukemia, and less frequent in immunosuppressed patients with aplastic anemia, lymphoma, multiple myeloma, organ transplantation, AIDS and solid tumors. Other nonimmunosuppressed patients have developed trichosporonosis associated with complications after cataract extraction, intravenous drug abuse, endocarditis after insertion of prosthetic cardiac valves, chronic ambulatory peritoneal dialysis, and septicemia in a renal transplant patient.

Etiologic agent

Trichosporon beigelii (Kuchenmeister et Rabenhorst) Vuillemin 1902, is the only species known to cause deep or disseminated trichosporonosis in humans.

Laboratory Procedures

Culture: See chapter 4 for more information on *T. beigelii*. Isolates from invasive clinical isolates produce two different colony types: a white powdery and white-rugose types. The powdery type has mostly budding yeasts and arthroconidia while the rugose type contains mostly hyphae on Emmon's modified Sabouraud glucose agar. Both types will change to smooth, gray colonies. This species does not ferment carbohydrates. The carbohydrates assimilated are glucose, lactose, maltose, xylose, and cellobiose. *T. beigelii* produces urease.

Microscopically the arthroconidia are rectangular in shape with rounded ends and the budding cells are spherical to oblong (3.5 to 7 by 3.5 to 14 μm in size).

In tissue the hyphae are 1.5 to 2.5 μm wide with small colonies frequently found in tissue. Occasionally hyphae and pseudohyphae are found (Figure 206).

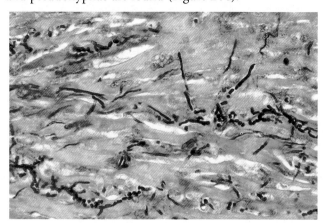

Figure 206. Trichosporonosis in tissue

3.   *Rhodotorula* Harrison

Definition: Infection with *Rhodotorula* species is not com-

mon at present. Case reports include fungemia, peritonitis, endocarditis, ventriculitis, and meningitis. Fungemia is more frequently found in patients with cancer, bacterial endocarditis and various debilitating disease with the indwelling intravenous catheters and chemotherapy for cancer.

Etiologic agent:

Rhodotorula rubra (Denne) Lodder 1934 (Synonym: *Rhodotortula mucilaginosa* Jorgensen) Harrison, 1928. The only species in humans is *R. rubra.* The other 7 species do not infect humans.

Laboratory Procedures

Rhodotorula rubra: See chapter 4 for more information on the culture. The colonies are deep coral to red or pink on mycological media.

This species assimilates glucose +, L-sorbose ±, sucrose +, maltose +, cellobiose ±, galactose ±, trehalose +, lactose -, melezitose ±, inositol -, D-xylose +, soluble starch -, raffinose +, and ethanol ±. Nitrate or nitrite are not assimilated.

4.   *Saccharomyces* Meyen ex Reess.

Definition

Saccharomyces cerevisiae, an ascomycetous yeast, has been reported in cases of fungemia, endocarditis, peritonitis, meningitis, ventriculitis, and with polymicrobial fatal pneumonia in AIDS patients.

Etiological agent

Other species of *Saccharomyces* may occur as normal flora in humans but *S. cerevisiae* is the only species involved in cases of infection.

Laboratory Procedures

The clinical specimens should be isolated on routine mycological media. See chapter 4 for information and illustrations of the yeast.

S. cerevisiae assimilates glucose +, maltose +, sucrose +, lactose -, galactose +, melibiose -, cellobiose -, inositol -, xylose -, raffinose +, trehalose ±.

5.   *Protothecosis* (hyaline algae)

Definition

Protothecosis is a rather rare infection in humans caused by species of *Prototheca.* The chronic localized infections occur as skin lesions, olecranon bursitis, and in the soft tissue infections located at the site of surgery or trauma in the extremity of the body. The species of *Prototheca* which are hyaline achlorophyllous algae are included with the yeast mycoses.

Etiologic agents

The two pathogenic species are: *Prototheca wickerhamii* Tubaki et Soneda, 1959, and *P. zopfii* Kruger, 1894.

Laboratory Procedures

Prototheca species grow readily on Sabouraud glucose agar and other mycologic media without cycloheximide. The colonies develop rapidly from skin scrapings or biopsy sections of infected lymph nodes, liver, lungs, or peritoneum for histologic study.

Culture:

P. wickerhamii Tubaki et Soneda, 1959, develops a moist, cream-colored yeast colony on Sabouraud glucose agar at 25° or 37°C. Thiamine is required for growth. *P. wickerhamii* assimilates glucose, galactose, glycerol, mannose, and ethanol, but sucrose is -. The spherical to ellipsoidal cells are 2 to 11 μm in diameter or smaller than *P. zopfii*. The thecae (sporangia) are 5.4 to 10.8 by 5.4 to 13.4 with up to 50 autospores (endospores) developed inside. *P. wickerhamii* develops a zone of inhibition around a 50 μm clotrimazole disk.

P. zopfii Kruger, 1894 produces a dull, white yeast colony at 25° to 37°C. Thiamine is required for growth and cycloheximide is inhibitory. This species assimilates glucose, galactose, levulose, ethanol, and n-propanol. The cells are spherical to elliptical and 9 to 11 μm in diameter. The thecae (sporangia) of *P. zopfii* (Figure 207) are larger, ranging from 8 to 16 by 10.8 to 22.3 μm, with more autospores than *P. wickerhamii*.

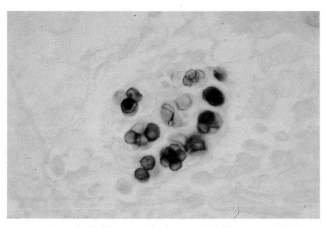

Figure 207. Thecae and autospores of *P. zopfii* in skin

6. Other yeasts

Blastoschizomyces capitatus (Didd. et Lood.) Salkin et al. 1985 (Synonym: *Trichosporon capitatum* Didens et Lodder, 1942).

A number of histologically proven cases due to this yeast include: neutropenic cases from leukemia or bone marrow transplantation for aplastic anemia, and other patients with an infected prosthetic valve, intravenous drug abuse, ovarian carcinoma, and bacterial wound infection.

Sarcinosporon inkin King et Jong (Synonym: *Trichosporon inkin*). Cases involve a scrotal dermatosis and a progressive pneumonia. The cells in tissue resemble *Prototheca* cells and sclerotic cells of chromoblastomycosis.

Hansenula anomala: This yeast developed in cases of fungemia from central venous catheters, nosocomial cerebral ventriculitis, and a urinary tract infection in a renal transplant recipient. Many cases were in neonates.

Other yeasts include: *Kluyveromyces marsianus*, *Debaryomyces hansenii*, *Pichia farinosa*, and *Sporobolomyces*.

For more detailed information on about 500 species of yeasts reference should be made to Kreger-van Rij (1984).

Selected References

Aucott JN, et al. 1990. Invasive infection with *Saccharomyces cerevisiae*: report of three cases and review. Rev. Infect. Dis. 12:406

Donald FE, et al. 1988. *Rhodotorula rubra* ventriculitis. J. Infect. 16:187

Doyle MG, et al. 1990. *Saccharomyces cerevisiae* infection in a patient with acquired immunodeficiency syndrome. Pediatr. Infect. Dis. J. 9:850

Gibb AP, Aggarwal R, Swanson CP. 1991. Successful treatment of *Prototheca* peritonitis complicating continuous ambulatory peritoneal dialysis. J. Infect. 22:183

Henwick S, et al. 1992. Disseminated neonatal *Trichosporon beigelii*. Pediatr. Infect. Dis. J. 11:50

Kenny RT, et al. 1990. Invasive infection with *Sarcinosporon inkin* in a patient with chronic granulomatous disease. Am. J. Clin. Pathol. 94:344

Kreger-van Rij NJW. (Ed.) 1984. The Yeasts: A Taxonomic Study. 3rd ed. Amsterdam, Elsevier Science Publishers

Larocco M, et al. 1988. Recovery of *Malassezia pachydermatis* from eight infants in a neonatal intensive care nursery: clinical and laboratory features. Ped. Infect. Dis. J. 7:398

Marcon MJ, Powell DA. 1992. Human infections due to *Malassezia* spp. Clin. Microbiol. Rev. 5:101

Sethi N, Mandell W. 1988. *Saccharomyces* fungemia in a patient with AIDS. NY State J. Med. 88:278

Tyring SK, et al. 1989. Papular protothecosis of the chest. Immunologic evaluation and treatment with a combination of oral tetracycline and topical amphotericin. B. Arch. Derm. 125:1249

Walsh TJ, et al. 1990. *Trichosporon beigelii,* an emerging pathogen resistant to amphotericin. B. J. Clin. Microbiol. 28:1616

Chapter 9

OPPORTUNISTIC INFECTIONS— MYCELIAL FUNGI

The opportunistic mycelial fungal infections include: aspergillosis, basidiomycosis, geotrichosis, hyalohyphomycosis, keratomycosis, pseudallescheriasis, penicilliosis marneffei, pythiosis, and zygomycosis.

The etiologic agents of hyalohyphomycosis normally occurring as ubiquitous saprophytes of soil, decomposing organic matter and growing on laboratory media as contaminants have in recent years become involved in clinical diseases as primary or secondary opportunistics mostly in the immunocompromised patients. This group of fungi develop in the tissue form as hyaline, septate mycelial elements that may be branched, and rarely toruloid. The term hyalohyphomycosis currently does not replace well established disease names such as adiaspiromycosis, pseudallescheriasis and aspergillosis. Until the many hundreds of filamentous fungi reported as causative agents of hyalohyphomycosis are reported more regularly in the future, these fungi are included together in this category. When these rarely reported fungal agents become more frequent in occurrence as etiologic agents, then these fungi will be assigned to a specific disease. Some of the well-established hyaline Hyphomycetes more frequently encountered in clinical specimens will be discussed in more detail, while the more rare fungal agents and unusual causative agents of hyalophomycosis will be listed in a table.

ASPERGILLOSIS

Definition

Aspergillosis is the name applied to any mycosis caused by a species of *Aspergillus*. The disease may be a localized infection involving the nail, foot (mycetoma), external auditory canal, or eye (Figure 208). Toxicity due to ingesting fungal-contaminated foods; may produce an allergic response, such as asthma or bronchopulmonary aspergillosis; may occur with colonization of the fungus in body cavities, also known as fungus ball, or aspergilloma; may develop into invasive granulomatous disease of the lungs; or may

develop into disseminated systemic infections in debilitated individuals or following extended use of antibiotics or steroids, a condition that usually is fatal unless treated.

Aspergillus has become increasingly important as an opportunist in severely debilitated patients with altered host defenses including leukemia, lymphoma, organ transplants, and bone marrow transplant patients. In cattle, abortion is an important symptom, while in birds, the disease frequently involves the air sacs.

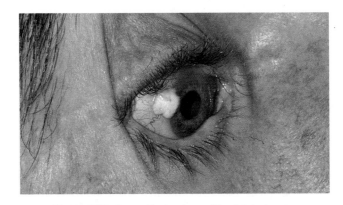

Figure 208. Aspergillosis, *Aspergillus fumigatus,* eye

Etiologic Agents

Aspergillus fumigatus Fresenius, 1850, is the most commonly isolated species in invasive and noninvasive aspergillosis. The second most common species is *A. flavus,* which is most likely to be isolated from invasive aspergillosis of immunosuppressed patients, and from nasal sinuses. The third most common agent of invasive pulmonary aspergillosis is *A. niger.* The former two species and *A. niger* are the most likely species to produce a "fungus ball" (aspergilloma). The fourth most common species to produce disease is *A. terreus.* Other species from aspergillosis cases are: *A. amstelodami, A. candidus, A. carneus, A. flavipes, A nidulans, A. neveus, A. ochraceus, A. oryzae, A. repens, A. restrictus, A. sydowi, A. ustus,* and *A. versicolor.*

Occurrence

Species of *Aspergillus* are commonly found in soil, farm homes, stables, barns, grain dust, and decaying vegetation. Threshing areas and mills for grinding grain have high concentrations of conidia.

Humans: Aspergillosis is found in all parts of the world. Reports of the disease as a secondary infection have increased following (1) prolonged antibiotic and corticosteroid treatments, (2) debilitating diseases such as organ transplants, tuberculosis, leukemia, bone marrow transplants, cytotoxin use, and AIDS, (3) injuries to the subcutaneous tissue and skin or cornea of the eye, and (4) prolonged exposure to cereal grains heavily contaminated with spores of species of *Aspergillus*.

Animals: Cow, horse, sheep, pig, cat, dog, rabbit, bison, deer, goat, monkey, and guinea pig. The birds include: budgerigar, canary, cormorant, duck, flamingo, goose, grouse, hawk, jay, ostrich, owl, parrot, peafowl, penguin, pheasant, pigeon, rook, seagull, sparrow, stork, swan, thrush, turkey, and chicken.

Laboratory Procedures

Specimen collection: Sputum, sinus drainage, or bronchial washings should be collected in a sterile container for laboratory identification. Skin and debris from the ear can be collected in the same manner as that given for the dermatomycoses and otomycosis. Repeated samples should be taken, in case of doubt, to try to eliminate the possibility of a contaminate in direct mounts and in culture. Biopsied material from invasive aspergillosis should be used for direct examination of small pieces microscopically and for culturing in addition to histological studies.

Direct examination: Drops of sputum, sinus drainage, or bronchial washings should be placed on a slide with a coverglass and examined under the microscope. It is important to find hyphae by direct examination of fresh clinical material to demonstrate clinic significance. In invasive aspergillosis ("fungus ball") cases hyphae are not likely to be seen in sputum. Small portions of biopsy material should be examined by mounting the material on a slide in 10% KOH along with 1 drop of fountain pen ink, then dissected with needles before being flattened and covering with a coverglass. The KOH will aid in digestion and clearing of the material around the fungus. Granulomatous lesions should be crushed in 10% KOH. The use of calcofluor white will enhance the appearance of the fungus on the slide.

Microscopically, the fungus appears as fragments of

dichotomously branched, septate hyphae, 4 to 6 μm in diameter as illustrated under histology (Figure 209). If conidiophores develop (aspergilloma) when sufficient oxygen and space is present in cavitary pulmonary cases for growth of these structures, it is possible to identify *A. fumigatus* in such preparations.

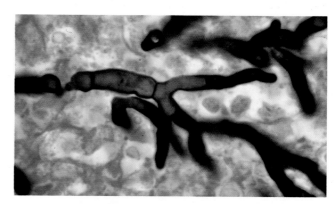

Figure 209. Aspergillosis, hyphae in lung. Gomori methenamine-silver stain. X1800

Culture: Colonies of *Aspergillus fumigatus* can be isolated readily on Sabouraud glucose agar or many media for fungi at temperatures of 30° to 37°C (up to 45°C for *A. fumigatus*), with antibacterial substances but not with cycloheximide. For surgical biopsy from an immunosuppressed patient the specimen should be put on media without any antibiotics to allow for isolation of *Nocardia* sp., and fungal opportunists. They develop rapidly as white filamentous growths on the surface of the medium, soon becoming green or gray-green in color (Figure 210). Conidiophores develop within 48 to 72 hours at temperatures of 30° to 37°C. Species identification is aided by preparing a slide culture for microscopic study of the conidiophores, vesicles, phialides (sterigmata), vesicles and conidial mass arrangement. Czapek agar is the medium of choice for identification of the species in case of doubt. Other species of *Aspergillus* that may develop may be identified by referring to Figure 217 in this section or Raper and Fennell's The Genus Aspergillus.

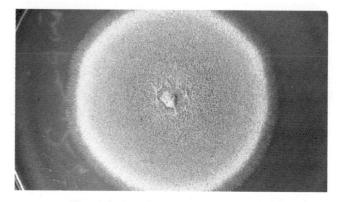

Figure 210. *Aspergillus fumigatus*, colony

Microscopically, all species of *Aspergillus* will show conidiophores with large terminal vesicles bearing many phialides which produce long chains of conidia. The conidiophores may be observed by placing the slant on the side underneath the low-power objective of the microscope. Slide cultures will show the undisturbed arrangement of chains of conidia. A direct mount from a colony may be made by cutting a thin sliver through the area where conidiophores are forming, placing this sliver on a slide with a drop of 70% alcohol, evaporating most of the alcohol, and adding a drop of lactophenol cotton blue and a coverglass. Slide cultures may be mounted for a study of the conidiophores. The **conidiophores** develop directly from a specialized foot cell in the vegetative hyphae and terminate in a bulbous head, the **vesicle**. The vesicle may be globose, hemispherical clavate or flask-shaped, covered or partially covered with a row of flask-shaped conidiogenous cells called **phialides**. The phialides may be in a single row (**uniserate**) around the vesicle or on a secondary row of *phialides* (**biseriate**) or a combination of both (as in *A. flavus*). The phialides develop long chains of conidia at their tips. The conidia are globose to subglobose with a variation in size, color, and wall texture, depending upon the species. Figure 211 shows the variations in the bulbous tip of the conidiophores. The four most commonly isolated species are described below. Table 17 has a comparison of the characteristics of these four species.

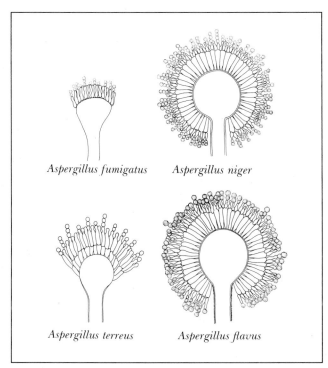

Figure 211. Conidiophores of uniseriate (*A. fumigatus*) and biseriate (*A. niger, A. terreus,* and *A. flavus*) aspergilli. (Reprinted with permission from J. W. Rippon.)

Aspergillus fumigatus Fresemius, 1863.

Characteristics of the species: *A. fumigatus* has a smooth-walled conidiophore up to 300 µm in length by 5 to 8 µm in diameter. The tip enlarges into a typical flask-shaped vesicle up to 30 µm in diameter. Phialides are in one series, uniserate, on the upper half of the vesicle with gray-green, round, usually echinulate conidia, 2.5 to 3 µm in diameter (Figure 212). The above characteristics, the bending of the phialides upward to produce a columnar mass of conidia, and the green to gray-green, dark-gray in older colonies are typical of the species (Figure 213). No cleistothecia with ascospores occur in this species. This species grows well at 45°C.

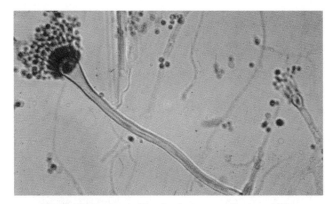

Figure 212. *Aspergillus fumigatus,* conidiophore X400

Aspergillus terreus Thom, 1918.

A. terreus produces smooth-walled conidiophores up to 250 µm in length. The vesicle is hemispherical or dome-like, up to 16 µm in diameter, with two series of phialides. The conidial heads are columnar with elliptical to nearly globose, smooth-walled conidia which are 1.8 to 2.4 µm in diameter. The colonies vary from brown to cinnamon in color (Figure 215).

Aspergillus flavus Link, 1809.

A. flavus develops thick-walled, nonpigmented, roughened conidiophores up to 1 mm in length. The globose to subglobose vesicle is up to 10 to 65 µm in diameter with phialides in one or two series. The globose conidia are 3.5 to 4.5 µm in diameter, with walls smooth to echinulate. The spore heads are radiate, splitting into loose columns with a deep-yellow to yellow-green colony color (Figure 214). Sclerotia may be produced.

Aspergillus niger Van Tieghem, 1867.

A. niger has smooth, colorless conidiophores up to 1.5 to 3.0 mm in length that have dark-colored walls near the vesicle. The globose vesicle is about 45 to 75 µm in diameter, phialides in two series, and brownish in color. The conidia are globose, 4 to 5 µm in diameter, thick, rough-walled with a brown to black color. The surface mycelium is white to yellow with the black mass of conidia on the colony (Figure 216). The conidial head radiates and at times splits into columns.

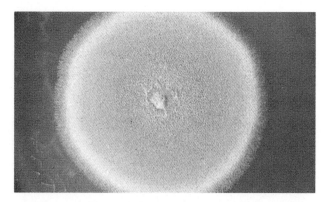

Figure 213. *A. fumigatus,* colony

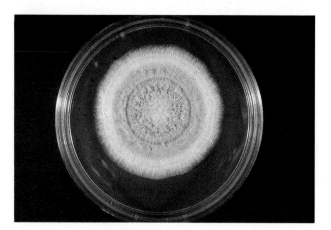

Figure 214. *A. flavus,* colony

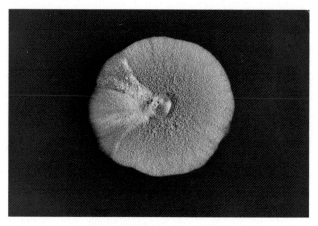

Figure 215. *A. terreus,* colony

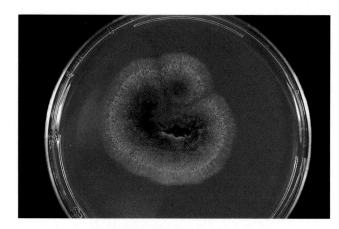

Figure 216. *A. niger,* conidiophore

The four most commonly isolated species and others are listed on the Table 17 to aid in tentative identification of the species.

A key for identification of some species of *Aspergillus.* See flow diagram, Figure 217. For tentative identification of unusual species, reference should be made to Raper and Fennell's The Genus Aspergillus (Raper and Fennell, 1965) for more detailed information.

Histopathology: In bronchial aspergillosis the fungus grows readily in the bronchial mucosa. Conidia and conidiophores may be present. The dichotomous branched hyphae are 3 to 4 µm in diameter with branches and septation. In disseminated lesions the fungus occurs in various locations, including brain, liver, kidney (Figure 218), myocardium, bone, and skin. In the lungs necrosis, inflammatory-cell infiltration and granulomatous reaction occur. Colony like formation may appear at first, later terminated by dichotomous branching. In chronic cases isolated lesions are walled off like a tubercle, the center becomes necrotic, forming a cavity where conidiophores and conidia may develop.

If material from a biopsy from humans, or granulomatous gray to yellow nodules from birds, is available, stained sections may be made for study of the histopathologic changes. The fungus can be demonstrated with Gridley, PAS, GMS, and usually H and E stains. Figures 219 and 209 illustrate the characteristic hyphae of aspergillosis in tissue. In tissue sections the hyphae are hyaline, septate, 3 to 6 µm in diameter, branched dichotomously at acute angles with smooth parallel walls.

Animal inoculation: Animal inoculation is not necessary for the identification of *A. fumigatus* or other species of *Aspergillus.* Experimental infections can be produced in newly hatched birds by exposing them to spores, which results in rapid infection in the air sacs. Pigeons were

Table 17. Characteristics of the four most commonly isolated species of *Aspergillus*

Group and organism	Colony color	Conidiophore	Vesicle	Seriation Uni	Bi	Conidial head	Conidia	Cleistothecia	Hülle cells	Comment
Fumigatus group *A. fumigatus*	White to green; slate gray with age; reverse side variable in color	Length, up to 300 µm); width 5-8 µm; smooth walled; greenish especially in upper portion	Dome shaped; conidiophore gradually enlarges, merging into vesicle; 20-30 µm in diameter; phialides on upper half only, with axes parallel to that of the conidiophore	+		Strongly columnar, compact	Globose to subglobose, elliptical in some isolates; echinulate to rarely smooth; most are 2.5-3.0 µm in diameter			Grows well at 45°C; one of the most commonly occurring moulds in nature; most common human pathogen
Flavus group *A. flavus*	Yellow to yellowish green to green with age	Length, 400-850 µm (rarely to 2.5 mm): uncolored; thick walled; coarsely roughened	Elongate, becoming subglobose to globose; 10-65 (commonly 25-45) µm in diameter	+	+	Radiate, splitting into columns with age	Globose; smooth to echinulate; 3-6 (most are 3.5-4.5) µm in diamter			Some strains produce toxins; enhanced at 37°C; small uniseriate vesicles; often produces dark-brown to black sclerotia; common human pathogen
Niger group *A. niger*	White, becoming black; reverse side occasionally pale yellow	Length, 1.5-3.0 mm; width, 15-20 µm; smooth walls; colorless with brownish shade on upper half	Globose; most are 45-75 µm in diameter		+	Globose, then radiate, splitting into columns with age	Globose; thick walls; brown; irregularly roughened; most are 4-5 µm in diameter			Frequent cause of otomycosis; sometimes associated with colonization of cavities
Terreus group *A. terreus*	Cinnamon buff to brown, rarely orange-brown	Length, 100-250 µm; width 4.5-6 µm; flexous; smooth walled; colorless	Hemispherical or domelike, merging into conidiophore; 10-16 µ, in diameter	+		Long, columnar; uniform in diameter through-out length	Globose to slightly elliptical; smooth; 1.8-2.4 µm in diameter			May form single globose conidia on submerged hyphae (aleurio-conidia, 6-7 µm)
				+						

(Swatek, et al., 1985)

Figure 217. Flow Diagram for the tentative identification of *Aspergillus* spp. commonly isolated from clinical specimens. From Rhodes JC, and Kwon-Chung KJ: Identification of agents of systemic mycoses and Clinical Mycology. Edited by Evans EGV, and Richardson, MD Oxford, I.R.L. Press.

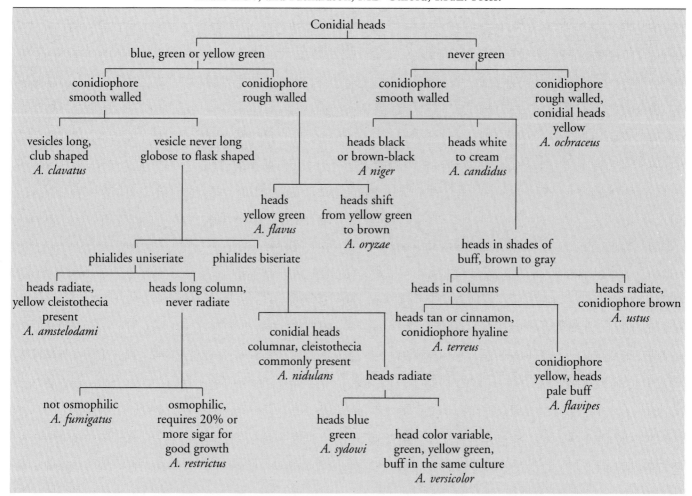

infected by Henrici (1939) when fed moldy grain. Intravenous injection of a small number of spores in pigeons produced tubercles in various organs.

will produce lesions in the brain and kidney. If mice receive steroids, then spores are injected, a fulminating disseminated aspergillosis develops.

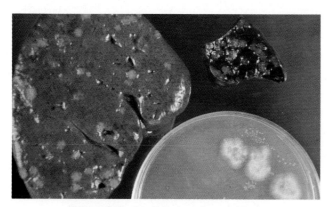

Figure 218. Candidiasis and aspergillosis, kidney and liver tissue

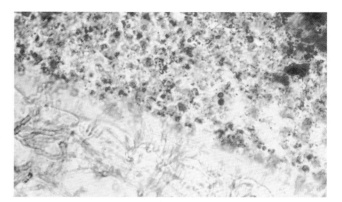

Figure 219. Aspergillosis, *Aspergillus fumigatus*, eye tissue, methenamine-silver stain X400

In rabbits, intravenous injection of a spore suspension will produce granulomatous lesions in internal organs, especially the kidneys. Intravenous injection of the spores in mice

Toxins: Endotoxins produced by *A. fumigatus* are apparently of importance in the acute hemorrhagic lesions that develop when numerous spores are present in birds and animals. It may be the cause of abortions in cattle and sheep.

A potent toxin, aflatoxin, is produced by *A. flavus* on peanuts and grain. This is of concern when eaten by humans or animals, but is not a component of the invasive disease process. Many problems are arising from toxins developed in storage of various grains for feeds. Fungi such as species of *Aspergillus* and many other species of the Deuteromycota are of concern. Further current information is listed under mycotoxicoses in the Review of Medical and Veterinary Mycology and in the books on mycotoxins.

Serology and Immunology: The immunodiffusion (ID) test has been especially useful for aspergillosis. Many researchers have reported that the ID test is an effective and specific method for the diagnosis of aspergillosis in patients with the immune systems intact (Kaufman and Reiss, 1992). The ID or micro ID test is performed with reference antigens of several species of *Aspergillus* (*A. fumigatus, A. flavus,* and *A. niger*) reference antisera, agar gel and patient's serum. Details may be found in Kaufman and Reiss (1992). One or more precipitin bands of identity by patient's serum with a reference serum and antigens indicate a positive reaction. A simple weak band may occur in sera from asthmatic patients. Three or more bands may occur in allergic aspergillosis with colonization of the bronchi and a maximum of 18 bands may appear in cases of aspergilloma (fungus ball). Invasive aspergillosis may show a few bands or none, as these patients have a defective immune system. Nonidentity lines should be investigated, as they would be due to the patient's C-reactive protein band, and may be eliminated by soaking the agar in a 5% sodium citrate solution for 45 minutes before the final reading.

For patients suspected of having invasive aspergillosis with serum negative for antibody, antigenemia tests should be carried out to attempt to obtain a specific antemortem diagnosis. Antigenemia in aspergillosis has been detected by counterimmunoelectrophoresis (CIE) and by radioimmunoassay (RIA).

Sources of commercial test kits for aspergillosis include: Greer Laboratories Inc., Lenoir, NC; Hollister-Stier Laboratories, Spokane, WA; Immuno-Mycologics Inc., Norman, OK; Meridian Diagnostics Inc., Cincinnati, OH; and M. A. Bioproducts, Walkersville, MD.

Questions

1. In what ways are *Aspergillus* and *Mucor* similar in tissue? Are there any differences?

2. Why is caution necessary in determining whether species of *Aspergillus* are pathogenic when these fungi are isolated in culture?

3. How does the shape of the vesicle of *A. fumigatus* differ from all other species of *Aspergillus?* What other characteristics of the conidiophore and conidia are used in determining species of *Aspergillus?*

4. Explain under what conditions aspergillosis may be considered a secondary infection rather than a primary infection.

Selected References

Aufauvre-Brown A, Cohen J, Holden DW. 1992. Use of randomly amplified polymorphic DNA markers to distinguish isolates of *Aspergillus fumigatus.* J. Clin. Microbiol. 30:2991

Austwick PK, Venn JA. 1961. Mycotic abortion in England and Wales 1954-1960. Proc. IVth Inter. Cong. On Reprod. The Hague, pp. 562-568

Baldo, L. 1992. Mortalita deitacchini in seguito ad un grave episodio di aspergillosi. Praxis Vet. (Milano). 13:25

Campbell G. 1972. Aspergillosis in captive penguins. Vet. Serv. Bull. Dept. Agr. Fish. [Dublin] 2:39

Chang ZN, et al. 1991. Allergenic components of *Aspergillus fumigatus* determined by radioimmunoprecipitation. J. Asthma 28:213

Coleman RM, Kaufman L. 1972. Use of immunodiffusion test in the serodiagnosis of aspergillosis. Appl. Microbiol. 23:301

Cox JN, et al. 1990. *Aspergillus* endocarditis and myocarditis in a patient with the acquired immunodeficiency syndrome (AIDS). Virchows Arch. (A) 417:255

Eggert MJ, Barnhart JV. 1953. A case of eggborne aspergillosis. J. Am. Vet. Med. Assoc. 122:225

Eisenberg HW. 1970. Aspergillosis with aflatoxicosis. New Engl. J. Med. 283:1348

Emmons CW. 1962. Natural occurrences of opportunistic fungi. Lab. Invest. 11:1026

Fairley CK, et al. 1991. Invasive aspergillosis in AIDS. Australian and N. Zealand J. Med. 21(5):747

Ford S, Friedman L. 1967. Experimental study of the pathogenicity of *Aspergilli* for mice. J. Bact. 94:928

Gray RL, et al. 1986. Aortic pseudoaneurysm with Aspergillus aortitis: an unusual complication of coronary by-pass surgery. Chest. 89:306

Hara K, et al. 1989. Disseminated *Aspergillus terreus* infection in immunocompromised hosts. May Clin. Proc. 64:770

Kaufman L, Reiss E. 1992. Serodiagnosis of fungal diseases. *In* Rose NR, et al. (eds). 4th ed. Manual of Clinical Immunology. Am. Soc. Microbiol. Ch 78

Kobayashi G. 1978. Fractionation of *Aspergillus* antigens. J. Aller. Clin. Immnunol. 61:230

Kurup VP, Fink JN. 1978. Evaluation of methods to detect antibodies against *Aspergillus fumigatus.* Am. J. Clin. Pathol. 69:414

Levy H, et al. 1992. The value of bronchoalveolar lavage and bronchial washings in the diagnosis of invasive pulmonary aspergillosis. Respir. Med. 86:243

Mahvi TA, Webb HM, Dixon CD, et al. 1968. Systemic aspergillosis by *Aspergillus niger* after open-heart surgery. J. Am. Med. Assoc. 203:520

Moore CK, et al. 1988. *Aspergillus terreus* as a cause of invasive pulmonary aspergillosis. Chest. 94:889

Pakes SP, New AE, Benbrook SC. 1967. Pulmonary aspergillosis in a cat. J. Am. Vet. Med. Assoc. 151:950

Paradise AJ, Roberts L. 1963. Endogenous ocular aspergillosis: Report of a case in an infant with cytomegalic inclusion disease. Arch. Ophthal. 69:765

Pepys J, et al. 1959. Clinical and immunologic significance of *Aspergillus fumigatus* in the sputum. Am. Rev. Resp. Dis. 80:167

Philips P, Radigan G. 1989. Antigenemia in a rabbit model of invasive aspergillosis. J. Infect. Dis. 159:1147

Raper KB, Fennell DL. 1965. The Genus *Aspergillus.* Williams and Wilkins Co., Baltimore.

Rowen JL, et al. 1992. Invasive aspergillosis in neonates. Report of five cases and literature review. Pediatric Infect. Dis. J. 11:576

Sabetta JR, Miniter P, Andriole VT. 1985. The diagnosis of invasive aspergillosis by an enzyme-linked immunosorbent assay for circulating antigen. J. Infect. Dis. 152:946

Samson RA, 1979. A compilation of the Aspergilli described since 1965. Stud. Mycol. 18:1

Sherertz RJ, et al. 1989. Impact of air filtration on nosocomial *Aspergillus* infections: unique risk of bone marrow transplant recipients. Am. J. Med. 83:709

Smith GR. 1972. Experimental aspergillosis in mice: Aspects of resistance. J. Hygiene 70:741

Wang JL, Patterson R, Rosenberg M, et al. 1978. Serum IgE and IgG antibody activity against *Aspergillus fumigatus* as a diagnostic aid in allergic bronchopulmonary aspergillosis. Am. Rev. Resp. Dis. 117:917

Witter JF, Chute HL. 1952. Aspergillosis in turkeys. J. Am. Vet. Med. Assoc. 21:387

Wogan GN (ed). 1964. *Mycotoxins in Foodstuffs.* MIT Press, Cambridge, MA

HYALOHYPHOMYCOSIS

There are many hundreds of fungi in the Hyphomycetes that are causative agents of hyalohyphomycosis that pro-duce hyaline hyphae in tissues of immunocompromised and other debilitated patients. These opportunistic fungi normally are not considered pathogens except when invasions occur in immunocompromised or other compromised hosts and then they are the etiologic agents of the disease. In such cases it is important to correlate the culture with the presence of hyaline hyphae in tissue from the patients.

The mycoses encompassed in the hyalohyphomycosis group are very heterogeneous with only the presence of hyaline hyphae in tissue as a common characteristic. Technically this group could include aspergillosis, basidiomycosis, keratinomycosis, pseudallescheriasis, and a few other diseases. However, these well established names will be considered separately from the hyalohyphomycosis group.

Table 18 contains a list of the most currently known agents of aspergillosis and hyalohyphomycosis as the more important causes of diseases in the debilitated patients. These 74 species belong to 20 genera distributed in the Ascomycota, Basidiomycota and phylum Deuteromycota. The majority of these species belong to phylum Deuteromycota (Fungi Imperfecti) in the form-class Hyphomycetes. Most of these fungi normally produce conidia or buds.

Occurrence

Humans: The portal of entry of agents of hyalohyphomycosis is either through the lungs or by trauma of the epidermis. In some cases entry is by means of contaminated surgical instruments, intraocular lenses, prosthetic devices, or contaminated solutions or equipment. In addition to invasive pulmonary or paranasal sinus infections, organs or tissues may be involved. Other types of infection may occur in the nail, ear canal, cutaneous and subcutaneous tissue, cornea, and other body locations such as cellulitis, bursitis, nephritis, endocarditis, peritonitis, and fungemia. In rare cases the CNS may be involved.

Laboratory Procedures

Specimen Collection: Specimens should be collected in sterile containers and processed as soon as possible in the laboratory. Types of specimens include: biopsies, transtracheal aspirates, and early morning sputum samples for microscopic examination and for isolation on media. Swabs of the mucous membrane, skin lesions, and blood cultures are usually of little value for diagnosis.

Cultures: Most hyaline fungi as causative agents of hyalohyphomycosis can be isolated on Sabouraud glucose agar or other media for fungi along with antibacterial agents such as: chloramphenicol, gentamicin, or penicillin and streptomycin. Most of the hyaline Hyphomycetes are sensitive or inhibited by cycloheximide. The inoculated media should be incubated at 25° and 37°C for up to 14 days.

Table 18. Currently known agents of aspergillosis and hyalohyphomycosis*

Acremonium	*Beauveria*	*Penicillium*
A. alabamensis	B. alba	P. casei
A. falciforme	B. bassiana	P. chrysogenum
A. kiliense		P. citrinum
A. potroni	*Chaetoconidium* spp	P. commune
A. recifei		P. expansum
A. roseogriseum	*Chrysosporium*	P. glaucum
A. strictum	*Chrysoporium* spp	P. marneffei
		(as a schizo-yeast
Anxiopsis	*Coprinus*	and mycelium in
A. fulescens	C. cinereus	tissue
A. sterocari	C. delicatulus	
		P. spinulosum
Arthrographis	*Coniothyrium fuckelii*	
		Phialenonium
A. kalrae	*Cylindrocarpon*	obevatum
	C. lichenicola	
Aspergillus	C. tonkinense	*Scedosporium*
A. amstelodami	C. vaginae	S. apiospermum
A. candidus		S. inflatum
A. carneus	*Fusarium*	
A. clavatus	F. chlamydosporum	*Schizophyllum*
A. conicus	F. dimerum	S. commune
A. deflectus	F. moniliforme	
A. fischeri	F. nivale	*Scopulariopsis*
A. flavipes	F. simifectum	S. acremonium
A. flavus	F. oxysporum	S. brevicaulis
A. fumigatus	F. proliferatum	
A. nidulans	F. roseum	*Scytalidium*
A. niger	F. solani	S. hyalinum
A. niveus	F. verticillioides*	
A. ochraceus		*Thermomyces*
A. oryzae	*Microascus*	T. amugisnosus
A. parasiticus	M. cinereus	
A. repens	M. desmosporus	*Trichoderma*
A. restrictus		T. viride
A. ruber	*Myriodontium*	
A. sydowi	M. keratinophylum	*Tritiarchium*
A. terreus		T. oryzae
A. ustus	*Neurospora*	
A. versicolor	Neurospora sitophila	*Volutella*
		V. cinerscens
	Paecilomyces	
	P. fumoso-roseus	
	P. javanicus	
	P. lilacinus	
	P. marquandii	
	P. variotii	

*Adapted from Rogers and Kennedy 1992.

Acremonium Link et Fries, 1821 (Cephalosporiomycosis)

Species of the genus *Acremonium* (Synonym: *Cephalosporium)* have been isolated from many cases of mycetoma, onychomycosis, mycotic keratitis, and colonizers of contact lens. Other cases have been reported describing the isolation of *Acremonium* species from various clinical sources including peritonitis and osteomyelitis, but without histological confir-

mation. Some of the more rare confirmed cases include: meningitis following after spinal anesthesia for a cesarean section, a fatal case in a patient undergoing dialysis, cases of dialysis fistulae in renal transplant patients, cerebritis in an intravenous drug abuser, endocarditis in a prosthetic valve operation, infection in an arthritic knee, osteomyelitis of the calvarium following trauma, and a pulmonary infection in a child.

Etiologic agents: Species of *Acremonium* in confirmed cases include: *A. alabamensis, A. falciforme, A. kiliensis, A. roseogriseum,* and *A. strictum.* Recently two other species have been reported: *A. potroni* and *A. recifei.* Some of the other cases were not speciated.

Occurrence: Species of *Acremonium* are commonly found in soil, decaying vegetation, and in decaying food.

Culture: *Acremonium* species can be cultured on Sabouraud glucose agar and other mycological media without cycloheximide. The colonies are white to gray or rose in color, with a velvety to cottony surface. The reverse side of the colony varies from colorless to yellow or pink. See sections on common contaminants (page 10), and mycetoma (page 103) for additional information.

Microscopically, many single unbranched tapering phialides develop from hyphae. At the apex balls of one or rarely two-celled, globose to cylindrical, hyaline conidia develop, 2 to 3 by 4 to 8 μm in diameter(see Figure 132, page 103). For speciation a specialist in mycology needs to be consulted or reference books on taxonomy.

Selected References

Boltansky H, et al. 1984. *Acremonium strictum* pulmonary infection in a patient with chronic granulomatous disease. J. Infect. Dis. 149:653

Fincher RE, et al. 1991. Infection due to the fungus *Acremonium* (*Cephalosporium*). Medicine 70:398

Szombathy SP, Chez MG, Laxer RM. 1988. Acute septic arthritis due to *Acremonium.* J. Rheumatol. 15:714

Beauveria Vuillemin, 1921

Beauveria spp. are common in soil and a well-known pathogen in silkworms and other insects. This fungus is occasionally recovered from bronchial aspirates and from lung tissue surgically removed from a patient with ulcerative, cervical lymphadenopathy, originally considered as having tuberculosis, and from keratinomycoses cases.

Etiologic agents: *Beauveria bassiana* and *B. alba.*

Culture: Species in this genus can be cultured on mycological media. The colonies, white to tan in color, become powdery on the surface.

Microscopically, dense clusters of hyaline, flask-shaped conidiogenous cells develop, inflating at the base and proliferating sympodically in a zigzag fashion (Figure 214). The conidiogenous cells may aggregate into sporodochia or *synnemata*. Conidia are one-celled, haline, globose to ovoid along the rachis at each bent point.

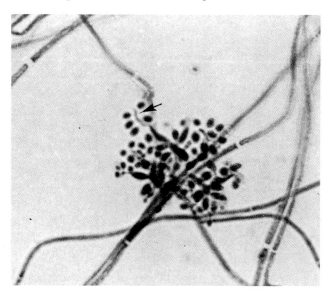

Figure 220. *Beauveria* species. Group of conidiogenous cells that produce zigzagging rachis (arrow) growth that is sympodial in development. A conidium is produced first on one side and then on the other.
(Reprinted with permission for use of the micrograph courtesy of Rogers and Kennedy.)

Selected References

Boltansky H, et al. 1984. *Acremonium strictum* pulmunary infection in a patient with chronic granulomatous disease. J. Infect. Dis. 149:653

Fincher RE, et al. 1991. Infection due to the fungus *Acremonium (Cephalosporium).* Medicine 70:398

Freour PM, et al. 1966. Une mycose nouvelle: etude clinique et mycologique d'une localization pulmonaire de "Beauveria." Bull. Soc. Med. Hop. Paris 117:197

Ishibashi Y, Honmura S. 1990. Keratomycosis and endogenous fungal endophthalmitis. Asian Med. J. 33(9):533

Rogers, AL, Kennedy, MJ. 1992. Opportunistic Hyaline Hyphomycetes. Chapter 63: 659–673. In Manual of Clinical Microbiology. 5th ed. 1991. Am. Soc. Microbiol.

Semalulu SS, et al. 1992. Pathogenicity of *Beauveria bassiana* in mice. J. Vet. Med. Series B39 (2):81

Szombathy SP, Chez MG, Laxer RM. 1988. Acute septic arthritis due to *Acremonium.* J. Rheumatol. 15:714

FUSARIUM

Link et Gray, 1821 (Fusariomycosis)

Species of *Fusarium* Link et Gray, 1821, have been reported as causative agents of keratomycosis, mycetoma, and onychomycosis. More recently *Fusarium* species have increasingly been reported in immunocompromised patients with severe underlying diseases, resulting in a high fatality rate. Infections in deeper tissues include: endophthalmitis, leg ulcers, facial granuloma, skin diseases (figs. 221, 222), osteomyelitis, infections of the central nervous system, transplants, fungemia, arthritis, peritonitis, bone marrow, and general dissemination.

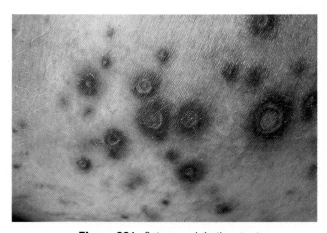

Figure 221. Cutaneous infection due to *Fusarium moniliforme*

Etiologic agents: *Fusarium* species most often reported from human infections are: *F. moniliforme, F. oxysporum,* and *F. solani.* Other less frequently reported species are: *F. chlamydosporum, F. dimerum, F. nivale, F. simifectum, F. proliferatum, F. roseum,* and *F. verticillioides.*

Occurrence: Species of *Fusarium* are well known as plant pathogens and as soil saprophytes.

Humans: *Fusarium* species occur in all parts of the world. Most of the human cases have been associated with trauma, burns, organ transplants, bone marrow transplants, facial granuloma, infection of the central nervous system, use of corticosteroids, immunosuppressed conditions, and catheters.

Animals: *Fusarium* infections occur in sea turtles, hatcheries, fish, poultry, shrimp, calves, and crocodiles.

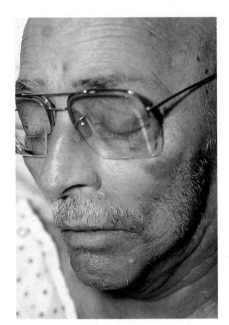

Figure 222. Face lesions due to
Fusarium oxysporum

Laboratory Procedures

Specimen collection: Procedures are similar as other subcutaneous or systemic infections: biopsies, pus, or blood should be collected under sterile conditions for immediate delivery to the laboratory.

Culture: *Fusarium* species grow rapidly on a number of different mycological media without cycloheximide which is inhibitory. Potato glucose agar or modified cornmeal is preferred for colony and microscopic characteristics needed for identification. On potato glucose agar *Fusarium* species produce white, lavender, pink, salmon or gray colored colonies with velvety to cottony surfaces. The reverse side varies depending upon the species.

Microscopically, the production of both fusoid macroconidia and microconidia are characteristic of the genus *Fusarium*. The macroconidia are hyaline, two to multicelled fusiform or sickle-shaped, 3 to 8 by 11 to 80 μm in size and usually develop in banana-like clusters. The presence of foot cells with a heel-like base are characteristic of the macroconidia. The fusiform macroconidia of *Fusarium* resemble those of *Cylindrocarpon* except this genus lacks foot cells. The microconidia are ovoid to cylindrical, hyaline, one to two celled, 2 to 3 by 4 to 8 μm in size, and are usually borne in mucous balls or occasionally in chains. On some media no macroconidia are produced, thus the fungus would resemble *Acremonium*.

Fusarium species

1. *F. moniliforme* Sheldon, 1904. Colony grows rapidly with white aerial mycelium, often tinged with purple. Reverse side of colony usually dark violet, occasionally lilac, vinaceous or cream (Figure 223). Tan to orange sporodochia may occur along dark blue sclerotia. Perithecia may occur on dead plant material.

Microscopically (Figure 224), microconidia are numerous, usually one-celled, oval to club-shaped with a flattened base, and formed in long chains. Macroconidia are formed, sometimes rare, slightly sickled-shaped to almost straight with nearly parallel, thin sidewalls, with 3 to 7 septa, and 2.5 to 4 μm by 25 to 60 μm in size. The basal cell is foot-shaped. Chlamydoconidia are absent. This species may resemble *F. oxysporum*.

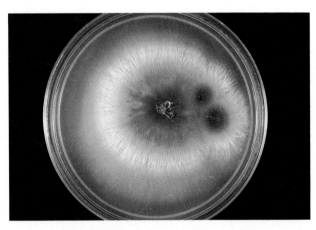

Figure 223. *Fusarium moniliforme*, colony

2. *F. oxysporum* Schlecht, 1824 ememd. Snyd. & Hans (1941). On PDA the colony grows fast with white aerial mycelium, tinged with purple or submerged by the blue color of the sclerotia if present. Cream, tan, or orange sporodochia may be present (Figure 225). The reverse side of the colony may be colorless, dark blue, or purple. These colors may be evident on the top surface. No perithecia have been reported.

Microscopically (Figure 224), microconidia are abundant, usually one-celled, oval to kidney-shaped, borne on false heads. Macroconidia are abundant, slightly sickled-shaped, thin-walled with 3 to 5 septations, with an attenuated apical cell and a foot-shaped basal cell. Chlamydoconidia are intercalary or terminal on the hyphae, solitary or in chains, hyaline, smooth to rough-walled.

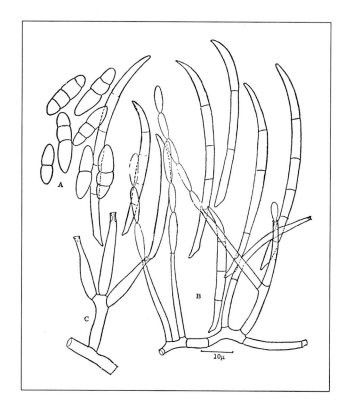

Figure 224. *Fusarium moniliforme* (*Gibberella fujikuroi*). a, ascospores; b, microconidia and conidiophores; c, macroconidia and conidiophores.

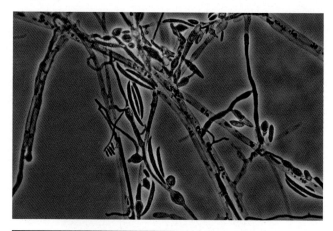

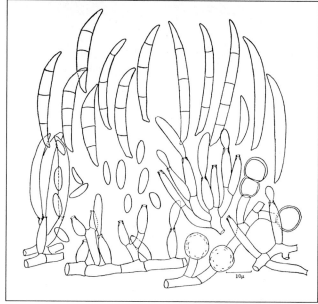

Figure 226. *Fusarium oxysporum.* Conidia, conidiophores and chlamydoconidia a. microscopic, b. diagram

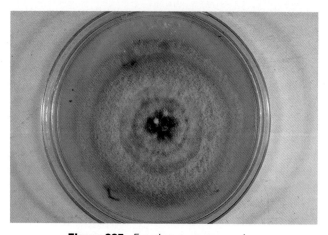

Figure 225. *Fusarium oxysporum,* colony

3. *F. solani* (Mart.) Appel & Wollenw. emend. Snyd. & Hans (1941). The colony develops rapidly with abundant aerial mycelium. The surface soon becomes covered with sporodochia that vary in color from cream, blue-green, or blue (never orange) (Figure 227). The under side of the colony is usually colorless or occasionally dark violet in color.

Microscopically (Figure 228), microconidia may be sparse or abundant, usually single-celled, 2 to 4 by 8 to 16 µm in size, oval to kidney-shaped and larger than *F. oxysporum.* The macroconidia are abundant, thick-walled, and usually cylindrical, with both cell walls parallel most of the distance on both sides. The apical cell is blunt and rounded, while the basal cell is rounded or foot-shaped, sometimes notched. Chlamydoconidia present, formed singly or in pairs, and usually abundant. A perfect state may form on a different host.

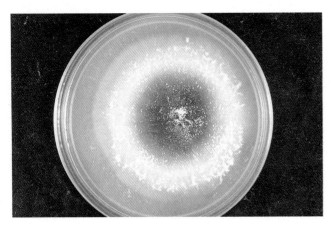

Figure 227. Colony of *Fusarium solani*

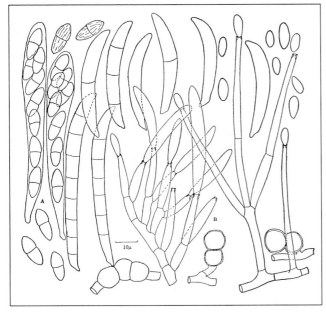

Figure 228. *Fusarium solani* (*Nectria haematococca*). A, asci and ascospores; B, conidia and conidiophores.

Key to the most important *Fusarium* spp. involved in human infections

A. Chlamydoconidia lacking

    1. Microconidia formed in chains—*F moniliforme*

B. Chlamydoconidia normally present
    1. Elongate phialides bearing microconidia—
                    F. solani

    2. short phialides bearing false heads of microconidia
                     F. oxysporum

The following Table lists some of the species of *Fusarium* that are the causative agents of invasive cutaneous and systemic infections.

Table 19. Diseseases caused by *Fusarium*

Fusarium spp.	Disease
F. chlamydosporum	Fungemia
F. moniliforme	Fungemia, dissemination, cutaneous lesions, arthritis, peritonitis
F. proliferatum	Dissemination
F. oxysporum	Dissemination, osteomyelitis, endophthalmitis, subcutaneous granuloma, skin lesions
F. roseum (*F. concolor*)	Burn wounds
F. solani	Dissemination, osteomyelitis, skin infection, fungemia, endophthalmitis
Fusarium spp.	Peritonitis, septic arthritis, urinary bladder, bone marrow, etc.

Fusarium species are difficult to identify. It is desirable to consult a mycologist who is a specialist in this group of fungi for determination of species. The references by Booth (1971), and Nelson, Toussoun, and Marasas (1983), are very useful for more detailed taxonomy of the *Fusarium* species.

Selected References

Ammari LK, Puck JM, McGowan KL. 1993. Catheter-related *Fusarium* solani fungemia and pulmonary infection in a patient with leukemia in remission. Clinical. Infect. Dis. 16(1):148.

Anaissie E, et al. 1988. The emerging role of *Fusarium* infections in patients with cancer. Medicine 67:77

Blazar BR, et al. 1984. Invasive *Fusarium* infection in bone marrow transplant recipients. Am. J. Med. 77:645

Booth C. 1971. The Genus *Fusarium*. Commonwealth Mycological Institute, Kew, England.

Chaulk CP, et al. 1986. Fungemia due to *Fusarium solani* in an immunocompromised child. Pediatr. Infect. Dius 5:363

Gamis AS, et al. 1991. Disseminated infection with *Fusarium* in recipients of bone marrow transplants. Rev. Infect. Dis. 13:1077

Gradon JD, Lerman A, Lutwick LL. 1990. Septic arthritis due to *Fusarium moniliforme*. Rev. Infect. Dis. 12:716

Jakle CJ, et al. 1983. Septic arthritis due to *Fusarium solani*. J. Rheumatol. 10:151

Nelson PE, Tousson TA, Marasas WFO. 1983. *Fusarium* species: An Illustrated Manual for Identification. Pennsylvania State University Press, State College, PA.

Peterson JD, Baker JJ. 1959. An isolate of *Fusarium roseum* from human burns. Mycologia 51:435

Vendetti M, et al. 1988. Invasive *Fusarium solani* infections in patients with acute leukemia. Rev. Infect. Dis. 10:653

PAECILOMYCES

Bainer, 1907

Paecilomyces Bainer. Most human cases have involved mycotic keratitis, endocarditis following valve replacement, cutaneous infections, pulmonary infections,chronic maxillary sinusitis, endophthalmitis, pyelonephritis, and corneal ulcers. Infection usually occurs in immunocompromised patients following trauma or occasionally from unopened packages containing intraocular lenses or from disinfectant used for surgical instruments.

Etiologic agents: Five species, commonly in soil, have been reported as causative agents of human infections: *Paecilomyces javanicus, P. lilacinus, P. marquandii, P. varioti,* and *P. viridis.*

Laboratory Procedures

Culture: Species of *Paecilomyces* grow well on Sabouraud glucose agar and many other fungal media but without cycloheximide. The colonies are at first floccose and white, then change color. Colonies of *P. lilacinus* are pink or vinaceous to lilac in color, while colonies of *P. variotii* are velvety and tan to olive-brown in color.

Microscopically, *Paecilomyces* resembles *Penicillium* species. The conidiophores are long (400 to 600 µm), with verticillate branches containing whorls of phialides that are flask-shaped with long tapering necks terminated by chains of ellipsoidal to fusiform conidia (1 to 2 by 2 to 3 µm). See Figures 14a, 14b and 14c, page 14 for illustration of the conidiophores.

Histopathology: The morphology of *Paecilomyces* in tissue is variable, ranging from *Aspergillus*-like hyphal forms with septate mycelium, 2 to 4 µm wide to chains of rounded cells, and in some cases yeast-like budding cells.

Selected References:

Allevato PA, et al. 1984. *Paecilomyces javanicus* endocarditis of native and prosthetic aortic valve. Am. J. Clin. Pathol. 82:247

Castro KGM, Salebian A, Sotto MN. 1990. Hyalohyphomycosis by *Paecilomyces lilacinus* in a renal transplant patient and a review of human *Paecilomyces* species infection. J. Med. Vet. Mycol. 28:15

Fagerburg R, et al. 1981. Cerebrospinal fluid shunt colonization and obstruction by *Paecilomyces variotii*: Case report. J. Neurosur. 54:257

Gordon MA, Norton SW. 1985. Corneal transplant infection by *Paecilomyces lilacinus*. Sabouraudia 23:295

Jade KB, Lyons MF, Gnann JW. 1986. *Paecilomyces liacinus* cellulitis in an immunocompromised patient. Arch. Dermatol. 122:1169

Miller GP, et al. Intravitreal antimycotic therapy and the cure of mycotic endophthalmitis caused by a *Paecilomyces lilacinus* contaminated pseudophokos. Ophthalmic Surg. 9:54

Sherwood JA, Dansky AS. 1983. *Paecilomyces pyelonephritis* complicating nephrolithiasis and review of *Paecilomyces* infection. J. Urol. 130:526

Silliman CC, et al. 1992. *Paecilomyces lilacinus* infection in a child with chronic granulomatous disease. J. Infect. 24(2):191

PENICILLIUM

Link ex Gray, 1821 (Penicilliosis)

Penicillium Link ex Gray. Species of *Penicillium* are very common contaminants in the environment and in the laboratory. Consequently the isolation of the fungus from a patient must be confirmed through examination of tissue sections. Among the many species of the genus *Penicillium, P. marneffei* is the only species known as a primary pathogen in human patients and in animals. This species has thermal dimorphism and at this time (1993) is restricted to the areas of Southeast Asia and in some areas of the Far East. *P. marneffei* will be described later in this chapter.

Etiologic agents: Some human cases have been associated with species of *Penicillium*. At autopsy a patient with acute leukemia had *P. commune* isolated from tissue studies of the lungs and brain with vascular invasion, thrombosis and infarction of the lungs. A case of urinary tract infection with uretheral catheterization established mycelial matts of *P. citrinum* was found to be present in the urine. More than four cases of endocarditis have been reported with the isolation of *P. chrysogenum* from a prosthetic valve while the others were unidentified species of *Penicillium*.

Two species, *P. citrinum* and *P. expansum* have been isolated from cases of keratinomycosis, and *P. decumbens*, a case of fungemia, in an AIDS patient. The following species of *Penicillium* although not established as primary etiologic agents have been reported: *P. crustaceum, P. glaucum, P. bertai, P. bicolor,* and *P. spinulosum.*

Laboratory Procedure

Culture: *Penicillium* species will grow on Sabouraud glucose agar, Czapek agar and other mycological media at 25°C. Czapek agar is useful for colony morphology and color development thus helpful in identification. The colonies grow rapidly, becoming downy, white at first, then change color with development of sporulation.

Microscopically, the hyphae are l.5 to 5 μm wide, hyaline, septate, and branched. The conidiophores are branched or unbranched, smooth to rough walls, hyaline to colored, and 100 to 250 μm long. The flask-shaped phialides are produced on unbranched or branched conidiophores. The branches on the conidiophores give a brush-like appearance and are designated as medulae. The unbranched conidiophore is designated as *Monoverticillata,* the conidiophore with symmetrical medulae, branched twice are termed *biverticillata-symmetrica,* or if the medulae are asymmetrical the designation is *Asymmetrica,* and a group or three or more medulae are designated as *Polyverticillata*. The conidia are round, smooth to finely roughened walls, in chains, 2 to 5 μm in diameter, and varied in color, commonly shades of green to blue green. See Figures 15b, 15c, and 15d, in Chapter 2 on contaminants for appearance of conidiophores. Sclerotia and sexual reproduction may occur. For species identification reference should be made to a specialist in mycology or to references by Raper and Thom (1949) and Samson and Pitt (1990).

Selected References

Del Rosii AJ, et al. 1980. Successful management of *Penicillium* endocarditis. J. Thorac. Cardiovasc. Surg. 80:945

Eschete M, et al. 1981. *Penicillium chrysogenum* endophthalmitis. Mycopathologia 74:1809

Liebler GA, et al. 1977. *Penicillium* granuloma of the lung presenting as a solitary pulmonary nodule. J. Am. Med. Assoc. 234:671

Ramirez C, Martinez AT. 1982. Manual and Atlas of the Penicillia. Elsevier Biomedical Press, Amsterdam, New York, Oxford.

Raper KB, Thom C. 1949. A Manual of the Penicillia. The Williams & Wilkins Co. Baltimore

Samson RA, Pitt JI. 1990. Modern Concepts in *Penicillium* and *Aspergillus* Classification. Plenum Publishing Corp. New York

Yoshida K, et al. 1992. *Penicillium decumbens.* A new cause of fungus ball. Chest. 101(4):1152

SCOPULARIOPSIS

Bainier, 1907(Scopulariopsosis)

Scopulariopsis Bainier. Infections with *Scopulariopsis,* usually *S. brevicaulis,* are at times found in nails. Occasionally invasion of deep tissue include fungus balls in preformed pulmonary cavities, pneumonia in a leukemic patient, and a subcutaneous infection in an ankle. A case of hypersensitivity pneumonitis in an intravenous opium addict was caused by *S. brumptii*. Three other species, *S. acremonium, S. fusca,* and *S. koningii* have been reported from toenails.

Laboratory Procedures

Culture: *S. brevicaulis* produces rather rapidly growing colonies that are powdery, and tan to beige. The reverse side of the colony is usually tan with a brown center.

Microscopically, The conidiogenous cells (annellides) are produced from unbranched or branched penicillate-like conidiophore. Conidia are in chains with the youngest conidium released from the annellide at the tip of the conidiophore. The conidia are thick-walled, round to lemon shaped, rough and spiny with hyaline or brown color. See Figures 16b, 16c, and 16d in Chapter 2 on Contaminants.

Selected References

Grieble HG, et al. 1975. *Scopulariopsis* and hypersensitivity pneumonitis in an addict. Ann. Intern. Med. 83:326

Onsberg P. 1980. *Scopulariopsis brevicaulis* in nails. Dermatologica 161:259

Sekhon AS, Williams DJ, Harvey JH. 1974. Deep scopulariopsis: a case report and sensitivity studies. J. Clin. Pathol. 27:837

Vaidya PS, Levine JF. 1992. *Scopulariopsis* peritonitis in a patient undergoing continuous ambulatory peritoneal dialysis. Peritoneal Dialysis Internat. 12:78

Wheat LJ, et al. 1984. Opportunistic *Scopulariopsis* pneumonia in an immunocompromised host. South Med. J. 77:1608

MISCELLANEOUS HYALINE HYPHOMYCETES

This list of etiologic agents involved in human infections continues to expand. These fungi have been isolated once to a few times (see Table 18, Chapter 10).

1. *Amxiopsis (Ahanoascus) fulvescens* and *A. stericoraria* have occurred in skin lesions resembling a dermatophyte infection. This keratinophilic fungus is found in the soil.

2. *Arthrographis kalrae (Oidiodendron kalrai)* has been cultured from sputum and corneal scrapings, but is of questionable significance. It has been converted into a dimorphic fungus and is pathogenic for mice (Wesari and Macpherson, 1968)

3. *Chaetoconidium* species have been cultured from biopsy specimens of a skin lesion in a renal transplant patient treated by immunosuppressive therapy. In tissue the hyphae were 3 to 5 µm in diameter. The colonies grow slowly on mycological media, developing a white to buff color. The chlamydoconidia are produced intercalary, round to oval in shape, with thick, verrucose walls, measuring 25 to 30 µm in diameter, and produced singly or in chains. Each conidiogenous branch terminates with a long, tapering hyaline tip.

4. *Chrysosporium* species have been isolated from a case of endocarditis and also from a case of osteomyelitis. The histological sections contained budding yeast cells and septate hyphae. *Chrysosporium panorum* has been cultured from infected toenails.

5. *Coniothyrium fuckelii* has been isolated from a patient with a liver infection and acute myelogenous leukemia. This fungus produces dark pycnidia similar to the *Phoma* species.

6. *Microascus desmosporus* and *M. cinereus* have been cultured from cases of onychomycosis. *M. cinereus* was cultured from a maxillary sinus and also from a section of lung tissue. Both cases had *Aspergillus* in the tissue too.

7. *Myriodontium keratinophilum* has been isolated from a frontal sinusitis secondary to nasal polyps. The hyphae are somewhat like *Aspergillus* except for the lack of dichotomous branching.

8. *Neurospora sitophila* has been isolated from a patient with endophthalmitis following cataract extraction.

9. *Phialenonium obovatum,* considered an opportunistic pathogen, was isolated from an infant who died of thermal burns. This fungus is intermediate between *Acremonium* and *Phialophora.* In tissue the hyphae of *P. obovatum* are hyaline with irregularly branched filaments, short chains of globose cells and pseudohyphae. This fungus in the disease state would be classified in the hyalohyphomycosis but in culture would be included in the phaeohyphomycosis.

10. *Scytalidium hyalinum* usually isolated from skin and nail infections, has been reported in a case of a subcutaneous cyst. This fungus with hyaline hyphae in tissue would have been considered in the hyalohyphomycosis group while in culture the dark hyphae indicates this fungus belongs with phaeohyphomycosis.

11. *Thermomyces lanuginosus* has been isolated from a patient with prosthetic valve endocarditis. This fungus produces hyaline hyphae with brown conidia similar to *Humicola* species except for rough walled conidia. This fungus may belong with phaeohyphomycosis.

12. *Trichoderma viride* was cultured from a case of peritonitis in a patient with renal failure secondary to amyloidosis and undergoing dialysis. *T. viride* was also isolated from a pulmonary fungus ball. See Figure 18a, 18b, and 18c for characteristic asexual reproduction under contaminants, chapter 2.

Selected References

Aznar C. et al. 1989. Maxillary sinusitis from *Micreascus cinereus* and *Aspergillus repens.* Mycopathologia 105:93

Blomquist K, Salonen A. 1969. *Oidiodendron cerealis* isolated from neurodermitis nuchae. Dermatologica 139:158

Booth C, Clayton YM, Usherwood M. 1985. *Cylindrocarpon* species associated with mycotic keratitis. Proc. Indian Acad. Sci. (Plant Sci.) 94:433

Carmichael JW. 1957. *Chrysosporium* and some other aleuriosporic hyphomycetes. Can. J. Bot. 40:1137

Gueho E, Villard J, Guinet R. 1985. A new human case of *Anixiopsis* sterocaria mycosis: discussion of its taxonomy and pathogenicity. Mykosen 28:430

Hay RJ, Moor MK. 1984. Clinical features of superficial

fungal infections caused by *Hendersonula toruloidea* and *Scytalidium hyalinum.* Br. J. Dermatol. 110:677

Kiehn TE, Polsky B. 1987. Liver infection caused by *Coniothyrium fuckelii* in a patient with acute myelogenous leukemia. J. Clin. Microbiol. 25:2410.

Lacey J. 1986. *Microascus cinereus* (Emile-Weil & Gaudin) Curzi: a human pathogen? Mycopathologia 96:137

Lesco-Bornet M, et al. 1991. Prosthetic valve endocarditis due to *Thermomyces lanuginosus* Tsiklinsky - first case report. J. Med. Vet. Mycol. 29:205

Loeppky CB, et al. 1983. *Trichoderma viride* peritonitis. South. Med. J. 76:798

Lomvardias S, Madge GE. 1972. *Chaetoconidium* and atypical acid fast bacilli in skin ulcers. Arch. Dermatol. 106:875

Maran AGD, et al. 1985. Frontal sinusitis caused by *Myriodontium keratinophilum.* Br. Med. J. 290:207

McAleer R, Froudist JH, Cherian GA. 1988. A dimorphic fungus *Arthrographis kalare,* implicated in two diseases. Abstract of the Tenth Congress of the Internat. Soc. for Human & Animal Mycol. Rev. Iber. Micol. 5:93

McGinnis MR, Gams W, Goodwin MN. 1986. *Phialemonium obovatum* infection in a burned child. Sabouraudia 24:51

Tewari RP, Macpherson CR. 1968. Pathogenicity and neurological effects of *Oidiodendron kalrai* in mice. J. Bacteriol. 95:1130

Todaro F, Criseo G, Urzi C. 1984. A propos d'un cas de tinea pedis par *Anixiopsis fulvescens* (Cooke) DeVries, var *fulvescens.* Bull. Soc. Franc. Mycol. Med. 13:239

Zaatari GS, Reed R. 1984. Subcutaneous hyphomycosis caused by *Scytalidium hyalinum.* Am. J. Clin. Pathol. 82:252

PSEUDALLESCHERIASIS

(Allescheriosis, Petriellidiosis, Monosporiosis, Scedosporiosis) and Scedosporium Infections

There is a wide range of types of infections caused by *Pseudallescheria boydii* (imperfect state: *Scedosporium apiospermum).* The following diseases caused by *P. boydii* are: sinusitis, brain abscess, meningitis, pulmonary colonization, fungus ball, invasive pneumonitis, endocarditis, arthritis, osteomyelitis, thyroid abscess, disseminated systemic disease, endophthalmitis, and cutaneous and subcutaneous granulomata. Mycotic mycetoma, usually involving the feet, is associated with *P. boydii,* and is discussed under mycetoma, page 99. *P. boydii* as one of the causative agents of keratomycosis and is discussed on page 200. The asexual state, *Scedosporium prolificans* has been

the etiologic agent of endocarditis, osteomyelitis, and arthritis in normal humans not debilitated.

Etiologic Agents: *Pseudallescheria boydii* (Negroni et Fischer) McGinnis, Padhye et Ajello, 1981 (Synonym: *Allescheria boydii* Shear, 1921; *Petriellidium boydii* (Shear) Malloch, 1970). Anamorph (asexual): *Scedosporium apiospermum* (Saccardo) Castellani et Chalmers, 1919 (Synonym: *Monosporium apiospermum* Saccardo, 1911). Another anamorph species has been more recently described: *Scedosporium prolificans* (Malloch et Salkin 1984) Gueho et de Hoog, 1991 (Synonym: *Scedosporium inflatum* Malloch et Salkin, 1984).

Occurrence

Humans: The fungus has been the causative agent in individuals throughout the world.

Animals: The fungus has been reported in the throats of normal donkeys, teats of cattle, a severe exophthalmos in the eye and as a nasal granuloma in a horse, a bovine mycotic abortion, in a case of mastitis in a cow, and several cases of uterine infections in horses.

Soil: *P. boydii* has been isolated from different saprophytic situations including soil, polluted streams, sewage sludge, and manure of poultry and cattle. Found world-wide.

Laboratory Procedures

Specimen collection: Material for the laboratory include: sputum, pus, bronchial washings, urine, or biopsy should be collected in sterile containers.

Direct examination: The hyphal strands of *P. boydii* in a slide mount appear like those of *Aspergillus.* Therefore culture isolation must be done for identification. The hyphae of *S. prolificans* in direct examination are indistinguishable from those of *P. boydii.*

Culture: Specimens from the patient should be spread over the surface of Sabouraud glucose agar with antibacterial antibiotics and incubated at 25° to 37°C. The colonies will grow in media with up to 8mg/ml of cycloheximide. The colonies grow rapidly, producing fluffy or tufted aerial mycelium, at first white, then becoming brownish-gray. The reverse side of the colony is gray to black in color. For colony appearance see Figures 133 and 134 under mycetoma (page 105).

Cleistothecia form in some strains of *P. boydii* on cornmeal agar, potato glucose agar or water agar. Isolates that do not produce cleistothecia are identified as *Scedosporium apiospermum.* Cleistothecia are brown in color, 100 to 200 μm in size, and develop around the periphery of the colony, maturing in 10 days. The asci are ovate to subglobose 12 to 18 by 8 to 13 μm in size, with 8 ascospores. The ascus wall disintegrates leaving free mature ascospores which contain internal oil droplets, a way to distinguish them from conidia.

Microscopically, the hyphae are hyaline (1 to 3 μm in diameter). The conidia borne singly or in small groups from annellides at the tips of the conidiophores or laterally on hyphae, are lemon-shaped, 4 to 9 by 6 to 10 μm, and light brown in color (see Figure 133 in the section on Mycetoma, page 105) Occasionally a second conidia form develops in some strains known as *Graphium* characterized by branched or unbranched synnemata or coremia with terminally developed conidia.

The second species, *Scedosporium prolificans,* can be differentiated from *S. apiospermum* by morphologic features of the conidiogenous cells. The conidiophores are brownish and unbranched. Unlike *S. apiospermum, S. prolificans* produces annellides with distinct swollen bases with conidial masses formed in wet spore balls. The conidia are hyaline, ovoid, smooth with a truncate base (Figure 229). In addition there is no *Graphium* conidial state, no cleistothecia, and does not grow in media containing cycloheximide.

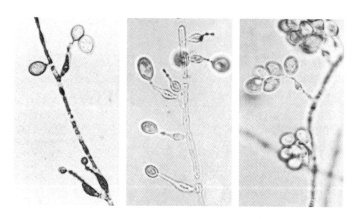

Figure 229. *Scedosporium prolificans.* a, b and c, Conidiogenous cells showing inflated bottoms and tapering tips with annellation and terminal conidia X850

S. prolificans is isolated more frequently from cases of osteomyelitis.

Histopathology: Hyphae of *P. boydii* have an affinity for blood vessels, growing into the lumen similar to *Aspergillus,* and are morphologically similar to Aspergillus. In cases of sinusitis a mycelial matt, conidia, and occasionally coremia may occur in cases of sinusitis. The coremia are brown and the hyphae are hyaline. When the fungus occurs as a ball in the lung, there are concentric rings of septate hyphae

(similar to *Aspergillus* fungus ball). The hyphae may have terminal or intercalary bulbous cells while some hyphae may be thick-walled, distorted in some cases, and produce swollen cells (Figure 230).

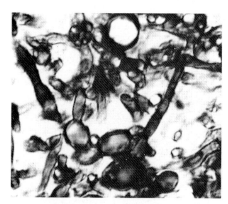

Figure 230. Pseudallescheriasis

Animal Inoculation: The virulence of *P. boydii* and *S. apiospermum* has been studies in mice. Cortisone-treated mice develop the infection by intravenous, intranasal, or intraperitoneal inoculation. Strains from human infections were more virulent than those from animals.

Selected References

Alsip SG, Cobbs CG. 1986. *Pseudallescheria boydii* infection of the central nervous system in a cardiac transplant recipient. South. Med. J. 79:383

Ansari RA, et al. *Pseudallescheria boydii* arthritis and osteomyelitis in a patient with Cushing's disease. South. Med. J. 80:90

Bell RG. 1978. Comparative virulence and immunodiffusion analysis of *Petriellidium boydii* (Shear) Malloch strains isolated from feed lot manure and a human mycetoma. Can. J. Microbiol. 24:856

Creitz S, Harris HW. 1955. Isolation of *Allescheria boydii* from sputum. Am. Rev. Tuberc. 71:126

Gari M, et al. 1985. *Scedosporium (Monosporium) apiospermum:* multiple brain abscesses. Sabouraudia 23:371

Gordon G, Axelrod JL. 1985. Case report: prosthetic valve endocarditis caused by *Pseudallescheria boydii* and *Clostridium limosum.* Mycopathologia 89:129

Gueho E, Hoog GS de. 1991. Taxonomy of the medical species of *Pseudallescheria boydii* infection after bone marrow transplantation. Ann. Intern. Med. 99:193

Lupan DM, Cazin J. 1976. Serological diagnosis of petriediosis (allescheriosis). I. Isolation and characterization of soluble antigens from *Allescheria boydii* and *Monosporium apiospermum.* Mycopathologia 58:31

Lupan DM, Cazin J.: Pathogenicity of *Allescheria boydii* for mice. Infect. Immun. 8:743

McGinnis MR, Padhye AA, Ajello L. 1982. *Pseudallescheria* Negroni et Fischer, 1943, and its later synonym *Petreillidium* Malloch, 1970. Mycotaxon 14:94

Morace G, Polonelli L. 1981. Exoantigen test for identification of *Petriellidium boydii*. J. Clin. Microbiol. 14:237

Raffanti SP, et al. 1990. Native valve endocarditis due to *Pseudallescheria boydii* in a patient with AIDS case report and review. Rev. Infect. Dis. 12:993

Rippon JW, Carmichael JW. 1976. Petriellidiosis (allescheriosis): four unusual cases and review of literature. Mycopathologia 48:117

Salitan ML, et al. 1990. *Pseudallescheria sinusitis* with intracranial extension in an immunocompromised host. Otolaryngol Head Neck Surg. 102:745

Salkin IF, et al. 1988. *Scedosporium inflatum:* an emerging pathogen. J. Clin. Microbiol. 26:498

Schwartz DA, et al. 1989. Cerebral *Pseudallescheria boydii* infection: unique occurrence of fungus ball formation in the brain. Clin. Neurol. Neurosurg. 91:79

Toy EC, et al. 1990. Endocarditis and hip arthritis associated with *Scedosporium inflatum*. South. Med. J. 83:957

Wilson CM, et al. 1990. *Scedosporium inflatum:* clinical spectrum of a newly recognized pathogen. J. Infect. Dis. 161:102.

ZYGOMYCOSIS

(Phycomycosis, Mucormycosis)

Definition: The term zygomycosis is preferred to mucormycosis or phycomycosis as the old classification was used when the zygomycetes, oomycetes and chytrids were in a single division. The term mucormycosis has been used for the mucoraceous fungi in the order Mucorales that are causative agents. Fungi in this group all are opportunistic in human cases associated with immunosuppression, metabolic acidosis, starvation, burns, trauma, or other forms of debilitation. These infections have a characteristic development of broad, sparsely septate hyphae and without an eosinophilic sheath in histopathology sections.

The term zygomycosis includes the second group of causative agents know as "entomophthoramycosis" for the mycoses caused by fungi in the order Entomophthorales. Two fungi, *Basidiobolus ranarum* and *Conidiobolus coronatus* are causative agents of diseases in physiologically and immunologically normal humans and animals in the warm climates. In tissue there is no vascular invasion or infarction but a prolific chronic inflammatory response occurs.

Even though the two groups of diseases are very distinctive, the term zygomycosis should be used for the mycoses caused by these zygote forming fungi.

Etiologic Agents: The causative agents in the Mucorales of zygomycosis in humans are: *Absidia corymbifera, Apophysomyces elegans, Cokeromyces recurvatus, Cunninghamella bertholletiae, Mucor circinelloides, M. ramosissimus, Rhizopus oryzae* (many cases identified as *R. arrhizus*), *R. microsporus* (or *R. microsporus* var *rhizopodiformis*), *Rhizomucor pusillus, Saksenaea vasiformis, Syncephalastrum racemosum.*

The more frequently isolated fungi from cases of zygomycosis are in the family Mucoraceae. *Rhizopus oryzae* is the most frequently causative agent of human zygomycosis, followed by *R. microsporus* var *rhizopodiformis.* Reports of *R. arrhizus,* considered a doubtful species are likely to have been *R. oryzae. Absidia corymbifera* previously more frequently isolated is now less common as a causative agent. *Rhizopus microsporus, R. microsporus* var. *oligosporum, Mucor ramosissimus, M. circinelloides, Apophysomyces elegans,* and *Rhizomucor pusillus* have been infrequently reported in human cases. *Mucor circinelloides* has been reported as a colonizing yeast form in the human vagina, bladder and intestine without producing a disease. There have been an increasing number of reports of *Cunninghamella bertholletiae* and *Saksenaea vasiformis* isolated from pulmonary and disseminated infections. The third and fourth most common agents of zygomycosis are *C. bertholetiae* and *Sakenaea vasiformis. Syncephalastrum racemosum* and *Cokeromyces recurvatus* are both rare etiologic agents. Rhinocerebral zygomycosis is the most common form in the United States, followed by an increasing number of pulmonary zygomycosis cases due to a complication of leukemia, lymphoma, or diabetes.

Invasion of the "Entomophthoramycosis" type fungi in the order Entomophthorales are usually *B. ranarum* and *C. coronatus.* These fungi usually occur in patients considered physiologically and immunologically normal. The mycelium in tissue is more regularly septate. This type of zygomycosis is characterized as an eosinophilic granulomatous disease involving deep tissues including muscles and lymph nodes, nasal polyps, invasion of the paranasal and frontal sinuses, and rarely as a massive subcutaneous invasion in the face.

Occurrence

The organisms causing zygomycosis are common worldwide in decaying vegetation, in soil, in house dust, air, and as contaminants in the laboratory. These fungi in the

Mucorales involved as agents of diseases usually occur in individuals with metabolic disturbances, such as uncontrolled diabetes, malnutrition, and other conditions are associated as acidosis. Other predisposing factors include increased use of corticosteroids, antibiotics, and antileukemic drugs.

The fungi in the order Entomophthorales, *Basidiobolus*, and *Conidiobolus* can occur in ordinarily normal people. *Conidiobolus* is found in plant detritus, feces of lizards, frogs, reptiles, and other animals. *Basidiobolus* occurs in plant detritus, a few insects, and on fruiting bodies of higher fungi.

Humans: These diseases are worldwide in distribution. The fungi in the Mucoraceae cause diseases as indicated above in individuals with metabolic disturbances or other debilitations, while the organisms in the Entomophthorales invade normal individuals. The primarily subcutaneous entomophthoramycosis caused by *Basidiobolus ranarum* occurs in Asia and Africa.

Animals: The disease has been reported in dogs, birds, horses, sheep, cows, pigs, mink, guinea pigs, and mice.

Laboratory Procedures

Specimen collection: There is considerable difficulty in obtaining material in most cases, except by biopsy, after autopsy, or from slides made for pathologic study. In case of suspected central nervous system zygomycosis, material should be taken from the nasal mucosa, sinuses, and cerebrospinal fluid for direct mounts. Scrapings or biopsy should be taken from cutaneous-type infections. Abscesses should be aspirated. Necrotic or purulent material or clear fluids such as cerebrospinal fluid should be centrifuged. And in pulmonary cases, sputum, and bronchial washings should be taken. Since zygomycosis is one of the most rapidly progressing diseases, rapid diagnosis is extremely important.

Direct examination: Direct KOH examination on slide mounts of sputum or scraped material should show mostly nonseptate mycelium and rarely rounded sporangia. Biopsied material should be teased apart before making a KOH mount. Stained sections on slides made from pathologic tissue will show the same structures as those found in direct examination of material (Figures 231 and 232). The hyphae are mostly nonseptate and average 10 to 15 µm in diameter. Swollen cells may be up to 50 µm in size. A biopsy specimen should be taken for examination from cases of entomophthoramycosis.

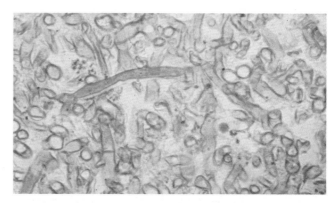
Figure 231. Mucormycosis, *Mucor* sp. hyphae in tissue, hematoxylin-eosin stain X400

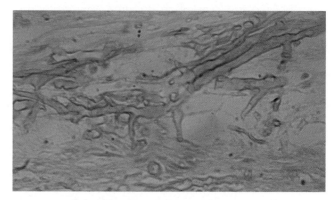
Figure 232. Mucormycosis, hyphae in sinus, hematoxylin-eosin stain X400

NOTE: Since species of all these genera except *Basidiobolus* and *Conidiobolus* are common laboratory contaminants, the isolation of these genera in culture becomes significant if mostly nonseptate hyphae are found in the specimen taken from the patient.

Culture: All of the organisms grow on Sabouraud glucose agar with or without the addition of antibacterial antibiotics. Other media may be used such as malt agar, modified cornmeal agar, or potato glucose agars. Cycloheximide should not be used in the media for isolation of any of these fungi. Streak the specimen over the surface of the medium in the plate and some into the medium. Incubate at 25° and 37°C. All colonies are fast growing, usually spreading over a plate in a couple of days, and have an abundance of aerial mycelium. If subcutaneous granulomatous tissue is available, a portion should be aseptically minced, inoculated into Sabouraud glucose agar, and incubated at 25° to 30°C.

Identification of genera and species: The agents of zygomycosis are located in 6 of the 13 families in the order Mucorales. The species identification of the organisms in the Mucorales are usually difficult, even for the experts. Several helpful references are useful for identification of the Mucorales: Gilman (1957); Zycha and Siepmann (1969); and Scholer et al (1983). Table 20 illustrates the key characteristic structures of the sporangia and describes the zygospores in the six families of the Mucorales.

1.   *Rhizopus* Ehrenberg ex Corda, 1838.

Two species and two varieties are recognized as causative agents in humans.

Growth is rapid, filling the plate with a cottony surface in a few days. See Chapter 2 on contaminant fungi (Figures 5a and 5b) for additional information and illustrations of the genus. All species usually produce sporangiophores that arise directly from a cluster of rhizoids. The sporangiophores expand at the apex into a spherical sporangium with a columella and spores filling the interior. Figure 233a shows colony characteristics and Figure 233b illustrates the rhizoids and sporangiophores.

R. oryzae Went and Prinsen-Geerlings, 1895, is the most frequently reported isolate of zygomycosis. This species is isolated in about 60% of the zygomycosis cases and about 90% of the rhinocerebral cases.

Colony: The fast growing white colonies fill a petri dish in a couple days, becoming yellowish-brown in color with dark-brown sporangia soon appearing.

Microscopically, the nonseptate hyphae have very long sporangiophores (up to 1 to 1.5 mm) with yellow-brown rhizoids. The gray-black sporangia, 150 to 175 µm in diameter, form light-brown, striated, irregularly formed spores, 6 to 8 by 5 to 6 µm in size. Zygospores form when two compatible strains are crossed on yeast extract agar.

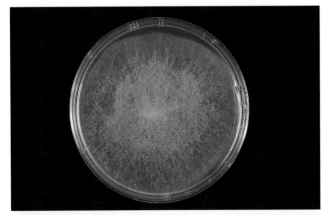

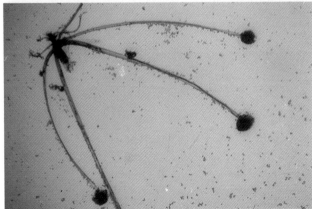

Figure 233. *Rhizopus* sp., a. Colony   b. Rhizoids, sporangiophores, sporangia, sporangiospores X150

Rhizopus microsporus var *rhizopodiformis* (Cohn) Schipper et Stalpers, 1984 (synonym: *Mucor rhizopodiformis* (Cohn) Zopf, 1890). This species is the second most frequently isolated fungus in zygomycosis cases, mostly from cutaneous cases and rarely from rhinocerebral form or subcutaneous abscesses.

Colony: The rapidly growing colonies range from gray to dark grayish-brown.

Microscopically, the sporangiophores are shorter than *R. oryzae,* up to 500 µm long, produced singly or up to four in

Table 20. Differential characteristics of five of the six families of Mucorales that include pathogenic species

Family	Sporangiosporogenous	Zygospores
Mucoraceae		Produced between equal or unequal suspensors.
Mortierellaceae		Produced between tongue-shaped suspensors. Zygospores are known only in a few species.
Cunninghamellaceae		Produced between equal or unequal suspensors.
Syncephalastraceae		Produced between equal suspensors.
Saksenaeaceae		Not known.

a group. The columellae are pyriform, with angular apophyses. The spores are subglobose to rhomboidal, with a smooth or finely spinulose surface. The colony grows at 50°C.

2. *Cunninghamella* Matruchot, 1903.

This fungus has been increasingly reported in recent years from immunocompetent patients in pulmonary and disseminated diseases. Earlier reports of *C. elegans* being isolated from clinical cases were determined to be *C. bertholletiae,* Stadel, 1911 after mating studies were made by Weitzman and Crist, 1979.

Colony (*C. bertholletiae*): Rapidly growing colonies at 37°C, white to gray with no color on the reverse side (Figure 234a)

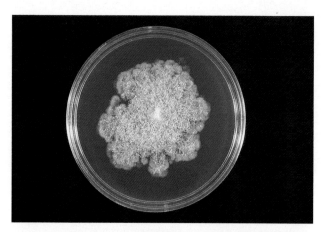

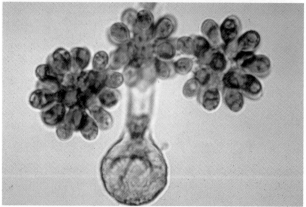

Figure 234. *Cunninghamella* sp., a. colony, b. conidiophore, vesicles, etc. conidiophore, vesicles, points of insertion, and conidia X330

Microscopically conidiophores are hyaline, straight or verticillately branched with terminal vesicles, and points of insertion on the vesicles for conidia. The conidia are spherical or oval and finely echinulate, 5 to 8 by 6 to 15 in size. Figure 234b illustrates the conidiophore structures.

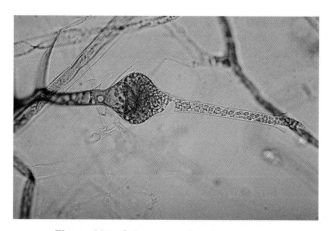

Figure 235. *Saksenaea vasiformis,* sporangum

3. *Saksenaea* Saksena, 1953.

This fungus has been increasingly reported since 1990, involving rhinocerebral infection, cranial infection, osteomyelitis, necrotizing cellulitis, subcutaneous lesions, and disseminated infections. The one species is *S. vasiformis* Saksena, 1953.

Colony: When the fungus is isolated on Sabouraud glucose agar or other media, this fast-growing hyaline colony ordinarily will not sporulate. The isolate should be transferred to a block of Sabouraud agar for 7 days at 25°C, then transferred into a petri dish with sterile distilled water (20 ml), supplemented with 0.2 ml of 10% filter-sterilized yeast extract solution and incubated for 7 to 10 days at 37°C. By this method described by Padhye and Ajello (1988) the isolates of *S. vasiformis* will readily sporulate.

Microscopically, the sporangia are flask-shaped, each containing a globose columella,and smooth, elongate spores, 3 to 4 by 1.5 to 2 µm in size. The generic name is easily determined due to the shape of the sporangia. More detailed information on the genus *Saksenaea* is found in Zycha and Siepmann, 1969. See Figure 235.

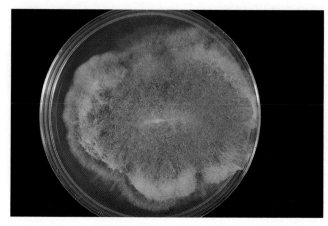

Figure 236. *Absidia,* Colony

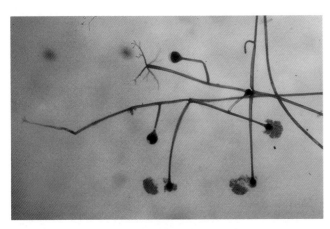

Figure 237. *Absidia*
Sporanges are formed on the intermodes.

The following fungi have been infrequently reported as causative agents of zygomycosis.

1. *Absidia corymbifera* Sachardo and Trotter, 1912 is a very infrequent causative agent of zygomycosis in humans. Several reports of this organism include a case of meningitis after a penetrating head injury and another case of a cutaneous infection, both in an immunocompromised patients. A recent report of zygomycosis was in an AIDS patient with a kidney infection.

Colony: The colony growth of the fungus gives a grayish brown to a greenish beige color, and a woolly appearance. The rate of growth is about the same as for *Rhizopus*. Figure 236 a shows a colony of *Absidia*.

Microscopically, the sporangiophores are formed between nodes on the internodes of the stolon instead of the nodes as in *Rhizopus*. The sporangia are somewhat pear-shaped with a columella in each. The spores are round to ellipsoidal, 2 to 3 by 3 to 4 μm in size. Zygospores may form. Figure 237 illustrates sporangiophores at the internodes and rhizoids at the nodes.

2. *Apophysomyces elegans,* Misra, Srivastava et Lata, 1979. This fungus has been the causative agent of several cases as a result of traumatic implantation or contamination of burn wounds. The organism has been isolated from soil.

Colony: Colonies of *A. elegans* grow rapidly on Sabouraud glucose agar, at first white, then becoming pale cream to yellow and will grow at temperatures up to 42°C. A simple method for inducing sporulation was described by Padhye and Ajello (1988).

Microscopically, sporangiophores develop singly on aerial hyphae, up to 300 μm long by 3 to 5 μm wide, topped by large pyriform shaped sporangia containing hemispherical columellae. The apex of the sporangiophore has funnel-shaped apophyses. Spores are oblong, smooth-walled, 5.4 to 8.0 by 4.0 to 5.7 μm in size. Figure 238 illustrates a mature sporangium.

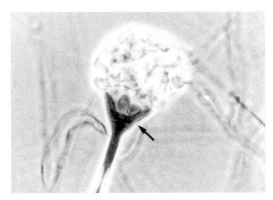

Figure 238. Mature sporangium of *Apophysomyces elegans* with sporangiospores and a clearly depicted apophysis (*arrow*) X1400. (*Courtesy of AA Padhye.*)

3. *Cokeromyces recurvatus* Poitras, 1950, has been isolated from a urine specimen of a cystitis patient. The fungus is dimorphic, producing yeastlike colonies at 37°C and mycelial colonies at 25° to 30°C.

Colony: The organism grows moderately fast on Sabouraud glucose agar, potato dextrose agar or cornmeal agar at 25°C, developing a thin radially wrinkled surface gray in color due to numerous sporangiophores (See Figure 239a). At 37°C a dry, cream colored yeast-like colony develops on YEPD (Yeast extract, peptone, dextrose agar).

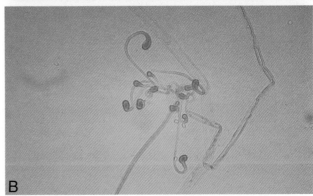

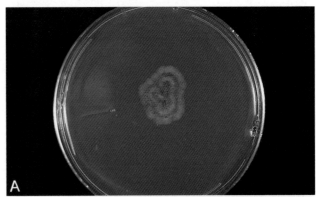

Figure 239. *Cokeromyces recurvatus.* a. Mycelial colony grown on potato dextrose agar for 1 week.
b. Spherical sporangioles containing multiple spores are produced at the tip of long, recurved stalks.

Microscopically, the hyphae are nonseptate in the growing tips later forming septations in the older part of the colony. Numerous zygospores are produced on PDA at 25°C. Sporangiophores are usually unbranched, producing many spherical sporangioles (8 to 11 μm in size), containing many spores. The sporangioles are on long, recurved, twisted stalks that arise from a terminal vesicle of sporangiphores. The spores are hyaline, smooth walled, 2 to 4 μm in size and oval to spherical in shape. - Figure 239b.

The yeast-like colony contains large, thin-walled yeast cells from 10 to 100 μm in size. The yeast cells produce from one to multiple buds, resembling *Paracoccidioides brasiliensis* when grown at 37°C.

4. *Mortierella* Coemans, 1863. This genus apparently has been isolated from a couple of cases in human infections, one from a subcutaneous infection and another from an ulcer on the leg. In both cases hyphae were seen in tissue, both cultures were gray or yellowish in color and neither one sporulated. Identification was based on colony characteristics. Ajello (1976) speculated that these two cultures may have been *Saksenaea vasiformis,* which requires special cultural techniques (see *Saksenaea*)

This genus is characterized by the production of a sporangium lacking a columella.The spores in the sporangium are small, 1 to 2 μm by 2 to 4 μm. Small one-celled conidia, called stylospores, with echinuate or spiny walls, are also formed. Figure 240 illustrates sporangia without columellas.

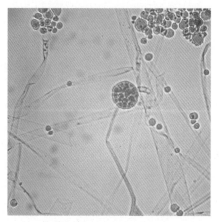

Figure 240. *Mortierella* sp.,
sporangia on sporangiophore X250

5. *Mucor* Micheli et Saint-Amans, 1822. Only a few species have been isolated from well-documented cases of zygomycosis. Infections from these species rarely occur. The colonies are rapidly growing, developing a gray to yellowish-gray surface. Sporangiophores are unbranched or branched, arising from aerial mycelium. No stolons or rhizoids are present. Sporangia are large and spherical with the wall usually dissolving (deliquescing) at maturity. Zygospores may develop. Figure 241 a shows a colony of Mucor spp., and Figure 242 shows a sporangium and dispersal of spores after wall dissolution.

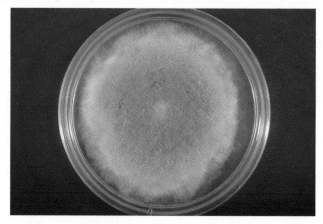

Figure 241. *Mucor* spp., colony

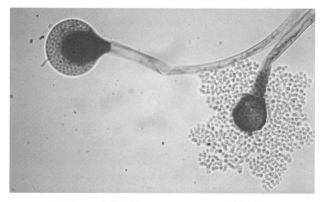

Figure 242. *Mucor* spp., sporongia X200

Mucor circinelloides van Tieghem, 1875 is the most common and variable species with several formae. *M. circinelloides f. circinelloides* has been isolated from a subcutaneous nodule and from urine. This species is dimorphic with globose, multiple buds as a yeast form found in the urine. The sporangiophores are usually short, circinate branches with brown sporangia and has the ability to assimilate ethanol and nitrates. Poor growth occurs at 37°C.

M. circinelloides f. lusitanicus (Bruderlein) Schipper, 1976 has been isolated form a raised erythematous skin lesion. This fungus is similar to *M. circinelloides f. circinelloides,* but grows more rapidly, with white-gray, fluffy colonies that become brownish when mature and is heterothallic, with orange-brown zygospores.

Mucor ramosissimus Samutsevitsch, 1927 has been reported from a chronic infection on the face, and from a case of rhinocerebral zygomycosis. The fungus is slow-growing, and light gray when grown at room temperature. The short sporangiophores become more narrow toward the apex along with a small constriction at the base, and is repeatedly branched sympodially with slightly roughened walls. Sporangia are black when mature, and does not assimilate ethanol.

Mucor hiemalis Wehmer F. *Luteus* (Linnemann) Schipper, 1973. This species commonly occurring in soil was isolated from a subcutaneous infection with verrucous lesion in the finger of a diabetic case. The fungus grows rapidly at 25°C, producing yellow, round sporangia up to 70 μm in diameter with globose columellae. Sporangial spores are ellipsoidal.

Mucor indicus Lendner, 1930 (Synonym: *M. rouxii* (Calmette) Wehmer, 1900) has apparently isolated from a gastric mucormycosis in a patient. The fungus grows at temperatures up to 42°C, requires thiamine for growth, and cannot assimilate nitrates. The colonies are a deep-yellow color.

6. *Rhizomucor* (Lucet et Costantin) Wehmer et Vuillemin, 1931. This genus includes the thermophilic species of *Mucor* that may at times produce stolons and rhizoids with dark sporangia.

Rhizomucor pusillus (Lind) Schipper, 1978 has been cultured from cutaneous infections, endocarditis, disseminated infections and pulmonary cases. The species is frequently reported from animals. The fungus develops rapidly, maturing into dark brown colonies. The sporangiophores are usually unbranched arising from hyphae that are occasionally anchored to the substratum by short rhizoids. The sporangia are globose, dark brown, measuring up to 100 μm in diameter containing subglobose to pyriform columellae and subglobose spores 3 to 4 μm in diameter. The range of temperatures for growth are 20° to 54° (rarely to 58°C).

7. *Syncephalastrum* Schroter, 1886. This genus forms cylindrical merosporangia (spores inside the sporangium) on a terminal swelling of the sporangiophore (see Figure 243).

Syncephalastrum racemosum Cohn et Schroter, 1886. A cutaneous zygomycosis case report indicated the identification of the culture was *Syncephalastrum* sp. The fungus produces a rapidly growing colony with merosporangia, a characteristic that distinguishes this genus from other members of the Mucorales.

Entomophthorales. This order includes the etiological agents *Conidiobolus coronatus* and *Basidiobolus ranarum* species that are causative agents of zygomycosis (Entomophthoramycosis). *Conidiobolus coronatus* is the causative agent of infections of the head and face, and designated as rhinofacial zygomycosis. The second genus and species, *Basidiobolus ranarum* causes diseases of the trunk and arms, rarely reported as a disseminated disease. In most cases the disease is reported in Africa, India and Asia, and recently the infections have been reported in the United States, Caribbean, and South America. Infection is by inhalation or inoculation of spores from the fungus. The patients do not have to be debilitated.

1. *Basidiobolus ranarum* Eidem, 1886 (synonym: *B. haptosporus*, Drechsler, 1947)

Colony: The colony is rapid in growth at 30°C, flat, folded, furrowed, grayish in color, and with a waxy surface. Large hyphae, 8 to 20 μm in size develop, becoming increasingly septate. In 7 to 10 days the colony is overgrown with mycelia containing masses of zygospores, chlamydoconidia, and conidia.

Microscopically, the large vegative hyphae shows masses of zygospores, 20 to 50 μm in diameter with usually smooth walls, chlamydoconidia, and conidia. Figure 244 illustrates zygospores. Conidiophores (sporangiophores) produce unicellular conidia at their apices. The apical portion of the conidiophore enlarges, becoming a vesicle beneath the conidium, then is blown out of the top of the swelling. The vesicle then emits a stream of fluid that propels the conidium, a characteristic of this genus.

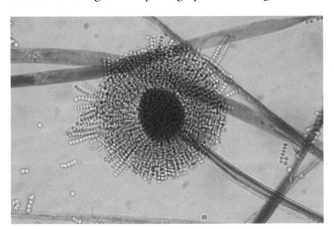

Figure 243. *Syncephalastrum* sp., sporangiophore, vesicle, merosporangia, sporangiospores (merospores) X825

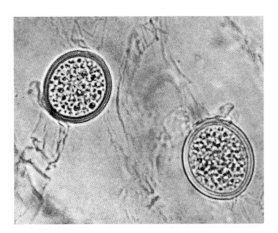

Figure 244. Zygospores of *B. ranarum*

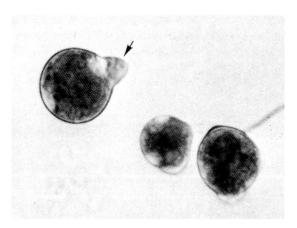

Figure 245. Conidia of *conidiobolus coronatus* with basal papilla

2. Conidiobolus coronatus (Costantin) Batko, 1964.

Colony: The colony grows rapidly, with a glabrous surface, then developing furrows and folding particularly at 37°C. The older colonies become covered with short aerial mycelium and conidiophores. The conidia are forcibly discharged from the conidiophores and adhere to the lid of a petri dish or test tube. Older colonies become tannish to light brown.

Microscopically, the organism produces short, erect unbranched conidiophores with single-celled, large conidia, 25 to 45 µm in diameter. When mounted on a slide the conidia may have been discharged from the conidiophores. The conidia (Fig 245) differ from those of *Basidiobolus* sp. as they have prominent papillae on the wall that can give rise to more secondary conidia, giving the original spore a corona appearance. A spore may also produce hairlike appendages called villae.

Histopathology: The hyphae causing the zygomycosis stain well with H and E, GMAS and PAS stains. Large, branched hyphae (branching at a 90° angle) are usually abundant in infected tissues where there is extensive polymorphonuclear infiltration and necrosis. The hyphae tend to invade the blood vessel walls to produce obstructive thrombi. The hyphae are usually nonseptate and wider than *Aspergillus,* or around 15 to 20 µm in diameter, and up to 200 µm in length.

In cases with chronic granulomatous lesions, that are usually subcutaneous and due to *Basidiobolus* sp. and *Conidiobolus* sp. the hyphae do not appear to infiltrate the walls or vessels, but go through the involved tissue and are surrounded by eosinophilia sleeves.

Animal inoculation: Cerebral and pulmonary zygomyco-

sis has been reported in rabbits (made diabetic with alloxan and injected with *R. oryzae* Baker, 1956). Mice inoculated intraperitoneally with 1 ml of 10% suspension of ground *R. oryzae* may develop inflammatory masses with hyphae in the peritoneum. Masses should be found in the upper quadrant binding the liver, spleen, pancreas, and stomach together. The animals recover in about four weeks. Animals are not sufficiently susceptible to be useful in determining pathogenicity.

Serology: At present an immunodiffusion (ID) test that is specific and sensitive for systemic zygomycosis (mucormycosis) has been developed with homogenate antigens by Jones and Kaufman (1978) and Kaufman and Reiss (1992). The 1992 report also indicates the Enzyme Immunoassay (EIA) has been evaluated. There are no commercial kits available.

Questions

1. What are the predisposing factors that aid in the development of zygomycosis ?

2. How does the tissue phase of zygomycosis differ from that of aspergillosis?

3. What are differences and similarities between, *Syncephalastrum, Saksenaea, Rhizopus, Mucor, Cunninghamella, Cokeromyces, Absidia,* and *Apophysomyces?*

Selected References

de Aguilar E, Moraes WC, Londero AT. 1980. Gastrointestinal entomophthoramycosis caused by *Basidiobolus haptosporum.* Mycopathologia 72:101

Ajello L, Dean DF, Irwin RS. 1976. The zygomycete *Saksenaea vasiformis* as a pathogen of humans, with a critical review of the etiology of zygomycosis. Mycologia 68:52

Axelrod P, et al. 1987. Chronic cystitis due to *Cokeromyces recurvatus.* J. Infect. Dis. 155:1062.

Brennan RO, et al. 1983. *Cunninghamella:* a newly recognized cause of rhinocerebral mucormycosis. Am. J. Clin. Pathol. 80:98

Carbone KM, et al. 1985. Mucormycosis in renal transplant patients: a report of two cases and review of the literature. Q. J. Med. 57:825

Clark R, Greer DL, Carlisle T. 1990. Cutaneous zygomycosis in a diabetic HTLV-I-seropositive man. J. Am. Acad. Dermatol. 22:956

Cockshott WP, Clark BM, Martinson FD. 1968. Upper respiratory infection due to *Entomophthora coronata.* Radiology 90:1016

Cooter RE, et al. 1990. Burn wound zygomycosis caused by *Apophysomyces elegans.* J. Clin. Microbiol. 28:2151

Corbel MJ, Eades SM. 1976. Experimental phycomycosis in mice: examination of the role of acquired immunity in resistance to *Absidia ramosa.* J. Hyg. (Camb.) 77:221

Ellis JJ, Ajello L. 1982. An unusual source of *Apophysomyces elegans* and a method for stimulating sporulation of *Saksenaea vasiformis.* Mycologia 74:144

Gams W. 1977. A key to the species of *Mortierella.* Persoonia 9:381

Ginsberg J, Spaulding AG, Laing VO. 1966. Cerebral phycomycosis (mucormycosis) with ocular involvement. Am. J. Ophthal. 62:900

Gilman JC. 1957. A Manual of Soil Fungi. 2nd ed. Ames, the Iowa State College Press.

Hesseltine CW, Ellis JJ. 1973. Mucorales. *In* Ainsworth GC, Sparrow FK, Sussman AS (eds). The Fungi, Vol. IVB. A Taxonomic Review with keys.- Basidiomycetes and Lower Fungi. Academic Press, New York

Hamdy MAG, et al. 1989. Fatal cardiac zygomycosis in a renal transplant patient treated with desferrioxamine. Nephrol. Dial. Transplant 4:911

Jaffey PB, Haque AK, El-Zaatari M. 1990. Disseminated *Conidiobolus* infection with endocarditis in a cocaine abuser. Arch. Path. and Lab. Med. 114:1276

Jones KW, Kaufman L. 1978. Development and evaluation of an immunodiffusion test for diagnosis of systemic zygomycosis (mucormycosis): Preliminary report. J. Clin. Microbiol. 7:97

Kamalam A, Thambiah AS. 1980. Cutaneous infection by *Syncephalastrum.* Sabouraudia 18:19

Kaufman L, Reiss E. 1992. Serodiagnosis of fungal diseases. *In* N. R. Rose, Friedman, Fahey, J. L. (ed). Manual of Clinical Laboratory Immunology. 4th ed. Am Society for Microbiology, Washington, D. C.

Kaufman L, Padhye AA, Parker S. 1988. Rhinocerebral zygomycosis caused by *Saksenaea vasiformis.* J. Med. Vet. Mycol. 26:237

King DS. 1977. Systematics of *Conidiobolus* (Entomophthorales) using numerical taxonomy. III. Descriptions of recognized species. Can. J. Bot. 55:718

Kitz DJ, Embree RW, Cazin J. 1983. The comparative virulence of thermotolerant Mucorales species in mice. Mycopathologia 82:17

Lombardi G, Padhye AA, Standard PG, Kaufman L, Ajello L. 1989. Exoantigen tests for the rapid and specific identification of *Apophysomyces elegans* and *Saksenaea vasiformis.* J. Med. Vet. Mycol. 27:113

Mackenzie DWR, Soothill JF, Millar JHD. 1988. Meningitis caused by *Absidia corymbifera.* J. Infect. 17:241

McGough DA, Fothergill AW, Rinaldi MG. 1990. *Cokeromyces recurvatus* Poitras, a distinctive zygomycete and potential pathogen: criteria for identification. Clin. Microbiol. Newsletter 12:113

Misra PC, Srivastava KJ, Lata K. 1979. *Apophysomyces,* a new genus of the Mucorales. Mycotaxon 8:377

Nimmo GR, Whiting RF, Strong RW. 1988. Disseminated mucormycosis due to *Cunninghamella bertholletiae* in a liver transplant recipient. Postgrad. Med. J. 64:82

Nui T, Takeda Y, Lizuka H. 1965. Taxonomical studies on the genus *Rhizopus.* J. Gen. Appl. Microbiol. Suppl. 11:1

Padhye AA, Ajello L. 1988. Simple method of inducing sporulation by *Apophysomyces elegans* and *S. vasiformis.* J. Clin. Microbiol. 26:1861

Queiroz Telles Filho, F., et al. 1985. Subcutaneous mucormycosis caused by *Rhizopus oryzae* probable nosocomial acquired infection. Rev. Inst. Med. Trop. Sao Paulo 27:201.

Rosenberger RS, West BC, King JW. 1983. Survival from sino-orbital mucormycosis due to *Rhizopus rhizopodiformis.* Am. J. Med. Sci. 286:25

Schipper MAA, 1984. A revision of the genus *Rhizopus* I. The *Rhizopus stolonifer* group and *Rhizopus oryzae.* Studies in Mycology No. 25 pp. 1-19

Schipper MAA. 1978. On certain species of *Mucor* with a key to all accepted species. Stud. Mycol. 17:1

Schofield RA, Baker RD. 1956. Experimental mucormycosis (*Rhizopus* infection) in mice. Arch. Pathol. 61:407

Scholer HJ, Muller E, Schipper MAA. 1983. Mucorales. *In* Howard, D. H. (ed.) Fungi Pathogenic for Humans and Animals. New York. Marcel Dekker. pp. 9-59

Smith AG, Bustamante CI, Gilmor GD. 1989. Zygomycosis (absidiomycosis) in an AIDS patient. Absidiomycosis in AIDS. Mycopathologia 105:7

Strastsma BR, Zimmerman CE, Gass JD, 1962. Phycomycosis: A clinicopathologic study of fifty-one cases. Lab. Invest. 11:963

Tintelnot K, Nitsche B. 1988. *Rhizopus oligosporum* as a cause of mucormycosis in man. Mycoses 32:115

Wadsworth JA. 1951. Ocular mucormycosis: Report of a case. Am. J. Ophthall. 34:405

Weitzman I, Crist MY. 1980. Studies with isolates of *Cunninghamella.* II. Physiological and morphological studies. Mycologia 72:661

Windus DW, et al. 1987. Fatal *Rhizopus* infections in hemodialysis patients receiving deferoxamine. An. Inter. Med. 107:678

Waldorf AR, Peter L, Polak A. 1984. Mucormycotic infections in mice following prolonged incubation of spores *in vivo* and the role of spore agglutinating antibodies on spore germination. J. Med. Vet. Mycol. 22:101

Zycha H, Siepmann, et al. 1969. Mucorales. Lehre, Verlag von J. Cramer, pp. 355

MISCELLANEOUS FUNGAL INFECTIONS

1. *Adiaspiromycosis* (Haplomycosis, Adiasporosis)

This rare self-limited fungal pulmonary disease of humans and animals is caused by inhalation of conidia which only enlarged (adiaconidia) with thick walls along with no reproduction in tissue. A sufficient number of adiaconidia in tissue may cause distress. The conidia eventually die and may become calcified.

Etiologic agents

There are two causative agents: *Emmonsia parva* (Emmons et Ashburn) Ciferri et Montemartini 1959 var. *parva* (Synonym: *Chrysosporium parvum* var. *parvum* Carmichael, 1962). *E. parva* (Emmons et Ashburn) Ciferri et Montemartini var *crescens* (Emmons et Jellison, 1960) van Oorschot, 1980.

Occurrence

Humans: Only a small number of cases have been reported since 1964, usually in the lung. When a large number of conidia are in the lung a severe respiratory distress may occur. The disease has occurred in Honduras, Venezuela, France, and Czechoslovakia.

Animals: The disease has been reported in mice, moles, rats, rabbits, ground squirrels, skunks, weasels, minks, opossums, aradillas and wallabies.

Laboratory Procedures

Specimen collection: Biopsy needs to be taken from the lungs for histological and laboratory studies.

Direct examination: Histological sections are needed to detect the adiaconidia which are usually 150 to 300 μm in diameter in tissue. Figure 246 shows two large adiaspores of *E. parva* var *crescens*. Microscopic examination of smears from excising small pieces of tissue on a direct mount should show the large adiaconidia in the smashed nodules, and will confirm the diagnosis.

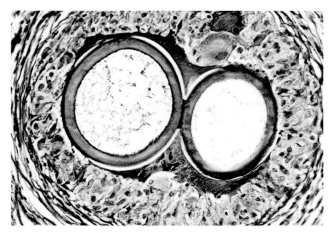

Figure 246. Two large Adiaconidia of *E. parva crescens*

Culture: Minced pieces of tissue on Sabouraud glucose agar or other media will allow the organism to grow within 2 to 3 weeks. Both varieties grow best at 20° to 25°C.

E. parva var. *parva.* The colonies are white to buff, thin, zonate and tufted. Aerial hyphae may form coremia. The reverse side is cream to light brown. When the hyphae and conidia of this variety are placed on media at 40°C the hyphae degenerate, while the conidia enlarge into uninucleate adiaconidia, and are up to 40 μm or greater with a thick wall.

Microscopically, the conidia are hyaline, finely roughened, and 3 to 3.5 μm in diameter. The conidia are produced on sides of hyphae or on conidiophores that branch at right angles from the hyphae.

E. parva var. *crescens.* The colonies of this variety resemble *E. parva* var. *parva* except for slightly larger conidia, measuring 2 to 4 by 2.5 to 4.5. When the fungus is grown at 37°C the hyphae usually disintegrate and the conidia enlarge to become multinucleate adiaconidia. This organism will not produce the enlarged conidia at 40°C. The adiaconidia produced in experimental animals may increase up to 200 to 700 μm in diameter with three-layered walls up to 70 μm thick. When cultured at 25°C, the adiaconidia may develop numerous bud like sprouts, resembling somewhat the multiple buds of *Paracoccidioides brasiliensis.*

Selected References

Bambirra EA, Nogueira AMMF. 1983. Human pulmonary granulomas caused by *Chrysosporium parvum* var *crescens (Emmonsia crescens)*. Am. J. Trop. Med. Hyg. 32:1184

Cavallari VM, et al. 1986. Adiaspiromycose pulmonar: relato de μm caso. J. Pneumol. 12:95

Ciferri R, Montemartini A. 1959. Taxonomy of *Haplosporangium parvum*. Mycopathol. Mycol. Appl. 10:303

Dvorak JM, et al. 1973. Adiaspiromycosis caused by *Emmonsia crescens* Emmons and Jellison, 1960. Prague, Ceskoslovenska Acad. Ved. pp. 1-120

Emmons CW. 1964. Budding in *Emmonsia crescens*. Mycologia 56:415

Emmons DW, Jellison WL. 1960. *Emmonsia crescens* sp. n. and adiaspiromycosis (haplomycosis in mammals). Ann. NY. Acad. Sci. 89:91

Jellison WL. 1969. Adiaspiromycosis (=Haplomycosis). Mountain Press, Missoula, Montana.

Kodousek R, et al. 1972. Pulmonary adiaspiromycosis in man caused by *Emmonsia crescens*: report of a unique case. Am. J. Clin. Pathol. 56:394

Menges RW, Habermann RT. 1954. Isolation of *Haplosporangium parvum* from soil and results of experimental inoculation. Am. J. Hyg. 60:106

2. *Basidiomycosis.*

Fungi belonging to the phylum Basidiomycota consists of many species of large fruiting bodies, pathogens in plants, saprophytes and yeast-like forms in their life history. Only a few species have been associated with human infections. The most well-known basidiomycetous pathogen is *Filobasidiella*, the teleomorphic state of *Cryptococcus neoformans*.

Emmons (1954) reported repeated isolation of *Coprinus micaceous* from a patient with bronchiectasis. Another mushroom, *C. cinereus*, well-documented as the etiologic agent of endocarditis, was isolated from an aortic valve and the adjacent aortic wall during surgery. The fungus which produced septate hyphae and oidia in culture, was crossed with a known monokaryotic hyphae and oidia of *C. cinereus*. Fruiting bodies developed typical of this species.

Schizophyllum commune has been reported as the causative agent in the following cases: onychomycosis in the cerebrospinal fluid in a patient with meningeal symptoms, and in a chronic lung disorder case. None of these cases had confirmation by biopsy. In 1973 (Restrepo, et al, 1973) *S. commune* was well documented as the causative agent of ulceration and perforation of the palate. Biopsy of the ulcer showed the submucosa had been penetrated by hyphae. Three more cases due to *S. commune* (Kern and Uecker, 1986 and Rosenthal, et al, 1992) were identified by cultures taken from surgically removed sinus contents. All cultures had hyphae with clamp connections.

Culture: *Schizophyllum commune* can be cultured on Sabouraud glucose agar, or potato flake agar without cycloheximide at 30° to 37°C. In about three weeks white, large, fan-shaped leathery basidiocarps (about 2.5 cm) with split gills have developed around the periphery of the colony. Figure 248 shows a basidiocarp in culture.

Microscopically, the hyphae produce clamp-connections usually at each septum. Characteristic spicules develop on the surface of the hyphae (Figure 247). Basidia produce elongate, tear drop basidiospores.

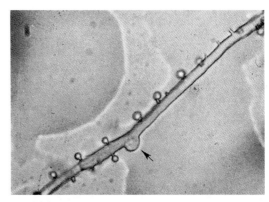

Figure 247. Mycelium in culture showing clamp connection (*arrow*) and series of spicules. The latter are characteristic of *Schizophyllum*.

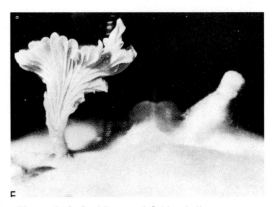

Figure 248. Basidiocarp of *Schizophyllum commune* from culture of lesion. (Courtesy of A. Restrepo-Moreno and D. Greer.)

Two species of *Ustilago* have been reported as causative agents of human infections. *U. maydis* was found in a cutaneous lesion, and *U. Zeae* was reported in a brain lesion. Neither case was confirmed by culture.

Selected References

Ciferri R, et al. 1956. Isolation of *Schizophyllum commune* from sputum. Atti. Inst. Bot. Lab. Crittogamico Univ. Pavia 14:118

Greer DL. 1978. Basidiomycetes as agents of human infections: a review. Mycopathologia 65:133

Kern ME, Uecker FA. 1986. Maxillary sinus infection caused by the homobasidiomycetous fungus *Schizophyllum commune*. J. Clin. Microbiol. 23:1001

Restrepo A, Greer DL, Robledo M. 1973. Ulceration of the palate caused by a basidiomycete *Schizophyllum commune*. Sabouraudia 11:201

Rosenthal J, et al. 1992. Chronic maxillary sinusitis associated with the mushroom *Schizophyllum commune* in a patient with AIDS. Clin. Infect. Dis. 14:46

Speller DCE, MacIver AC. 1971. Endocarditis caused by a *Coprinus* species: a fungus of the toadstool group. J. Med. Microbiol. 4:370

3. *Geotrichosis*

Definition

Geotrichosis is a fungus infection that may produce lesions in the mouth, intestinal tract, bloodstream, bronchi, and vagina. Pulmonary involvement is the most frequently reported form for this disease. There have been numerous isolations of the fungus from stool specimens, sputum, feces, urine and vaginal secretions with the organism being found in 18 to 31 percent of the individuals. These isolates have never been associated with any specific disease. This fungus is considered opportunistic. It is important to carefully check for the presence of budding cells on arthroconidia and assimilate patterns as *Trichosporon beigelii* is likely to be the causative agent. *Geotrichium candidum* does not have budding cells on arthroconidia. Another similar fungus *Blastoschizomyces capitatus* needs to be considered.

Etiologic Agent

Geotrichum candidum Link, 1809 (Synonym: *Oidium pulmoneum* Bennett 1842).

Perfect (Teleomorph) state: *Galactomyces geotrichum* (Butler et Petersen) Redhead and Malloch, 1978 (synonym: *Endomyces geotrichum* Butler and Petersen, 1972).

Occurrence

Geotrichum sp. may be found in the mouth, skin, and intestinal tract of normal people. The more filamentous *Geotrichum* occurs as a contaminant in sputum, cottage cheese, milk, decaying food-stuffs, tomatoes, and soil. The organism is ubiquitous in nature.

Humans: There are too few reports of isolations of the fungus from tissue. Since a diagnosis of geotrichosis is very difficult without elimination of other similar organisms.

Geotrichosis has been reported a number of times in North America and occurs worldwide in distribution.

Geotrichum is part of normal flora in 18% to 31% of healthy humans.

Animals: The disease is also quite rare in animals although there are reports of cases in pigs, dogs, fowl, cattle (mastitis), and an intestinal disease in an ocelot.

Laboratory Procedures

Specimen collection: Sputum, pus, or bloody stool should be placed in sterile containers for laboratory examination.

Direct examination: Pus or sputum, with or without the addition of 10% KOH, should be placed on a slide with a coverglass. Bloody feces also may be examined on a slide. A smear of infected material may be stained by Gram's method.

Microscopically, the cells of *Geotrichum* are rectangular, 4 by 8 μm, with ends somewhat rounded, or are spherical and 4 to 10 μm in diameter (Figure 249 shows arthroconidia and hyphae from a sputum smear). Stained cells are Gram positive.

Culture: Infected material should be streaked on Sabouraud glucose agar plates, with the addition of antibacterial agents if desired, and maintained at room temperature for one or more weeks. Growth is not as rapid at 37°C.

Colonies: At room temperature the fungus develops rather fast as a flat, membranous- or mealy-surfaced colony, yeast-like in consistency, and white to cream in color (Figure 250).

At 37°C colonies have only a small surface growth and extensive subsurface growth. Microscopically, the wide septate hyphae segment into rectangular arthroconidia, which are variable in size and rounded on the ends. Look for arthroconidia that are segmenting on the slide mount (Figure 251).

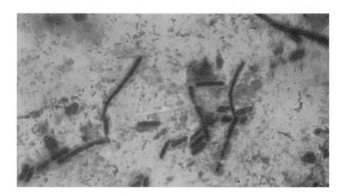

Figure 249. *Geotrichum candidum,* sputum, Gram stain X200

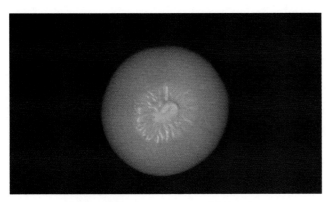

Figure 250. *Geotrichum candidum,* colony

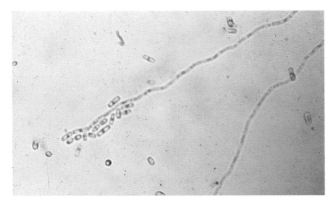

Figure 251. *Geotrichum candidum,*
arthroconidia from culture X200

When self-sterile strains of *G. candidum* are paired on malt extract agar or potato dextrose agar, oval to spherical naked, hyaline asci with single or rarely two ascospores are produced. The globose to oval ascospores are uninucleate. The outer wall of the ascospore is rough while the inner wall is smooth.

Animal inoculation: Infection has not been successfully achieved in laboratory animals.

Special nutritional requirements: This organism can assimilate glucose, galactose, lactose, and xylose, but not sucrose or maltose. It grows well on ethanol medium. The organism does not ferment glucose, galactose, sucrose, maltose, or lactose.

Questions

1. Compare the colonial and microscopic characteristics of *Coccidioides immitis* with *Geotrichum candidum.* Any similarities?

2. How does *Geotrichum candidum* differ from common yeasts such as baker's yeast-*Saccharomyces cerevisiae, Trichosporon beigelii,* and *Blastoschizomyces capitatus?*

Selected References

Butler EF, Petersen LJ. 1972. *Endomyces geotrichum,* a perfect state of *Geotrichum candidum.* Mycologia 64:365

Carroll JM, Jasmin AM, Baucom U. 1968. Intestinal geotrichosis (*Geotrichum candidum*) in the ocelot (*Relis pardalis*). Am. J. Vet. Clin. Pathol. 2:257

Heinic GS. et al. 1992. Oral *Geotrichum candidum* infection associated with HIV infection. A case report. Oral Surg., Oral Med. & Oral Path. 73:726

Hoog GS de, Smith MT, Gueho E. 1986. A revision of the genus *Geotrichum* and its teleomorphs. Stud. Mycol. 29:1

Jagirdar J, Geller SA, Bottone EJ. 1981. *Geotrichum candidum* as a tissue invasive human pathogen. Hum. Pathol. 12:668

Lincoln SD, Adcock JL. 1968. Disseminated geotrichosis in a dog. Path. Vet. 5:282

Minton R, Young RV, Shanbrom E. 1954. Endobronchial geotrichosis. Ann. Intern. Med. 40:340

Oblack DL, Rhodes JC. 1983. Use of the rapid diazonium blue B test to differentiate clinically important species of *Trichosporum* and *Geotrichum.* Sabouraudia 21:243

Restrepo A, Uribe L de. 1976. Isolation of fungi belonging to the genera *Geotrichum* and *Trichosporum* from human dermal lesions. Mycopathologia 59:3

Quadri SM, Nichois CW. 1978. Tube carbohydrate assimilation method for the rapid identification of clinically significant yeasts. Med. Microbiol. Immunol. 165:19

Redhead SA, Malloch DW. 1977. The Endomycetaceae: New concepts, new taxa. Can. J. Bot. 55:1711

Ross JD, Reid KD, Speirs CF. 1966. Bronchopulmonary geotrichosis with severe asthma. Br. Med. J. 1:1400

Salkin IF, et al. 1985. *Blastoschizomyces capitatus,* a new combination. Mycotaxon 22:375

Torheim BJ. 1963. Immunochemical-investigations in *Geotrichum* and certain related fungi. II. Introduction and description of the strains. Sabouraudia 2:146

Tricerri R, et al. 1990. Esophageal ulcer caused by *Geotrichum candidum* in a case of AIDS. Pathologica 82:187

Weijman ACM. 1979. Carbohydrate composition and taxonomy of *Geotrichum, Trichosporon,* and allied genera. Antonie Van Leeuwenhoek. 45:119

KERATOMYCOSIS

(Mycotic keratitis)

Definition

Fungus infection of the cornea is usually initiated by trauma. A white plaque develops after the spores germinate, and mycelial growth occurs in the area of the trauma. Ulceration develops in the cornea around the opacities (Figure 252). Keratomycosis is more frequent since the extensive use of antibacterial antibiotics and topical corticosteroid therapy has been used for eye injuries and diseases. Corneal trauma, corneal disease, and glaucoma are predisposing factors. Usually the cases of eye infections caused by *Blastomyces dermatitidis*, *Candida* spp., *Coccidioides immitis*, *Cryptococcus neoformans*, *Rhizopus* spp., and *Sporothrix schenckii* are causative agents of endophthalmitis and not keratitis.

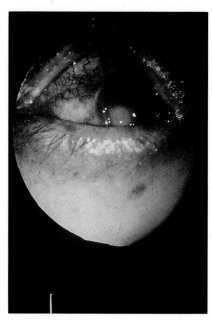

Figure 252. Keratomycosis, eye infection

Etiologic Agents

Many different fungi may be the etiologic agents of keratomycosis ranging from yeastlike organisms to many other fungi that are often soil saprophytes. Examples of the genera with species isolated and/or histologically proven cases from corneal scrapings are: *Acremonium* spp., *Aspergillus* spp., *Beauveria* spp., *Botrytis* spp., *Botryodiplodia* spp., *Bipolaris* spp., *Cephaliophora* spp., *Cladorrhinum* spp., *Cladosporium* spp., *Colletotrichum* spp., *Curvularia* spp., *Cylindrocarpon* spp., *Diplosporium* spp., *Exophiala* spp., *Exserophilum* spp., *Fusarium* spp., *Geotrichum* spp., *Gibberella* spp., *Gliocladium* spp., *Glomerella* spp., *Lasiodiplodia* spp., *Macrophoma* spp., *Myrothecium* spp., *Paecilomyces* spp., *Penicillium* spp., *Periconia* spp., *Phaeltrichoconis* spp., *Phialophora* spp., *Pleospora* spp., *Pseudallescheria* spp., *Pullularia* spp., *Pythium* spp., *Rhizoctonia* spp., *Scopulariopsis* spp., *Sphaeropsis* spp., *Tetraploa* spp., *Trichophyton* spp., *Tritirachium* spp., *Ustilago* spp., and *Volutella* spp. A large number of cases are due to species in the genus *Aspergillus*, especially the

species *A. fumigatus*, *A. flavus*, and *A. niger*. In the genus *Fusarium*, the species *F. solani* is the most common isolate.

Occurrence

Humans: Worldwide in distribution. The incidence of mycotic infections of the cornea has increased following more extensive use of antibiotics or topical cortisones.

Animals: Intracorneal necrosis in the rabbit eye has been established under laboratory conditions.

Laboratory Procedures

Specimen collection: Scrapings should be taken deep in the ulceration around the opacities. Occasionally a corneal biopsy is necessary for diagnosis. Surface swabbing is not sufficient to remove the organisms.

Direct examination: Corneal scrapings of the filamentous fungi should be placed on a sterile microscope slide in 10% KOH solution or lactophenol. The fungus should appear as septate, branching, hyphal fragments. Fungal elements may be difficult to find. Giemsa stain is useful and rapid to help differentiate the fungal structures in the small amount of tissue.

Culture: Sabouraud glucose agar with chloramphenicol is suitable for most of the organisms likely to be isolated. The infected material should be placed on the medium and kept at 24° to 30°C, and checked in about three days, and if negative, held for a couple of weeks to check for slow growing organisms. A temperature of 37°C will inhibit most of the organisms causing mycotic keratitis. The presence of more than one colony is a good indicator of the etiologic agent, especially if the histologic section has fungal hyphae.

Identification of the fungus is based on colony morphology and color and the arrangement and types of spores. For a description of some of the various etiologic agents, reference should be made to the section on contaminant fungi (page 8) in this manual or to the literature cited at the end of this section. Many of these genera are difficult to speciate, requiring a mycologist specializing in the taxonomy of these fungi.

Histopathology: Sections of the infected cornea should be stained with PAS, Gridley, or the Gomori methenamine-silver stain. In the PAS and Gridley stained sections, the fungal structures will appear red, while in the Gomori methenamine-silver stain the structures will be black.

Animal inoculation: Corneal infections have been established in rabbits by the use of cortisone and oxytetracycline or following trauma and inoculation of the organism.

Selected References

Anandi V, et al. 1988. Corneal ulcer caused by *Bipolaris hawaiiensis.* J. Med. Vet. Mycol. 26:301.

Barnett HL, Hunter BB. 1987. *Illustrated Genera of Imperfect Fungi.* 4th Edition. MacMillan Publishing Co., New York.

Barron GL. 1968. *The Genera of Hyphomycetes From Soil.* Williams and Wilkins Co., Baltimore.

Berson EL, Kobayashi GS, Oglesby RB. 1965. Treatment of experimental fungal keratitis. Arch. Ophthal. 74:403

Bulmer C. 1977. The ocular mycoses. Contrib. Microbiol. Immunol. 4:56

Chick EW, Conant NF. 1962. Mycotic ulcerative keratitis; a review of 148 cases from the literature (abstr). Invest. Ophthal. 1:419

Ernest JT, Rippon JW. 1966. Keratitis due to *Allescheria boydii (Monosporium apiospermum).* Am. J. Ophthal. 62:1202

Forster R, et al. 1975. Dematiaceous fungal keratitis: clinical isolates and management. Br. J. Opthalmol. 59:372

Halde C, Okumoto J. 1966. Ocular mycoses: A study of 82 cases. Amsterdam Excerpta Med. Intern. Congress p. 705

Ishibashi V, Kaufman HE. 1986. Corneal biopsy in the diagnosis of keratomycosis. Am. J. Opthalmol. 101:228

Ishibashi V, Hommura S, Matsumoto V. 1987. Direct examination vs culture of biopsy specimens for diagnosis of keratomycosis. Am. J. Opthalmol. 103:636

Jones DB, Sexton R, Rebel TG. 1970. Mycotic keratitis in South Florida: a review of 39 cases. Trans. Ophthal. Soc. UK. 89:78

Kirkness CM, et al. 1991. *Sphaeropsis subglobosa* keratomycosis, first reported case. Cornea 10(1):85

Krachmer JH, Anderson RL, Binder P, et al. 1978. *Helminthosporium* corneal ulcers. Am. J. Ophthal. 85:666

McDonnell PJ, et al. 1985. Mycotic keratitis due to *Beauvaria alba.* Cornea. 3:213

Naumann G, Green WR, et al. 1967. Mycotic keratitis: A histopathologic study of 73 cases. Am. J. Ophthal. 64:668

O'Day DM. 1977. Fungal endophthalmitis caused by *Paecilomyces ilacinus* after intraocular lens implantation. Am. J. Ophthal. 13:130

Okabe S, Matsuo N, Okuda K, et al. 1977. A case of keratomycosis caused by *Fusarium* light and electron microscopic observations. Fol. Ophthal. Jap. 28:80

Polack FM, Kaufman HE, et al. 1971. Keratomycosis,

medical and surgical treatment. Arch. Ophthalmol. 85:41

Suie T, Havener WH. 1963. Mycology of the eye: a review. Am. J. Ophthalmol. 56:63

Thomas PA, Kuriakose T. 1990. Keratitis due to *Arthrobotrys oligospora* Fres 1950. J. Med. Vet. Mycol. 28:47

Zapater RC. 1986. Opportunistic fungus infections: *Fusarium* infections. Jpn. J. Med. Mycol. 27:68

PENICILLIOSIS AND PENICILLIOSIS MARNEFFEI

Definition

Penicillium species are well established as agents of external ear infection but their role in rare cases as causal agents of pulmonary infection in severely immunosuppressed patients or barrier breaks has not occurred until recently. The exception is *P. marneffei* which has become increasingly important in immunosuppressed patients as a causative agent of invasive mycoses.

Etiologic Agent

Penicillium marneffei Segretain, 1959.

Occurrence

Humans: The most frequent sites of infection by *P. marneffei* are lymph nodes, lung, liver and skin. Other sites include: spleen, bone marrow, bowel, pericardium, kidney, meninges, finger, and nasopharynx.

Animals: The fungus has been isolated from burrows of bamboo rats in China. Most of the bamboo rats contain *P. marneffei* in their internal organs with no external lesions. The fungus is found as small yeastlike cells, 4.5 μm in diameter, somewhat like *Histoplasma,* within macrophages. These yeast cells reproduce by plantae division and not by budding.

Laboratory Procedures

Specimen collection: Biopsies from skin, bone, or liver are necessary for histopathologic study.

Culture: The sputum or aspirates of pulmonary abscesses or skin nodules should be spread on Sabouraud glucose agar with antibacterial antibiotics. The cultures should be incubated at 25° and 37°C to develop the dimorphic characteristics. The colony develops rapidly at 25°C, becoming grayish with a floccose surface. The under surface produces a soluble pigment, brownish-red to wine in color. The surface becomes blue-green when the conidiophores mature. At 37°C the colonies develop a soft, white to tan, yeast-like colonies within 2 weeks.

Microscopically, at 25°C the conidiophores are smooth with terminal verticils with 3 to 5 metulae. Several phialides are produced on each metula (9 to 11 by 2 to 5 μm). The phialides produce chains of smooth, globose to subglobose conidia, 2 to 3 μm in diameter. At 37°C the cultures contain shortened hyphal cells with many septa and extensive branching. After conversion the yeast-like cells are oval to elliptical (2 to 6 μm in diameter) with reproduction by fission.

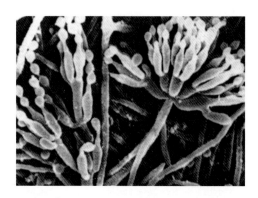

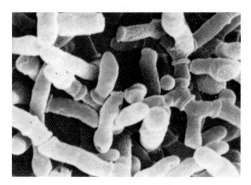

Figure 253. *Penicillium marneffei*. a, SEM showing conidiophores produced in a colony grown at 25°C. b. Early stages of conversion from mycelial to yeast form. From Deng, Z., et al.: Rev. Infect. Dis. *10*. 640–652, 1988

Histopathology: Histopathologic features of the lesions are similar to histoplasmosis with granulomatous inflammation, necrosis, and the presence of yeastlike cells inside the phagocytes. The cells of *P. marneffei* are well-stained with either PAS or GMS. The yeast cells are about 3 to 4.5 μm in diameter with some elongated cells up to 8 μm in length with cross walls.

Question

1. What are several important differences between *Penicillium marneffei* and other species of *Penicillium?*

Selected References

Chan YF, Woo KC. 1990. *Penicillium marneffei,* osteomyelitis. J. Bone Joint Surg. (Br) 72:500

Chiewchanvit S, et al. 1991. Cutaneous manifestations of disseminated *Penicillium marneffei* mycosis in five HIV infected patients. Mycoses 34:245

Deng AL, Conner DH. 1985. Progressive disseminated penicilliosis caused by *Penicillium marneffei:* report of eight cases and differentiation of the causative organism from *Histoplasma capsulatum.* Am. J. Clin. Pathol. 84:323

Deng A, Yun M, Ajello L. 1986. Human penicilliosis marneffei and its relation to the bamboo rat (*Rhizomys pruinosus*). J. Med. Vet. Mycol. 24:383

Deng A, et al. 1988. Infections caused by *Penicillium marneffei* in China and Southeast Asia: review of eighteen published cases and report of four more Chinese cases. Rev. Infect. Dis. 10:640

Droughet E, et al. 1988. Mycological ultrastructural and experimental aspects of *Penicillium marneffei* isolated from a disseminated penicilliosis in AIDS. Bull. Soc. Fr. Mycol. Med. 17:77

Estrada JA, et al. 1992. Immunohistochemical identification of *Penicillium marneffei* by monoclonal antibody. Internat. J. Dermat. 31:410

Hulshof CMJ, et al 1990. *Penicillium marneffei* infection in an AIDS patient. Eur. J. Clin. Microbiol. Infect. Dis. 9:370

Jayanetra P, et al. 1984. Penicilliosis marneffei in Thailand: report of five human cases. Am. J. Trop. Med. Hygf. 33:637

Pautler KB, et al. 1984. Imported penicilliosis marneffei in the United States: report of second human infection. Sabouraudia 222:433

Peto TEA, et al. 1988. Systemic mycosis due to *Penicillium marneffei* in a patient with antibody to human immunodeficiency virus. J. Infect. 16:285

Ramirez C. 1982. Manual and Atlas of the Penicillia. Elsevier Biomedical Press. New York.

Raper KB, Thom C. 1949. A Manual of the Penicillia. Williams & Wilkins. Baltimore.

Tsui WMS, Ma KF, Tsang DNC. 1992. Disseminated Penicillium marneffei infection in HIV infected subjects. Histopathology 20:287

Wei X, sd G, et al. 1985. Report of the first case of penicilliosis marneffei in China. Natl. Med. J. China 65:533

PYTHIOSIS INSIDIOSI

(Swamp cancer, hyphomycosis destruens)

Definition

Pythiosis insidiosi was considered an animal disease until the first human cases were reported in 1987. The majority of the patients had alpha- or beta-thalassemia as the underlying condition along with severe arteritis. There is gradual onset of symptoms related to vascular insufficiency of the lower extremities, resting calf pain and leg coldness. Some of the patients had amputation or died and others recovered. One patient had an orbitofacial infection after an eye injury (see Figure 254).

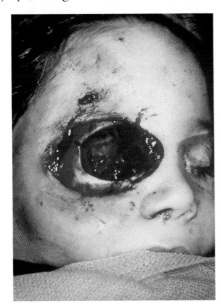

Figure 254. Orbitol infection in right eye caused by *Pythium insidiosum*

The disease in animals develops granulomatous and necrotic lesions mostly on the head and lower portions of the legs. Less frequently the animals develop infections of the lung, lymphatic vessels, nasopharynx, and bone. The animal disease has several synonyms including "swamp cancer," hyphomycosis destruens, "Florida horse leech," and "equine phycomycosis."

Etiologic agent

Pythium insidiosum De Cock, Mendoza, Padhye, Ajello et Kaufman 1987. (Synonym: *Hyphomyces destruens* Bridges et Emmons, 1961; *Pythium gracile* Schenk 1859 (sensu Middleton); *Pythium destruens* Shipton, 1987. This fungus belongs in the phylum Oomycetes.

Occurrence

Humans: Most of the patients with pythiosis insidiosi have been farmers with exposure areas to swamps. Eight cases have been reported in Thailand and a case of orbitofacial infection in Texas.

Animals: The disease has been reported most commonly in horses and mules. Occasionally cattle, dogs, and cats have been infected. In the United States most of the cases have been reported from Florida and Texas.

Laboratory Procedures

Specimen collection: Biopsies or material from ulcers, granulomatous or necrotic lesions should be available for laboratory and histology studies.

Direct examination: Material should be teased apart and mounted in 10% KOH to look for fungal hyphae 3 to 10 μm in diameter around the small arterial branches in the necrotic lesions. The usually nonseptate hyphae are very thin-walled and may collapse.

Cultures: Colonies of the fungus grown on Sabouraud glucose agar are white to yellowish-white, covering the plate in 4 to 5 days. On Sabouraud glucose agar *P. insidiosum* does not sporulate. Zoosporangia are filamentous and are produced from hyphae when a block of agar medium and colony are placed in water or grown in water agar culture.

Microscopically, the development of the vesicle and release of the zoospores may be observed with water and hyphae from the water culture mounted on a slide with a coverglass. The zoosporangium develops a thin-walled discharge tube up to 700 μm in length and 3 to 4 μm in width. The protoplasm moves through the discharge tube to form a spherical vesicle. Cleavage of protoplasm occurs inside the vesicle to form biflagellate zoospores, with the shorter anterior flagella of the tinsel type and the longer posterior flagella of the whiplash type. With more movement the zoospores break the vesicles and swim away, later encysting and germinating under favorable conditions. See vesicle in Figure255.

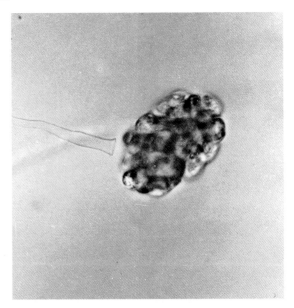

Figure 255. Vesicle formation by *Pythium insidiosum*

Globose smooth-walled oogonia (19 to 36 μm in diameter) may develop on cornmeal agar at 24° to 30°C. Antheridia arise from the same or different hyphae and attach to the oogonium. Usually one round, thick-walled oospore (17 to 27 µm in diameter) forms in the oogonium. Sometimes oogonia form in old water cultures.

Histopathology: Sections of tissue show infiltration by neutrophils, eosinophils, and on rare occasions multinucleate giant cells. The aseptate hyphae, 4 to 20 µm in diameter, are readily seen at the periphery and around small arterial branches in the necrotic lesions. Figure 256 shows nonseptate hyphae in a bone biopsy.

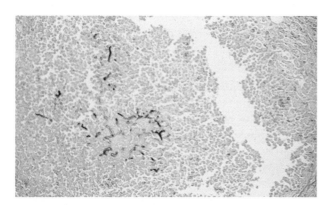

Figure 256. Nonseptate hyphae of *Pythium insidiosum* from a bone biopsy.

Serology: An immunodiffusion test has been developed with a culture filtrate antigen to detect antibody to *P. insidiosum* (Pracharktam, R, et al. 1991).

Selected References

Ader PL. 1974. Phycomycosis in fifteen dogs and two cats. J. Am. Vet. Med. Assoc. 174:1216

Austwick PKC, and Copland JW. 1974. Swamp cancer. Nature 250:84

Bridges CH, Emmons CW. 1961. A phycomycosis of horses caused by *Hyphomyces destruens*. J. Am. Vet. Med. Assoc. 138:579

Chaiprasert A, et al. 1990. Induction of zoospore formation in Thai isolates of *Pythium insidiosum*. Mycoses 33:317

De Cock A.W. A. M., et al. 1987. *Pythium insidiosum* sp. nov. the etiologic agent of pythiosis. J. Clin. Microbiol. 25:344

Dick MW. 1990. Keys to Pythium. Dept of Bot; School Plant Sci, Reading, United Kingdom.

Mendoza L, Prendas J. 1988. A method to obtain rapid zoosporogenesis of *Pythium insidiosum*. Mycopathologia, 109:59

Mendoza L, et al. 1992. Evaluation of two vaccines for the treatment of pythiosis insidiosi in horses. Mycopathologia 119(2):89

Pracharktam R, et al. 1991. Immunodiffusion test for diagnosis and monitoring of human *Pythiosis insidiosi*. J. Clin. Microbiol. 29:2661

Renaldi MG, et al. 1989. *Pythium insidiosum* as an agent of devastating orbital-facial mycosis: mycological and management aspects. Abst Am Soc Microbiol Ann Meeting F-11. New Orleans.

Shipton WA. 1987. *Pythium destruens* sp. nov. an agent of equine pythiosis. J. Med. Vet. Mycol. 79:15

Chapter 10

ACTINOMYCETES

The actinomycetes are a group of filamentous microorganisms with many of the characteristics of bacteria and some appearance of fungi. The group is usually classified with the bacteria in the Phylum Schizomycota. The rudimentary mycelium is very thin, being about 1 μm in diameter, and when fragmented, resembles coccoid or bacillary forms. Some of the organisms in this group are sensitive to the same antibiotics as the Gram-positive bacteria. Other bacteria-like characteristics are: muramic acid in the cell wall structure, lack of a structural nucleus, lack of mitochondria, and motile forms similar in structure. The actinomycetes are included in this manual for comparison with fungi.

Since some of the families in the actinomycetes produce branched filaments, conidiophores, and conidia, the organisms causing diseases are listed among those causing mycotic diseases. These are: *Actinomyces, Nocardia, Actinomadura,* and *Streptomyces.* It is important to recognize the similarities to bacteria. The term "actinomycete" usually includes all of the Actinomycetales except the Mycobacteriaceae. The somatic filaments or cells of all members of the group are approximately 1 μm in diameter. The order is separated into three families. The Mycobacteriaceae have rudimentary or no mycelium and contain the well-known genus *Mycobacterium.* The Actinomycetaceae have a freely branched mycelium that becomes septate and breaks up into bacillary or coccoid forms. In this family the genus *Actinomyces* is anaerobic or microaerophilic, obligate, not acid-fast, and catalase-negative. The genus *Nocardia* is aerobic, partially acid-fast or acid-fast, a saprophyte or a facultative parasite, and catalase-positive. The third genus of medical importance in this family is *Actinomadura,* which is not acid-fast, does not fragment into bacillary or coccoid forms, but produces chains of oval to round conidia. There is no "lipid characteristic" present in members of the *Actinomadura* genus, the wall contains mesodiaminopimelic acid (meso-DAP), and the organism is catalase-positive.

The members of the third family, Streptomycetaceae, have well-branched filaments and reproduce by sporangia or conidia in chains or singly at tips of conidiophores. Spiral conidiophores may be present. The genus *Streptomyces,* containing species that produce most of the commercially important antibiotics, is in this family. This genus reproduces by means of conidia from the ends of filaments, it is catalase positive, L-diaminopimelic acid (DAP) and glycine are in the cell wall of members. There is no "lipid characteristic," as in *Nocardia* species, *Micromonospora* produces conidia singly at the ends of short conidiophores, and the cell wall has meso-DAP as well as glycine.

The actinomycetes are usually Gram-positive. In smear preparations of the pathogenic forms, the mycelium is extensively broken up into bacillary forms. The properties of colonies vary in the actinomycetes. A wide variety of nitrogen and carbon compounds can be utilized, and many colonies show proteolytic activity. Differentiation of species of the actinomycetes is based on morphologic and physiologic characteristics (Tables 21 and 22 on page 212).

ACTINOMYCOSIS

(Lumpy Jaw)

Definition

Actinomycosis is a chronic suppurative and granulomatous filamentous bacterial infection with lesions or draining sinuses discharging the characteristic "sulfur granules." The disease is most common in the head and neck but may spread to the abdominal organs, thoracic organs, and other parts of the body (Figure 257, and Figure 258). The filamentous hyphae are much smaller than fungus hyphae found in tissue. It is useful to be able to recognize the difference. Actinomycosis is common in cattle but much less common in humans due to the extensive use of antibiotics.

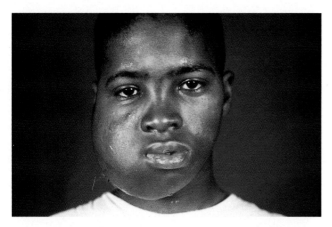

Figure 257. Actinomycosis, *Actinomyces israelii*

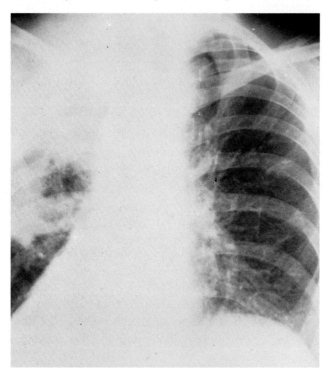

Figure 258. Pulmonary actinomycosis,
Actinomyces israelii, X-ray film

Etiologic Agents

Actinomyces israelii (Kruse) Lachner-Sandoval, 1898, is the usual organism isolated from human lesions or from normal human tissues. A part of the normal flora of humans.

Actinomyces bovis Harz, 1877. Regularly is the cause of actinomycosis in cattle and other animals. The organism is in the normal flora of the oral cavity in various animals. Rarely a disease in humans.

Actinomyces odontolyticus Batty, 1958. In the oral cavity of humans, rats, and hamsters. Frequently cause of human and animals actinomycosis and other types of infections such as endocarditis.

Actinomyces meyeri (Prevot) Cato, Moore, Mygaard, Holdeman, 1982. This organism has only been reported in human flora.

Actinomyces naeslundii Thompson and Lovestedt, 1951 has caused many cases of human actinomycosis. A part of the normal flora of the human oral cavity.

Actinomyces viscosus (Howell, Jordan, Georg, and Pine) George, Pine, and Gerencser, 1969. Frequently causes human and animal actinomycosis and other types of infections such as endocarditis.

Arachnia propionica (Buchanan and Pine) Pine and Georg, 1969. This organism is part of the flora in the human mouth, and encountered as a cause of actinomycosis and lacrimal canaliculitis.

Bifidobacterium dentium Scardovi and Crociani, 1974 (synonym Georg, Roberstad, Brinkman, and Hicklin, 1965). A few human cases.

Occurrence

Actinomyces israelii has been isolated from the surface of carious teeth, tonsillar crypts, various areas of the mouth, and sputum by various investigators (Emmons, 1938, Rosebury et al, 1944). The organism has not been isolated from soil or plant sources. Frost (1940) first reported *A. bovis* in the mouths of normal cattle. The endogenous origin for all of the above organisms is indicated with the main locations being in the tonsillar crypts and the teeth.

Humans: Actinomycosis is worldwide in occurrence.

Animals: Most of the cases have been reported in turkeys, cattle, sheep, pigs, dogs, horses, deer, and cats.

Laboratory Procedures

Specimen collection: Pus should be collected in a sterile container (test tube or bottle) as it drains out of sinus or be removed from unopened lesions with a syringe. Sputum, urine, or biopsy or autopsy material may be available for laboratory examination.

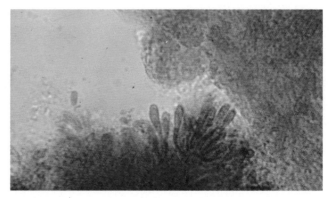

Figure 259. *Actinomyces* sp., Granule with clubs, direct mount, cotton blue lactophenol X1000

Direct examination: Place a loopful of pus containing one or more "sulfur granules" on a slide and lightly crush it with a coverglass. Eosin, lactophenol cotton blue, or trypan blue may be added to the pus to color the granules (Figure 259). Another granule should be smeared on a slide and stained by Gram's method.

Microscopically, the unstained granule is composed of fine, branching, interwoven hyphae (1 μm in diameter). In some strains the ends of the hyphae are frequently surrounded by gelatinous sheaths which give the appearance of club-shaped structures around the edges of the granule (Figure 259). The granule is apparently cemented together by a polysaccharide-protein complex containing about 50% calcium phosphate (Pine and Overman, 1966). On the Gram-stained slide, under immersion oil lens, note the Gram-positive branched hyphae. Some old hyphae may be short, rod-shaped, and bacteria-like and may appear Gram-negative. If material contains no granules, pus, or sputum from possible cases of actinomycosis should be smeared, stained, and examined for Gram-positive branched hyphal forms. If an acid-fast stain is made, the organisms will show nonacid-fast branched forms.

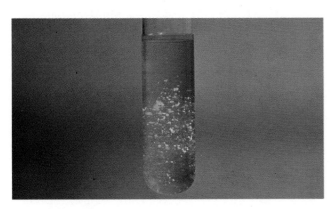

Figure 260. *Actinomyces israelii*, thioglycolate culture

Culture: Gram-positive, nonacid-fast branching hyphal forms from granules or from cases without granules should be cultured under anaerobic conditions. All *Actinomyces* spp. are anaerobic and catalase-negative. If the material is uncontaminated, the organisms can be grown in thioglycollate broth, deep-shake cultures of brain-heart infusion glucose agar, sealed up for anaerobic conditions at 37°C. In four to five days colonies appear about 1.5 cm below the surface of the medium (Figure 260).

Contaminated material should be washed several times in sterile distilled water or sterile saline solution to remove contaminating organisms before granules are crushed and streaked on the agar surface. A number of media may be used for isolation of species of *Actinomyces:* brain-heart

infusion agar (BHI) with 10% rabbit blood, chocolate agar, BHI with 0.2% glucose, casitone-starch medium (Howell and Pine), or trypticase soy agar. The appearance of the colonies on BHI at the end of about seven days and a negative catalase test are important in identification of the species (Figure 261). The above culture media should be incubated at 37°C under 95% nitrogen and 5% CO_2 for two to seven days.

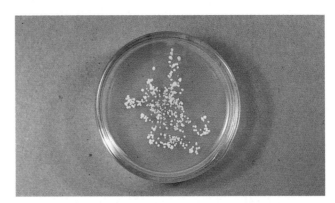

Figure 261. *Actinomyces israelii*, brain-heart infusion agar

Identification of species: The transfer of colonies resembling *A. israelii*, *B. dentium* (formerly *eriksonii*), or *A. bovis* to broth culture is useful to show the characteristic growth pattern. Branching forms are usually abundant. Colonies appear in four to six days about 5 mm below the surface, with the broth remaining clear. The saprophytic species, *A. naeslundii*, grows and spreads rapidly throughout the medium.

Culture: On streaked plates the colonies appear as a small, white, smooth to rough convex surface with a fuzzy or smooth edge, depending on the species (Figure 261). The colonies develop in seven to ten days. The central portion of the colonies may give a concave, molar-tooth appearance due to lysis.

Microscopically, colonies crushed in a drop of water on a slide with a coverglass show tangled masses of branching hyphae 1 μm in diameter. Stained smears show Gram-positive branching hyphae (Figure 262) and/or pleomorphic diphtheroid-like rods, depending upon species (Figure 263).

Identification based on morphologic and physiologic characteristics: Two references by Georg, et al (1964, 1965) separate the microaerophilic and anaerobic *Actinomyces* species on the basis of morphologic, biochemical, and immunologic differences. Reference should be made to these papers for detailed information. Some of the distinguishing features are given in Tables 21 and 22. The physiologic characteristics, including results of biochemical tests, are useful in the separation of species of *Actinomyces*.

B. dentium (*eriksonii*) resembles *A. israelii* and *A. naeslundii* morphologically but differs from them in biochemical reactions and oxygen requirements (Table 22). The agar gel precipitin reactions are reported by Georg, et al, 1965 to be antigenically distinct for *B. dentium*. All of the physiologic tests are available commercially from various manufacturers (such as: API 20 anaerobes, and API Zym test).

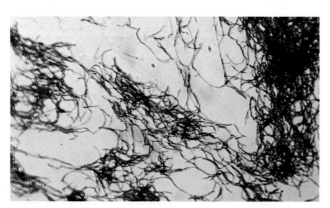

Figure 262. *Actinomyces israelli,* branching hyphae. Gram stain X600

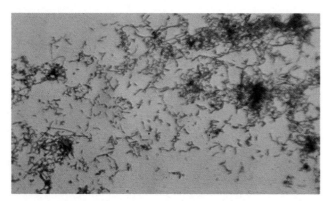

Figure 263. *Actinomyces israelli,* diphtheroids. Gram stain X600

Media for biochemical tests:

Catalase Test: A small amount of the colony is placed on a slide and a drop of peroxide (fresh H_2O_2) is added. No bubble formation should occur for the *Actinomyces* species (negative).

Gelatin Liquefaction: Check the gelatin liquefaction reaction on gelatin-heart infusion casitone medium (see page 42 for preparation). Use pyrogallol-carbonate seal (page 41), incubate four weeks at 37°C.

Nitrate Reduction: Inoculate the medium, add pyrogallol-carbonate seal, and incubate at 37°C. Test small amounts two or three times during a two-week interval for nitrate reaction (a few drops of both sulfanilic acid solution

[glacial acetic acid, 100 ml; water, 250 ml; sulfanilic acid, 2.8 g] and 158 Actinomycetes dimethyl-alpha-naphthylamine solution [glacial acetic acid, 100 ml; water, 250 ml; dimethyl-alpha-naphthylamine, 2.1 ml], which should show a red to brown color if nitrates are reduced to nitrites. Zinc may be used to reduce the remaining nitrates or see if the organisms did not reduce nitrates.

Starch Hydrolysis: Use plates or tubes or casitone starch medium (see section on "Media for Specific Use," page 43) and streak the culture on the surface. Use an anaerobic jar for plates or seal the tubes with the pyrogallol carbonate seal, and maintain at 37°C. Test the surface at the end of five or ten days with Gram iodine. A clear area around the colony indicates hydrolysis; deep-blue would mean no hydrolysis.

Sugar Fermentation: After the organism has been growing in heart infusion broth (or sugar-free medium), transfer to sugar fermentation tubes and seal with pyrogallolicarbonate seals. Incubate for one month at 37°C, checking for acid formation periodically. See page 41 for preparation of medium.

Characteristics of species of the Actinomyces:

1. *Actinomyces israelii* (Kruse) Lachner-Sandoval 1898.

Colony Morphology: On brain-heart infusion (BHI) blood agar plates after 1 to 2 days serotype 1 *A. israelii* develops minute, spiderlike colonies with branching "mycelial" elements radiating from the center. This can be observed by holding the plate at an angle above a light source. In 10 days the colony is hard, lobulated, gray-white and glistening. The other serotype 2 is small, entire, shiny in 1 to 2 days and smooth, entire, convex, and shiny in 10 days.

Microscopically short rods with branches and coccoid forms are present in young cultures, becoming more elongate in older colonies and in tissue. The genus *Actinomyces* is gram positive and nonacid-fast (Table 21).

Physiologic Characteristics: Table 22.

2. *A. bovis* Harz, 1877.

Colony Morphology: On BHI blood agar plates in 1 to 2 days under anaerobic incubation the colony is small, smooth, entire, white, and glistening. In 10 days it remains smooth, opaque, white, and grainy. This species is similar to *A. israelii* serotype 2.

Microscopically short diphtheroid-like rods, and coccoid bodies are seen in young colonies. In older colonies there are short, branching rods and fragmentation to coccoid bodies present (in both culture and tissue). Gram-positive, nonacid-fast. (Table 21).

Physiologic Characteristics: Table 22.

3.   *A. naeslundii* Thompson and Lovestedt, 1951.

Colony Morphology: On BHI blood agar plates in 1 to 2 days under anaerobic conditions small, smooth colonies develop with mycelium radiating around edge. In 10 days the colonies have an entire edge, with a raised, rough, grainy surface.

Microscopically short rods, branching, diphtheroid forms and small coccus-like cells should be seen in young colonies. In older colonies more fragmentation and coccoid bodies develop. (Table 21).

Physiologic Characteristics: Table 22 lists the characteristics.

4.   *A. viscosus* (Howell, Jordan, George, and Pine) Georg, Pine, and Gerencser, 1969.

Colony Morphology: On BHI blood agar plates grown aerobically with CO_2 the colonies form a dense center with a filamentous fringe, and are opaque, cream to white color, soft, with a viscous to mucoid consistency.

Microscopically, this organism has a mixture of coccoid, diphtheroid, and long sinuous branching filaments (Table 21)

Physiologic Characteristics: Refer to Table 22 for characteristics.

5.   *Bifidobacterium dentium* Scardovi and Crociani, 1974 (Synonym: *Bifidobacterium eriksonii* Georg 1974).

Colony Morphology: The colonies on BHI blood agar plates in 1 to 2 days under anaerobic conditions develop a dense filamentous appearance. The colonies are flat and granular with a conical center. In 10 days it is convex or conidial, soft, and entire with a white color.

Microscopically, smears of the young colonies show branching diphtheroid-like rods. Fragmentation and coccoid bodies develop in time. Gram-positive, nonacid-fast. (Table 21).

Physiologic Characteristics: Table 22 lists the characteristics.

6.   *Arachnia propionica* (Buchanan and Pine) Pine and Georg, 1969.

Colony Morphology: After 1 to 2 days the organisms on BHI blood agar plates develop a spiderlike colony like *A. israelii*. Ten days later the colony becomes smooth, round, and flat to convex more like *A. bovis.*

Microscopically typical *Actinomyces* morphology occurs in culture. Young colonies develop short-branching, diphtheroidlike forms and later develop fragmented to coccoid bodies (Table 21).

Physiologic Characteristics: Table 22 lists the characteristics.

Other less important species of the Actinomyces and other genera such as *Actinomyces odontolyticus, A. meyeri,* and *Rothia dentocariosa* may be found in more comprehensive references.

Histopathology: If material is available from biopsy, prepare sections and stain with H and E, PAS, or Gridley stains for showing the granules (Figure 264 and 265). The use of Gram-stain or Gomori methenamine-silver stain will bring out the mycelium better and not the granules.

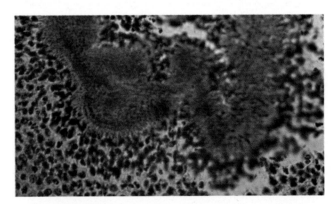

Figure 264. *Actinomyces* sp., granule, in tissue X600

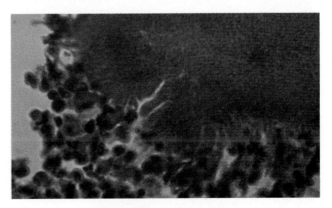

Figure 265. *Actinomyces* sp., granule with clubs, in tissue X1250

Table 21. Morphologic Characteristics of *Actinomyces* Spp.

Characteristic	*Actinomyces israelii*	*A. bovis*	*A. naeslundiii*	*A viscosus*	*Bifidobacterium dentium* *	*Arachinia propionia*
Colonies on BHI agar, 7-10 days, 37°C	Rough ("R") form starts as "spider" or granularlike, with lacelike border. Later lobulate, molar-tooth, glistening. "S" or smooth form transparent, like *A. bovis*	Dewdroplike, then entire edge convex cream color (S forms). Rare R forms resemble *A. israelii*, with scalloped border, lumpy surface	Similar to those of *A. bovis* or *A. israelii*. S forms most common	Similar to *A. bovis*, entire edge, raised, rough surface	Similar to those of *A. bovis*; white to cream, convex, to conical, smooth or pebbly surfaced with scalloped edge	Similar to those of *A. israelii* in 48 hrs., to those of *A. bovis* in 10 days. Smooth and flat
Colinies in thioglycollate broth, 37°C	Rough lobulate, or with fuzzy edges, broth clear, not broken readily	Soft, diffuse or crumblike, readily broken-up	Fast growing, granular or floccose, diffuse, somewhat cloudy	Soft, diffuse crumblike	Soft, lobular, diffuse growth, broth cloudy if shaken	Diffuse or turbid growth
Microscopic (all Gram-positive)	Rods and branched forms, some with clubbed ends. Long hyphae at times. Diptheroid in S form	Diptheroid forms usual, branching rare. Rare R strains with long, branched hyphae.	Short hyphae with branches. Irregular, long hyphae vary in thickness. Some diphth-eroidlike forms.	Diphtheroid forms, branching, fragment to coccoid forms.		Short branching rods, becoming long branching filaments with age. Grains in tissue

*Formerly *eriksonii*

Table 22. Physiologic Characteristics of *Actinomyces* Spp.

Reactions (37°C)	*Actinomyces israelii*	*A. bovis*	*A. naeslundiii*	*A viscosus*	*Bifidobacterium dentium* *	*Arachinia propionia*
O₂ Requirements	Anaerobic to microaerophilic	Anaerobic to microaerophilic	Facultative with increased CO$_2$	Anaerobic to microaerophilic	Obligate anaerobe	Anaerobic to microaerophilic
Biochemical						
Catalase	0	0	0	+	0	0
Gelatin liquefaction	0	0	0	0	0	0
Nitrate reduction	+ (80%)	+	+ (90%)	+	0	+
Starch hydrolysis	0 (usually)	+	0 (usually)		+	0
Propionic acid production	0	0	0	0	0	+
Sugar fermentation (acid formation only)						
Glucose	+	+	+	+	+	+
Mannitol	+ (80%)	0	0	0	+	±
Mannose	+	0 or ±	+	+	+	+
Raffinose	Varies	0	+ (80%)	+	+	+
Xylose	+ (80%)	0	0	0	+	0
Ribose	+	0	±	±	+	±
Maltose	+	+	+	+	+	+
Glycerol	0	0	±	+	0	0
Lactose	+	+	+	+	+	+
Sucrose	+	+	+	+	+	+

*Formerly *eriksonii*   0 = no reaction; + = positive ± = variable.

Microscopically, these sections or other prepared slides will show variations in appearance of the lesions from an abscess with polymorphonuclear cells to proliferation of connective tissue.

Commonly found in histologic sections are many leukocytes in necrotic areas surrounded with granulation tissue. The granule has well-branched mycelium loosely or compactly formed, usually with clubs on the surface of the granule, varying from 30 to 400 µm in size (see Figure 264). The sulfur granule is characteristic of some, but not all, species of *Actinomyces*. *Bifidobacterium dentium* does not produce granules.

NOTE: The demonstration of the typical sulfur granule in tissue or pus of a specimen is sufficient to indicate the diagnosis of actinomycosis in humans.

Animal inoculation: Occasional pathogenicity has been established in male hamsters and mice with *A. bovis*. Meyer and Verges (1950) demonstrated progressive infection of actinomycosis in young mice injected with cultures suspended in 5% gastric mucin (hog).

Behbehani et al (1983) achieved experimental infections in mice with pure cultures of *A. israelii* and *Arachnia propionica*. In experimental disease the essential features of a natural infection occurred, including the formation of typical granules with clubs.

Serology: Agglutinins, precipitins, and complement-fixing antibodies can be demonstrated in individuals with the disease. However, at the present time methods are not sufficiently standardized for ˌpractical use. Fluorescent (FA) procedures have been developed that are specific for staining *A. israelii*, Group D; *A. naeslundii*, group A; *A. bovis*, group B; *A. odontolyticus*, group E; and *A. viscosus*, group F; from smears of tissue, exudates, or cultures (Happonen, and Viander, 1982). The standard FA antisera can be used for identity of an unknown isolant.

Special requirements: Species of *Actinomyces* are difficult to maintain in culture for stock supply. One of the best methods is lyophilization of a brain-heart infusion broth culture by taking the spun-down culture and sterilized milk, adding both to the lyophilization tubes, and lyophilizing the tubes. Pine and Watson (1959) have developed an *Actinomyces* maintenance medium. After the organism has grown in the liquid medium under pyrogallol-carbonate seal, the tube is kept in a deep freeze. If the tube is kept in the refrigerator, transfers should be made about every six months.

Questions

1. List some similarities and differences between *Actinomyces* and *Nocardia*.

2. What are some differences between *Mycobacterium*, diphtheroids, and *Actinomyces?*

3. In what ways do the Actinomycetes resemble the bacteria? The fungi?

Selected References

Avery RJ, Blank F. 1954. On the chemical composition of cell walls of the Actinomycetales and its relation to their systematic position. Can. J. Microbiol. 1:140

Behbehani MJ, Heeley JD, Jordan HV. 1983. Comparative histopathology of lesions produced by *Actinomyces israelii*, *Actinomyces naeslundi* and *Actinomyces viscosis* in mice. Am. J. Pathol. 110:267

Blank CH, Georg LK. 1968. The use of fluorescent antibody methods for the detection and identification of *Actinomyces* species in clinical material. J. Lab. Clin. Med. 71:283

Boone CJ, Pine L. 1968. Rapid method for characterization of actinomycetes by cell wall composition. Appl. Microbiol. 16:279

Brock DW, Georg LK. 1969. Determination and analysis of *Actinomyces israelii* serotypes 1 and 2. J. Bacteriol. 97:581

Brown JM, Georg LK, Waters LC. 1969. Laboratory identification of *Rothia dentocariosa* and its occurrence in human clinical materials. Appl. Microbiol. 17:150

Cato EP, et al. 1984. *Actinomyces meyeri* sp. nov. specific epithetrer. In J. Syst. Bacteriol. 34:487

Coleman RM, Georg LK, Rozzell A. 1969. *Actinomyces naeslundii* as an agent of human actinomycosis. Appl. Microbiol. 18:420

Duguid HI, et al. 1982. *Actinomyces* and intrauterine devices. J. Am. Med. Assoc. 248:1579

Georg LK, Roberstad GW, Brinkman SA. 1964. Identification of species of *Actinomyces*. J. Bacteriol. 88:477

Gereneser MA, Slack JM. 1976. Serological identification of *Actinomyces* using fluorescent antibody techniques. J. Dent. Res. 55:184

Gillis TP, Thompson JJ. 1978. Quantitative fluorescent immunoassay of antibodies to, and surface antigens of, *Actinomyces viscosus*. J. Clin. Microbiol. 7:202

Happonen RP, Viander M. 1982. Comparison of fluorescent antibody techniques and conventional staining methods in diagnosis of cervico-facial actinomycosis. J. Oral. Pathol. 11:417

Jordan HV, Kelley DM, Heeley JD. 1984. Enhancement of experimental actinomycosis in mice with *Eikenella corrodens*. Infect. Immun. 46:367

King S, Meyer E. 1963. Gel diffusion technique in antigen-antibody reactions of *Actinomyces* species and "anaerobic diphtheroids." J. Bacteriol. 85:186

Lénnette EH, Barlows A, Hausler W, Shadomy HJ. 1985. Manual of Clinical Microbiology. 4th ed. Am. Washington. Soc. Microbiology

Li Y, Georg LK. 1968. Differentiation of *Actinomyces propionicus* from *Actinomyces israelii* and *Actinomyces naeslundii* by gas chromatography. Can. J. Microbiol. 14:749

Marucha PT, Keyes PH, Wittenberger CL, et al. 1978. Rapid method for identification and enumeration of oral *Actinomyces*. Infect. Immun. 21:786

Meyer E, Verges P. 1950. Mouse pathogenicity as a diagnostic aid in the identification of *Actinomyces bovis*. J. Lab. Clin. Med. 36:667

Pine L, Howell A, Watson SJ. 1960. Studies on the morphological, physiological, and biochemical characteristics of *Actinomyces bovis*. J. Gen. Microbiol. 23:403

Pine L, Overman JR. 1966. Differentiation of capsules and hyphae in clubs of bovine sulfur granules. Sabouraudia 5:141

Pine L, Watson SJ. 1959. Evaluation of an isolation and maintenance medium for *Actinomyces* species and related organisms. J. Lab. Clin. Med. 45:107

Pine L, Bradley-Malcolm, Cirtis EM, Brown JM. 1981. Demonstration of *Actinomyces* and *Arachnia* species in cervicovaginal smears by direct staining with species specific fluorescent antibody conjugate. J. Clin. Microbiol. 13:15

Slack JM, Landfried S, Gerencser MA. 1969. Morphological, biochemical, and serological studies on 64 strains of *Actinomyces israelii*. J. Bacteriol. 97:873

Sohler A, Romano AH, Nickerson WJ. 1958. Biology of Actinomycetales. III. Cell wall composition. J. Bacteriol. 75:283

Staneck JL, Roberts GD. 1974. Simplified approach to the identification of aerobic actinomycetes by thin-layer chromatography. Appl. Microbiol. 28:226

Valicenti JK, Papas AA, Graber C, Williamson HO. 1982. Detection and prevalence of IUD associated *Actinomyces* colonization and related morbidity. A prospective study of 69,925 cervical smears. J. Am. Med. Assoc. 247:11490

NOCARDIOSIS

Definition

Nocardiosis is an infection similar to actinomycosis in symptoms, with suppuration and granuloma in the subcutaneous tissues resulting in swelling, abscesses, and draining sinuses. The disease may be a primary pulmonary infection (Figure 266) later involving other organs, especially the brain and at times the kidneys, spleen, liver, and adrenals through hematogenous spread. Invasive pulmonary and disseminated nocardioses are considered true opportunistic infections. These may occur due to various clinical and therapeutic factors. Individuals with a T-cellular immune deficiency as a result of hematologic malignancy, antirejection therapy for organ allograft, drug abuse or acquired immunodeficiency are more susceptible to actinomycotic infection. Some species may develop subcutaneous mycetomas in the extremities (see mycetoma, chapter 6 page 99, Figure 129) with the skin as the portal of entry.

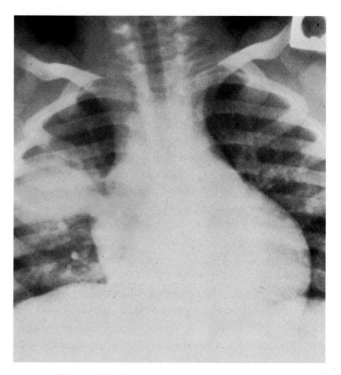

Figure 266. Pulmonary nocardiosis, X-ray film

Nocardia asteroides is the causative agent of 81% to 91% of the serious pulmonary and systemic infections. *N. brasiliensis* is second with a small number of the remaining cases. The most common agents of actinomycotic mycetoma are *N. brasiliensis, Streptomyces somaliensis,* and *Actinomadura madurae.* These aerobic actinomycetes are catalase positive, and diphtheroid-like to branching filamentous bacteria.

Etiologic Agents of Nocardiosis and Actinomycotic Mycetoma:

Nocardia asteroides (Eppinger, 1891) Blanchard, 1896, is the most common cause of nocardiosis throughout the world. A second agent, *N. brasiliensis* (Lindenberg, 1909) Castellani and Chalmers, 1913, may cause nocardiosis on occasions in the United States but is more common in

Central and South America. Both organisms may also be the cause of mycetomas.

These two *Nocardia* species and a third species, *N. caviae* (Erickson) Gordon and Mihm, 1962, as well as species of *Actinomadura, Streptomyces,* and *Actinomyces,* may cause actinomycotic mycetoma. In all cases the mycelial elements in the mycetoma are 1 µm or less in diameter in contrast to hyphae in the eumycotic mycetoma granules. Species of *Actinomadura* and *Streptomyces* causing mycetomas are: *A. madurae* Lechevalier, 1970; *A. pelletierii* Lechevalier, 1970; *S. somaliensis* (Brumpt) Mackinnon and Artagaveytia-Allende, 1956; and *S. paraguayensis* (Almeida) Mackinnon and Artagaveytia-Allende, 1956.

Occurrence

N. asteroides has been isolated from soil a number of times. Gonzales-Ochoa (1964) reported *N. brasiliensis* from a soil sample in Mexico. The infection is exogenous and introduced through injury or inhalation of the fungus.

Humans: Nocardiosis due to *N. asteroides* occurs throughout the world, while the disease due to *N. brasiliensis* has been reported in Mexico, Central America, South America, North America, India, and Africa.

Animals: A number of infections due to *N. asteroides* have been reported in dogs, cows, and rainbow trout (Snieszko et al, 1964).

Laboratory Procedures

Specimen collection: Pus, sputum, or tissue should be collected in a sterile container. Cerebrospinal fluid should be brought to the laboratory for centrifugation to concentrate sediment for examination. Biopsy or autopsy specimens may be available for laboratory study. The material should contain branching Gram-positive hyphae and fragmented bacillary forms in nocardiosis cases. Actinomycotic mycetomas of the foot contain grains.

Direct examination of agents of nocardiosis: Prepare smears of pus, sputum, or centrifuged sediment and stain with Gram stain or the modified Kinyoun acid-fast stain for examination. The decolorization that occurs with acid alcohol should not exceed five to ten seconds.

Microscopically, the smears are always Gram-positive with branching hyphae 1 µm in diameter or bacillary and coccoid forms. The results of the acid-fast stain will vary according to species.

Culture: The organism infected materials will grow on Sabouraud glucose agar, Sabouraud yeast extract agar, or Lowenstein-Jensen medium, all without antibiotics. The species of *Nocardia* are sensitive to antibacterial antibiotics. Digestion of contaminated material may increase the chance for isolation of *N. asteroides* by reducing competition of contaminating microorganisms. Cultures should be incubated at 25° and 37°C. Species are separated on the basis of colony characteristic, morphology, acid-fastness, hydrolysis of casein, amylolytic activity, and reactions to tyrosine, xanthine, and other biochemicals (Table 23). Hyphae of these species are less than 1 µm in diameter. Isolation by paraffin bait technique is useful (page 42). All are catalase-positive.

In the laboratory compare *N. asteroides* with *N. brasiliensis.* Stain slides with Gram and acid-fast stains to check microscopic appearance. Compare cultural and biochemical characteristics for both species. The first three species following are etiologic agents of nocardiosis as well as actinomycotic mycetomas on occasion. The last three are causes of actinomycotic mycetomas (see section on mycetomas, page 99). Slide cultures are useful for study of morphology of these organisms.

Agents of nocardiosis

1.   *Nocardia asteroides*

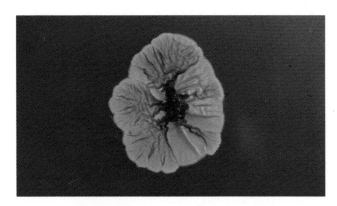

Figure 267. *Nocardia asteroides,* colony

Colony: On Sabouraud glucose agar, the colonies are glabrous, chalky, folded or wrinkled, white, pink, brown to orange-pink in color, and have aerial hyphae. On Czapek agar the color is yellow to orange (Figure 267), 37°C is optimum. The colony grows at 46°C.

Microscopically, smears show Gram-positive, branched hyphae fragmenting into bacillary and coccoid forms (Figure 268). Partially acid-fast or acid-fast. Chains of squarish conidia may form.

Physiologic characteristics: See Table 23.

Table 23. Characteristics of *Nocardia*, *Actinomadura*, and *Streptomyces* spp.

Species	Granula	Fragmentation hyphae	Acid-fast	Cell wall type*	Casein hydrolysis	Decomposition of tyrosine	Decomposition of xanthine	Amylolytic activity	Utilization of paraffin	Liquification of gelatin	Urease test
N. asteroides	White to yellow if present, about 1 mm; absent if systemic	+	+	IV	−	−	−	−	+	−	+
N. brasiliensis	Like above, granules more common, with or without clubs	+	+	IV	+	+	+	−	+	+	+
N. caviae	Like *N. asteroides*	+	+	IV	−	−	−	−	+	−	+
A. madurae	White to yellow or red, large, 1-10 mm, soft, lobulated	−	−	III	+	+ (−for 14%†)	−	+	−	+	−
A. pelletierii	Red, smooth-edged, hard, 0.3-0.4 mm	−	−	III	+	+	+	−	+ for (13%†)	+	−
S. somaliensis	Yellow to brown, hard, 1-2 mm, round	−	−	I	+	+	+	−	−	+	−
Streptomyces spp. (saprophytes)	—	—	*Spores usually* +	I	+ (or) −	+	+	(or) +	(usual)	(usual)	+

+ = growth; − = no growth — = trace of growth.
*Cell walls of actinomycetes have glucosamine, muramic acid, glutamic acid, and alanine. Individual groups contain the following components:
(I) L-diaminopimelic acid (DAP) and glycine; (III) meso-DAP; (IV) meso-DAP, arabinose, and galactose (Becker, 1965).
†Gordon (1966).

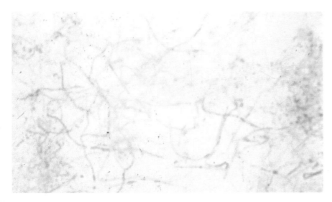

Figure 268. *Nocardia asteroides,* filamentous, bacillary, partially acid-fast X600

2. *N. brasiliensis*

Colony: On Sabouraud glucose agar, the colonies are folded, cerebriform, white, yellow, tan to orange in color, dry and chalky, or glabrous usually with an earthy odor (Figure 269). On Czapek agar the colonies are similar in appearance. 30°C is optimum. Terminal conidia may be present. Does not grow at 46°C.

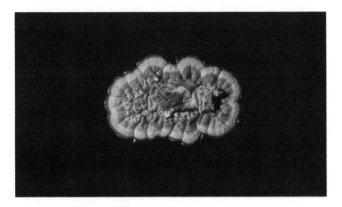

Figure 269. *Nocardia brasiliensis,* colony

Microscopically, stained slides are Gram-positive with mycelium fragmenting into different length bacillary forms. Partially acid-fast or acid-fast. On slide culture the branching filaments of *N. brasiliensis* separates it from *N. asteroides*. *N. brasiliensis* grows as spherical colonies on the sides of the tube (with 0.4 per cent gelatin) while *N. asteroides* does not.

Physiologic characteristics: See Table 23.

3. *N. caviae*

Colony: On Sabouraud glucose agar, the white to orange colored colonies are glabrous, folded, wrinkled or granular, and resemble both *N. asteroides* and *N. brasiliensis*. Growth varies at 46°C. On Bennett's medium, *N. caviae* is cream to

peach in color. Tufts of short aerial mycelium may develop. Microscopically, the organism is Gram-positive and is partially acid-fast with branched hyphae fragmenting into bacillary and coccoid forms.

Physiologic characteristics: See Table 23.

Agents of Actinomycotic Mycetoma

4. *A. madurae*

Colony: Colonies on Sabouraud agar are glabrous, waxy, wrinkled, moist, granular, cream to occasionally red in color (Figure 270). On Czapek agar the colonies are cream colored at first and later pink to red in color. 37°C is optimum.

Microscopically, smears are Gram-positive with delicate hyphae that do not fragment. Chains of spherical conidia may be formed in some isolates. Not acid-fast (Figure 271).

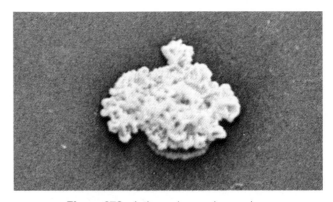

Figure 270. *Actinomadura madurae,* colony

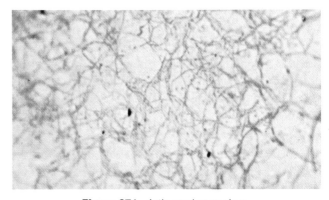

Figure 271. *Actinomadura madurae,* filaments, not acid-fast stain X600

Physiologic Characteristics: Found in Table 22.

5. *A. pelletieri*

Colony: On Sabouraud glucose agar, colonies develop slowly with a wrinkled, heaped, glabrous surface and a coral pink to red color. On Czapek agar the colonies are coral red. 37°C is optimum.

Microscopically, stained slides are Gram-positive and have delicate, branched hyphae that do not fragment. Not acid-fast.

Physiologic characteristics: See in Table 23.

6. *S. somaliensis*

Colony: Colonies grow slowly with a creamy, wrinkled or folded, leathery surface. A white to tan aerial hyphal growth may develop. Older colonies may become dark gray to brown. 30°C is optimum.

Microscopically, stained slides have nonfragmenting, delicate branched hyphae. Conidia may be present. Not acid-fast. At times spores may be acid-fast.

Physiologic characteristics: Table 23.

Techniques for *Nocardia* and *Streptomyces* identification

Stains: For procedure and preparation of stains for Gram and acid-fast stains (Kinyoun's modification) see section on staining methods, page 34.

Casein Medium: For preparation of this medium to check proteolytic activity, see page 40. Streak or make single point inoculations of each organism on the plates, and at the end of one and two weeks check for clearing of casein. *N. asteroides* will not hydrolyze casein.

Bennett's agar: This medium is useful for sporulation of aerobic actinomycetes. The medium consists of: yeast extract, 1 g; beef extract, 1 g; casamino acid, 2 g; dextrose, 10 g; and distilled water, 1,000 ml. The pH is adjusted to 7.3 and the medium is autoclaved at 15 psi for ten minutes. After cooling to 50°C, 35 ml is poured into petri dishes.

Gelatin Liquefaction: Check the gelatin liquefaction reaction on the nutrient broth gelatin medium (see page 41 for preparation). Inoculate the organisms slightly below the surface of the medium and incubate either at 24° or 37°C, along with a control. After growth occurs, refrigerate until control solidifies and check for liquefaction.

Other tests: Organisms should be inoculated into tyrosine

(see page 45) and xanthine and starch-agar plates for characteristic species reactions. Urease test broth should be used to determine the reaction for urease. Utilization of paraffin may readily be determined.

Slide Cultures: Useful for the study of morphology.

Histopathology: If biopsy or autopsy material is available, sections should be made and stained by Gram stain to demonstrate branching hyphae or granules, if present. The hyphae are also readily shown by the Gomori methenamine-silver stain. Periodic acid-Schiff stain is not satisfactory, nor is H and E stain, for demonstrating nocardiosis. The branching hyphae are shown in Figure 272 in a case of nocardiosis in the lung. A suppurative tissue reaction is usually evident in most cases. The separate hyphae or granules containing hyphae usually are found in the abscesses. For additional information see references.

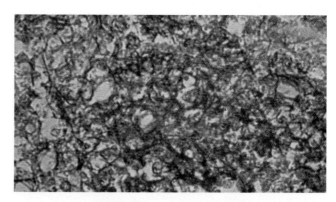

Figure 272. *Nocardia asteroides*, lung tissue, Brown-Hopps stain X400

Animal inoculation: For routine diagnostic work it is not necessary to check animal pathogenicity, as identification is based on morphology and biochemical activity. The virulence among strains varies considerably, making it necessary to select strains and inoculate larger numbers of animals for demonstration of pathogenicity. The use of 5% gastric mucin is of value in increasing the susceptibility of the animal. The guinea pig, rabbit, and mouse have been reported to be susceptible to experimental nocardiosis.

Pathogenicity test for *Nocardia* species (Georg, et al, 1961): After a heavy colony growth has developed in several tubes of Sabouraud glucose agar (about one to two weeks), scrape the growth from the slant into a mortar and add an equal amount of 5% gastric mucin before grinding. Inject 1 ml intraperitoneally into at least two guinea pigs. If the animal dies, or at the end of two and four weeks, autopsy the animals and examine for the presence of lesions with acid-fast hyphae.

Male mice may be inoculated intravenously with 0.2 ml of a 0.1% suspension of the pathogenic species of *Nocardia* and at the same time a 0.5 ml amount of a 5% gastric mucin suspension injected intraperitoneally. In two weeks the organism should be isolated from the spleen if it is pathogenic. (Mohapatra and Pine, 1963). Both *N. asteroides* and *N. brasiliensis* can maintain viability in tissues for up to three weeks. A mouse model for pulmonary nocardiosis was developed by Sugar, et al (1983).

Special tests for presumptive identification: Gordon and Mihm (1962) have suggested a presumptive identification of several *Nocardia* species as follows: An actinomycete with aerial hyphae that does not utilize casein, L-tyrosine, or xanthine may tentatively be considered *N. asteroides.* If a similar organism is acid-fast and utilizes casein and tyrosine but not xanthine, it should be *N. brasiliensis.* Similar forms that decompose xanthine but not casein or tyrosine may be considered *N. caviae.* Acid-fastness may vary in all three.

Serology: Immunodiffusion and counterimmunoelectrophoresis tests using serum can be used to aid in diagnosing mycetomas. The immunodiffusion tests differentiate forms of actinomycetoma from eumycetoma as well as distinguishing the several specific agents of actinomycetoma with some cross-reaction between *A. madurae* and *A. pelletierii.* The intensity and number of precipitin bands are directly related to the size of the lesions; these lines disappear as the patient responds to treatment.

The diagnostic serology for nocardiosis has not been developed in humans but has been developed for dogs and for nocardial mastitis of cattle (Pier, et al, 1975).

Questions

1. What are the characteristics used to separate species of *Nocardia?*

2. Compare *Nocardia* with *Actinomyces* and *Streptomyces.*

3. What true fungi may cause mycetomas (maduromycosis)?

Selected References

Avery RJ, Blank F. 1954. On the chemical composition of the cell walls of the Actinomycetales and its relation to their systematic position. Can. J. Microbiol. 1:140

Beadles TA, Land GA, Knezek. 1980. An ultrastructural comparison of cel envelopes of selected strains of *Nocardia asteroides* and *Nocardia brasiliensis.* Mycopathologia 70:25

Beaman BL, Sugar AM. 1983. *Nocardia* in naturally acquired and experimental infections in animals. J. Hyg. 91:393

Berd D. 1973. Laboratory identification of clinically important aerobic actinomycetes. Appl. Microbiol. 25:665

Blumer SO, Kaufman L. 1979. Microimmunodiffusion test for nocardiosis. J. Clin. Microbiol. 10:308

Boncyk LH, Millstein CH, Kalter SS. 1976. Use of CO_2 for more rapid growth of the *Nocardia* species. J. Clin. Microbiol. 3:463

Calegari L, Asconeguy F, Conti-Diaz IA. 1982. Patogenicidad experimental de cepas de *Nocardia asteroides, Nocardia brasiliensis,* y *Nocardia caviae* de differentes procedencias. Sabouraudia 20:195

Georg LK, Ajello L, McDurmont C, et al. 1961. The identification of *Nocardia asteroides* and *Nocardia brasiliensis.* Am. Rev. Respir. Dis. 84:337

Gonzales-Mendoza A, Mariat F. 1964. Sur l'hydrolyze da la gelatine comme caractere differentiel entre *Nocardia asteroides* et *N. brasiliensis.* Ann. Inst. Pasteur (Paris) 107:560

Goodfellow M, Cross T. 1984. Classification, p. 7-164. *In* M. Goodfellow, Mordarski, M., Williams, S. T. (ed). Biology of the actinomycetes. Academic Press, Inc. (London) Ltd, London.

Gordon MA, 1985. Aerobic pathogenic Actinomycetaceae, p. 249-262. In E. H. Lennette, A. Balows, W. J. Hausler, and H. J. Shadomy (ed.) Manual of clinical microbiology. 4th ed. American Society for Microbiology. Washington, DC.

Gordon RE, Mihm JM. 1962. Identification of *Nocardia caviae* (Erickson) Nov. comb. Ann NY Acad Sci 98:628

Gordon RE, Smith MM. 1955. Proposed group of characters for the separation of *Streptomyces* and *Nocardia.* J. Bact. 67:147.

Huppert M, Wayne LG, Juarez WJ. 1957. Characterization of atypical *Mycobacteria* and *Nocardia* species isolated from clinical specimens. II. Procedures for differentiating between acid-fast microorganisms. Am. Rev. Tb. Pul. Dis. 76:468

Jimenez T, Diaz A, Zlotnik H. 1990. Monoclonal antibodies to *Nocardia asteroides* and *Nocardia brasiliensis* antigens. J. Clin. Microbiol. 28:87

Land GA, Staneck J. 1988. The aerobic actinomycetes. p. 271-302. *In* B.B. Wentworth, M.S. Bartlett, B.E. Robinson, and I.F. Salkin (ed). Diagnostic manual for mycotic and parasitic infection. 7th ed. American Public Health Association, Washington, DC.

Law BJ, Marks MI. 1982. Pediatric nocardiosis. Pediatrics. USA. 70:560

Lechevalier MP, Lechevalier H. 1970. Chemical composition as a criterion in the classification of aerobic actinomycetes. Int. J. Syst. Bacteriol. 20:435

Mishra SK, Randhawa HS. 1969. An application of paraffin bait technique to the isolation of *Nocardia asteroides* from clinical specimens. Appl. Microbiol. 18:686

Mohapatra LN, Pine L. 1963. Studies on the pathogenicity of aerobic actinomycetes inoculated into mice intravenously. Sabouraudia 2:176

Pier AC, Gray DM, Fossatti MJ. 1958. *Nocardia asteroides,* a newly recognized pathogen of the mastitis complex. Am. J. Vet. Res. 19:319

Presant CA, Wiernik PH, Serpick AA. 1973. Factors affecting survival in nocardiosis. Am. Rev. Respir. Dis. 108:1444

Shadomy HJ, Warren NG, 1988. Nocardiosis p. 671-677. *In* A. Balows, W.J. Hausler, Jr., M. Ohashi and A. Turano (ed.). Laboratory diagnosis of infectious diseases: principles and practices. Vol. I. Springer-Verlag. New York

Snieszko SF, Bullock GI, Dunbar CE, et al. 1964. Nocardial infection in hatchery-reared fingerling rainbow trout *Salmo gairdneri).* J Bacteriol 88: 1809

Shawar RM, Moore DG, LaRocco MT. 1990. Cultivation of *Nocardia* spp. on chemically defined media for selective recovery of isolates from clinical specimens. J. Clin. Microbiol. 28:508

Singh M, Sandhu RS, Randhawa HS. 1987. Comparison of paraffin baiting and conventional culture technique for isolation of *Nocardia asteroides* from sputum. J. Clin. Microbiol. 25:176

Stevens DA, Pier AC, et al. 1981. Laboratory evaluation of an outbreak of nocardiosis is immunocompromised hosts. Am. J. Med. 71:928

Wilson JP, et al. 1989. Nocardial infections in renal transplant patients. Medicine 68:38

DERMATOPHILOSIS

(streptotrichosis, strawberry foot rot, epidemic eczema)

Definition

Dermatophilosis is an exudative pustular dermatitis of the skin followed by the formation of scabs and crusts in animals and rarely in humans. Alopecia may be evident after scabs and crusts fall off in healed areas. It may be highly contagious, causing severe economic loss in animals.

Etiologic Agent

Dermatophilus congolensis Van Saceghem, 1915, emend. 1916. Isolates from cattle, sheep, horses, and deer have been assigned other names. Gordon (1974) considers these variations of *D. congolensis*. The etiologic agent is an actinomycete of the Actinoplanaceae (those with motile cells in the life cycle).

Occurrence

Humans: The organism has been reported in persons living in Texas, Iowa, New York, and South America.

Animals: The disease is frequently found in cattle and sheep, and at times in goats, horses, antelopes, deer, zebras, swine, giraffes, foxes, lizards, monkeys, and domestic cats. The disease in cattle is commonly known as "mycotic dermatitis," in sheep as "lumpy wool" or "strawberry foot rot."

Laboratory Procedures

Specimen collection: Crusts and scabs from the animal should be placed in containers and brought to the laboratory for examination and culture.

Direct examination: Smears may be prepared from the scabs or crusts and suspended in saline. Giemsa or methylene blue are useful for staining. For tissue sections, hematoxylin and eosin, Giemsa, or Grocott silver stain may be used (Gordon, 1974).

Microscopically, the organism may be seen in any of the various stages of its life cycle in the cellular serous exudate or keratinizing cells of the superficial epithelia or hair follicle epithelia. The characteristic branched filaments divide both transversely and longitudinally to develop packets of coccoid forms. The branched filaments are 2 to 5 μm in diameter. Motility is usually evident, and clusters of spores may be germinating.

Culture: The organism may be isolated in pure culture by streaking the exudate (taken from a closed pustule) on blood agar plates. If the crust or scab is contaminated, immerse in a bottle of distilled water for 3- hours at 24°C, expose to CO_2 in a candle jar for 15 minutes, and streak the surface film of the water containing the zoospores onto the agar medium (Haalstra, 1965).

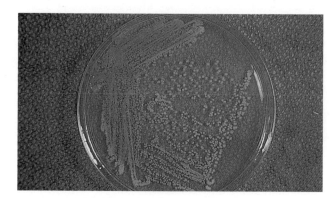

Figure 273. *Dermatophilus congolensis,* colony

On blood agar at 37°C the colonies develop in 24 hours. They are small; round, square, or irregular; grayish-white;

raised; rough; hard; adherent; and usually form pits in the medium. In two to five days an orange pigment usually develops (Figure 273), Betahemolysis develops on beef-heart infusion-horse blood agar. Colonies vary in color from white to orange and may be granular or membranous on brain-heart infusion slants at 37°C, depending on the strain. In beef infusion-peptone broth at 37°C there is a thick sediment while the supernatant fluid is clear.

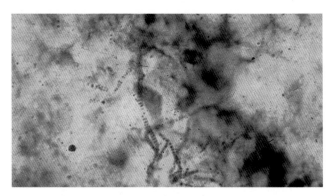

Figure 274. Segmentation state of filaments of *D. congolensis*

Microscopically, in wet, unstained mounts or with methylene blue stain, look for branched filaments, segmentation stage (see Figure 274) , cocci arranged irregularly in cube-shaped packets or the clusters of germinating spores, which release flagellated, motile zoospores. Check for motility of coccoid spores, about 0.5 to 1.0 µm in diameter.

Biochemical reactions: The organism is catalase-positive, and the urease test is positive. Casein and starch are decomposed while xanthine is not. Gelatin is liquefied and nitrates are reduced while indole is not produced. Starch is hydrolyzed but not xanthine or tyrosine. In broth the organism produces acid but no gas from glucose and fructose. There is no fermentation in sucrose, lactose, xylose, mannitol, dulcitol, sorbitol, and salicin.

Animal inoculation: This is not necessary for identification of *D. congolensis,* but may be helpful in detecting and isolating the organism from specimens brought in for study in the laboratory.

The abraded skin of a rabbit, guinea pig, or mouse is inoculated with the organism. Acute ulcerative pustular dermatitis should develop mostly around the hair follicles.

Question

Compare *Dermatophilus* with *Nocardia* microscopically, in culture, and on/or in the animal or in the human.

Selected References

Albrecht R, Horowitz S, et al. 1974. *Dermatophilus congolensis* chronic nodular disease in man. Pediatrics. 53:907

Dean DJ, Gordon MA, Severinghaus CW, et al. 1961. Streptotrichosis: A new zoonotic disease. NY State. J. Med. 61:1283

Erickson EL. 1975. *Dermatophilus congolensis* infection in man. Cutis. 16:83

Gordon MA. 1964. The genus *Dermatophilus.* J. Bacteriol. 88:509

Haalstra RT. 1965. Isolation of *Dermatophilus congolensis* from skin lesions in the diagnosis of streptotrichosis. Vet. Rec. 34:824

Kaplan W. 1966. Dermatophilosis - a recently recognized disease in the United States. S. West Vet. 20:140

Le Riche PD. 1968. The transmission of dermatophilosis in sheep. Aust Vet J 44:64

Lloyd DH, Sellers KC. 1976. *Dermatophilus* infection in Animals and Man. Academic Press, New York

McKenzie RA. 1977. Dermatophilosis of horses and cattle: An early Australian report. Aust. Vet. J. 53:352

Moreira EC, Barbosa M, Moreira YK. 1974. Dermatophilosis in South America. Arqui de Escola de Vet de Univer Fed de Minas Garais. 26:77

Salkin IF, Stone WB. 1981. *Dermatophilus congolensis* infection in wildlife in New York State. J. Clin. Microbiol. 14:604

Sercy GP, Hulland TJ. *Dermatophilus dermatitis* (streptotrichosis) in Ontario. I. Clinical observations. II. Laboratory findings. Can. Vet. J. 9:7

Weber A. 1978. Zür Dermatophilose bei Tier und Mensch. Ber Munch Tierarzt Wochenschrift 91:341

Fungal Cultures

Some of the saprophytic and pathogenic fungi and other organisms may be ordered from the following sources:

American Type Culture Collection, 12301 Parklawn Dr, Rockville, MD 20852. Phone: 301-881-2600; 800-638-6597. FAX: 612-633-6073

Carolina Biological Supply Co, 2700 York Rd., Burlington, NC 27215. Phone: 919-584-0381; 800-334-5551. FAX: 919-584-3399

Central bureau Voor Schimelcultures, Oosterstraat I, Baarn, Netherlands

Chrisope Technology, 3941 Ryan, Lake Charles, Louisiana 70605. Phone: 1-800-256-GERM. FAX 318-479-1006

Clinical laboratories and universities where cultures of the various saprophytic and pathogenic fungi are maintained.

Department of Health, Education and Welfare, Public Health Service, Center for Disease Control, Atlanta, GA 30333.

Triarch, Inc., N8028 Union St., P. O. Box 98, Ripon, WI 54971. Phone:1-800-848-0810. FAX: 414-748-3034

Turtox, P.O. Box 92912, Rochester, N:. Y. 14692. Phone: 800-826- 6164

Immunodiagnostics: Kits and Serological tests.

Microscan Div., Baxter Health-Care Corp. 1584 Enterprise Blvd. West Sacramento, CA 95691

Difco Laboratories, P. O. Box 1058. Detroit, MI 48232. Phone 800- 521-0851. FAX 313-5911-3530

Eiken Chemical Co., Tokyo, Japan.

Gibson Laboratories, Inc., 1040 Manchester St., Lexington, KY 40508. Phone: 800-477-4763. FAX 606-253-1476

Immuno-Mycologics, Inc, PO Box 1151, Norman, OK 73070. Phone: 800- 654-3639. FAX 405-288-2383

Meridian Diagnostics, Inc, PO Box 44216, Cincinnati, OH 45244 Phone: 800-543-1980. FAX 513-271-0124

Microbiological Associates, 4733 Bethesda Ave, Bethesda, MD 20014.

Ramco Laboratories, Inc., 13801 Kirby Dr., Suite 170, Houston, TX, 77098. Phone: 800-231-6238

Wampole Laboratories, P. O. Box 1001. Cranbury, N. Y. 08512. Phone 800-257-9525

Media (prepared and dried)

Becton-Dickinson Microbiology Systems, P. O. Box 243. Cockeysville, MD 21030. Phone: 800-638-8663

BioMerieux, Marcy-l'Etoile 69752 Charbonnieres-les-Bains Cedex/France. Phone: 78 87 81 10. Telex 330967

Difco Laboratories, Inc., P. O. Box 1058, Detroit, MI 48232. Phone: 800-521-0851

Hana Media, Inc., 626 Bancroft Way, Berkeley, CA 94710. Phone: 510-549-0874

Mycogel Labs, Inc., P. O. Box 6548, West Palm Beach, FL 33405. Phone 407:689-6490

Flow Laboratories, Inc., 7655 Old Springhouse Rd., McLean, VA 22102. Phone: 800-368-3569. FAX: 703-893-6727

Gibco/BRL, Inc., P. O. Box 6009, Gaithersburg, MD, 200877. Phone: 800-492-5663

REMEL, 120076 Santa Fe Dr., Lenexa, KS 66215. Phone: 800-255-6730

Sabhi, Inc., 1303 Riverwood Dr., Jackson, MS 39211.

Probe Systems

Gen-Probe Inc, 9880 Campus Point Dr., San Diego, CA 92121. Phone: 800-523-5001, 619-546-8000

Supplies for the Laboratory

The following list contains some of the sources where materials may be procured for teaching of courses and for the clinical laboratories in medical mycology.

Arthur H. Thomas Co., P. O. Box 779, Vine St at Third, Philadelphia, PA 19105.

American Laboratory Supply, Inc., P. O. Box 11, Gibsonville, N C. 27249. Phone: 919-449-6102

Baxter Scientific Products Div., 1430 Waukegan Rd., McGaw Park, IL 60085. Phone 708-689-8410. FAX: 708-473-0804

Becton Dickinson Microbiology Systems, P. O. Box 243, Cockeysville, MD 29030. Phone 800-638-8663

Carolina Biological Supply Co., Inc, 2700 York Rd, Burlington, NC 27215. Phone 800-334-5551. FAX 919-584-3399

Curtis-Matheson Scientific, 9999 Veterans Memorial Dr., Houston, TX 77038. Phone: 800-231-3100

Colab Laboratories, Inc, 3 Science Rd, Glenwood, IL 60425.

Fisher Scientific Co, 711 Forbes Ave., Pittsburgh, PA 15219. Phone: 412-562-8300

Gibco/BRL, Inc., P. O. Box 6009, Gaithersburg, MD 20877. Phone: 800-492- 5663

Matheson Scientific, 850 Greenleaf Ave, Elk Grove Village, IL 60007.

Pfizer Diagnostics Division, Chas. Pfizer and Co, Inc, 235 E 42nd 3 St, New York, NY 10036

Polysciences, Inc. Paul Valley Industrial Park, Warrington, PA 18976 (Fungi-Fluor Kit). Phone 215-343-6484

Sargent-Welch Co, 7400 N Linder Ave, Skokie, IL 60077. Phone: 800- 323-4341

Scientific Products, 1430 Waukegan Rd, McGraw Park, IL 60085.

Arthur H. Thomas Co, PO Box 779, Vine St at Third, Philadelphia, PA 19105.

Turtox, P. O. Box 92912, Rochester, N. Y. 14692. Phone 800-826-6164

Visual Aids

The following films are available on a short-term rental basis from the American Society for Microbiology, 1913 I St., N.W., Washington, DC 20006:

(1) The Diagnosis and Management of Cutaneous Blastomycosis (Gilchrist's Disease)
(2) The Treatment of Moniliasis with Nystatin
(3) Mississippi Valley Disease—Histoplasmosis

Association Films, Inc., 512 Burlington Ave., LaGrange, IL 60525, has the following films:

Treatment of Moniliasis with Nystatin Griseofulvin, Treatment of Superficial Fungus Infection
Fungus Infection of the Foot

Bayer Film Service, Bayer subsidiary in country of the individual: Mycoses of Internal Organs

Institut für den Wissenshaftlichen Film, Nonnenstieg 72, D-3400 Gottingen, Federal Republic of Germany. The following films are on medical mycology :

(1) Aspergillaceae—Asexual Development in *Aspergillus fumigatus* (H. Rieth), E475
(2) Dermatophyta—Asexual Development of *Microsporum gypseum* (H. Rieth), E476
(3) Dermatophyta—Asexual Development of *Microsporum canis* (H. Rieth), E477
(4) Dermatophyta—Pathological Growth Forms by Griseofulvin in *Microsporum canis* (H. Rieth), E478

Color Slides

American Registry of Pathology, Armed Forces Institute of Pathology, Washington, DC 20305.

American Society of Clinical Pathologists, 2100 W. Harrison St., Chicago, IL 60612.

Kaminskis Teaching Slides on Medical Mycology. 540 color transparences and 70 pages of text. Address: Adelaide Children's Hospital, South Australia.

Medical Mycology Teaching Slides. 12 sets of slides and cassettes, Instructional Media Center, Michigan State University, E. Lansing, MI. 48824.

Medical Mycology: 13 sets of slides and/or cassettes. Audio-Visual Library for loan only. South Central Association for Clinical Microbiology, 3901 N. Meridian St., Suite #235, Indianapolis, IN 46208.

Medical Mycology: Software program for teaching mycology and review covering laboratory and clinical aspects with line drawings. IBM or compatible computer with Microsoft Windows. Warlock Productions, 28½ Maple St, Hanover, New Hampshire 30755. Phone: 802-649-8434

Yeast Identification Media and Kits

Analytab Products, Inc, 200 Express St. Plainview, NY 11803 (API 20C, Yeast-Ident).

Becton Dickinson Microbiology Systems, PO Box 243, Cockeysville, MD 21030 (Microtek).
Phone 800-638-8663.

Microscan Div., Baxter Health Care Corp, l584 Enterprise Blvd., West Sacramento, CA 9569l (Enzyme-fluorescent scan).

REMEL, l2076 Santa Fe Dr., Lenexa, KS 662l5 (Uni-Yeast-Tek). Phone: 800-255-6730

Vitek Systems, 595 Anglum Dr., Hazelwood, MO 63042 (automated). Phone: 800-MD-VITEK

ACICULAR: needle-shape.

ACROGENOUS: borne at the tip of a conidiophore.

ACROPETAL: produced in succession toward the apex (youngest conidium at the tip).

ACUMINATE: tapering to a narrow tip.

ADIACONIDIUM (pl. adiaconidia): a conidia that greatly enlarges in the host or at high temperatures without reproduction.

AEROBIC: requiring the presence of molecular oxygen to grow.

ALEURIOCONIDIUM (pl. aleurioconidia): a terminal or lateral conidium developed by expansion of the end of a conidiophore or hypha, and detaches by lysis or fracture of the wall.

ANAEROBIC: living in the absence of molecular oxygen.

ANAMORPH: A somatic or reproductive structure without nuclear recombination in the asexual cycle.

ANNELLIDES: a conidiogenous cell that produces a succession of conidia and bears ring-like scars around the tip left by released conidia as in *Scopulariopsis.*

ANNELLOCONIDIUM (pl. annelloconidia): a conidium formed from an annellide.

ANTHERIDIUM (pl. antheridia): male gametangium.

ANTHROPOPHILIC: fungi that usually infect humans only. Example: *Microsporum audouinii.*

ANTIBODY: serum immunoglobulin that interacts only with a specific antigen.

ANTIGEN: the substance introduced into the body that induces formation of antibodies.

APICULUS: a short projection at one or both ends of a spore or conidium.

APOPHYSIS; the swelling of a sporangiophore immediately below the columella.

ARTHROCONIDIUM (pl. arthroconidia): a conidium resulting from segmentation of a hypha, as in *Geotrichum.*

ASCOCARP: a fruiting body containing ascospores.

ASCOSPORE: a spore formed as a result of sexual reproduction developed in a saclike cell known as an ascus.

ASCUS (pl. asci): a saclike structure containing usually eight ascospores developed during sexual reproduction in the Ascomycetes.

ASEPTATE: lacking cross-walls. Example: *Rhizopus.*

ASEXUAL: reproduction in an organism without nuclear fusion. Development by mitosis.

ASSIMILATION: the ability to utilize carbon or nitrogen as a source for growth in the presence of oxygen. Assimilation is indicated by the growth of the fungus.

AUXANOGRAPHIC TECHNIC: a method for determination of carbon or nitrogen utilization by placing the substrate onto the surface of a basal agar medium seeded with a test organism such as a yeast.

BASIDIOSPORE: a haploid spore borne on the outside of a basidium as a result of sexual reproduction in the Basidiomycetes.

BASIDIUM (pl. basidia): a cell frequently club-shaped usually bearing four external basidiospores as a result of sexual reproduction.

BLASTIC: development of a conidium by enlargement at first by de novo growth prior to prior to delimitation by a septum.

BLASTOCONIDIUM (pl. blastoconidia): the production of a small outgrowth (bud) from a parent cell or hypha. Example: *Candida.*

BUD: a small outgrowth (bud) from a parent cell. Asexual reproduction.

CHLAMYDOCONIDIUM (pl. chlamydoconidia): a thick-walled cell formed intercalary or terminal in a hypha, separating to function as a resting spore.

CLAVATE: club-shaped.

CLEISTOTHECIUM (pl. cleistothecia): a closed ascocarp or fruiting body containing asci with ascospores.

COENOCYTIC: hyphae with many nuclei and few or no septa. Example: hyphae of *Rhizopus.*

COLUMELLA (columellae): a sterile structure inside the sporangium, often an extension of the sporangiophore.

CONIDIOPHORE: a simple or branched hypha with conidiogenous tips bearing conidia.

CONIDIUM (pl. conidia): asexual spores produced at the tip or side of conidiogenous cells of the conidiophore.

COREMIUM (pl. coremia): a cluster of erect conidiophores cememted together producing conidia at the apeces.

DEMATIACEOUS: fungi with dark olivaceous gray or black hyphae and/or spores.

DERMATOMYCOSIS: any fungus infection in the skin of animals and humans.

DERMATOPHYTOSIS: an infection produced by a dermatophyte in the nails, hair, and skin.

DERMATOPHYTE: a group of keratinophilic fungi that can grow in nails, hair, and skin.

DICHOTOMOUS: branching into two approximately equal branches with further repetition in some cases.

DICTYOCONIDIUM (pl. dictyoconidia): a conidium with horizontal and verticle septa (a muriform spore).

DIMORPHIC: having two forms, the hyphal and yeast forms,or spherules. Example: *Histoplasma capsulatum*. Having two morphological forms.

DIPLOID: contains 2n chromosomes.

ECHINULATE: surface covered with spiny surfaces.

ECTOTHRIX: a sheath of arthroconidia on the outside of a hair and fungus growth inside the hair shaft.

ENDOSPORE: a spore formed within a cell or spherule.

ENDOTHRIX: a fungus growing inside the hair shaft producing arthroconidia.

FAVIC CHANDELIERS: spherical hyphae that branch with curved and irregular ends resembling antlerlike branches. In some dermatophytes, especially *Trichophyton schoenleinii*.

FISSION: division of a cell into two cells by splitting.

FLOCCOSE: woolly appearance on the colony surface.

FLUORESCENCE: light of a characteristic color from certain fungi when exposed to filtered ultraviolet light.

FRAGMENTATION: breaking or segmenting of the hypha, each of which is capable of forming a new organism.

FRUITING BODY: any large and complex fungal structure that bears spores.

FUSEAU: a fusiform or spindle-shaped, multiseptate macroconidium.

FUSIFORM: a spindle-shaped structure tapering at the ends.

GEOPHILIC: fungi whose natural habitat is in the soil.

GERM TUBE: a short tube or hypha produced by a germinating spore, conidium or yeast cell.

GLABROUS: smooth.

GYMNOTHECIUM (pl. gymnothecia): a cleistothecium-like ascocarp with loosely woven hyphae with asci loosely distributed throughout.

HAPLOID: having n or reduced number of chromosomes.

HETEROTHALLIC: requires the mating with another thallus for sexual reproduction.

HILUM: a scar between the conidium and the conidiophore or at both ends of the conidium if in chains.

HOMOTHALLIC: self-compatible so sexual reproduction can take place in one thallus.

HYALINE: colorless, transparent.

HYPHA (pl. hyphae): a branching tubular structure of most fungi.

IMPERFECT STATE: the asexual stage or anamorph, usually conidia, of a fungus.

KERATINOPHILIC: fungi that use keratin as a substrate. Example: Dermatophytes.

LANOSE: woolly.

MACROCONIDIUM (pl. macroconidia): the larger, multicelled conidium in those fungi with smaller conidia (microconidia) or conidia of two sizes. Example: *Fusarium*.

MEROSPORANGIUM (pl. merosporangia): a cylindrical small sporangium containing a few spores in a row.

MICROCONIDIUM (pl. microconidia): the smaller, usually one-celled conidium, of the two types produced by some fungi. Example: *Fusarium*.

MURIFORM: a multicelled, transverse and longitudinal septate conidium.

MYCELIA STERILIA: an order of the Fungi Imperfecti consisting of fungi that do not produce conidia or spores.

MYCELIUM (pl. mycelia): a large mass of hyphae forming the vegetative (somatic) portion of the fungus.

NODULAR BODY: one or more closely intertwined hyphae forming a rounded ball-like form.

NONSEPTATE: lacking septa or cross-walls (coenocytic).

PECTINATE BODY: hyphal branch with projections on one side like a comb.

PERFECT STATE (teleomorph state): sexual state of a fungus in which spores are formed after nuclear fusion.

PERITHECIUM (pl. perithecia): a flask-shaped ascocarp or fruiting body with a pore on top and asci inside.

PHIALIDE: a conidiogenous cell that produces a succesion of blastic conidia (phialoconidia) with no increase in length of the phialide.

PHIALOCONIDIUM (pl. phialoconidia): a conidium produced by a phialides.

PLEOMORPHISM: having two or more colony forms, the second form developing as a cottony, sterile mutant usually without spore production. Pleomorphism normally is irreversible.

PSEUDOHYPHA (pl. pseudohyphae): a series of elongated budding cells remaining attached, resembling hyphae.

PYCNIDIUM (pycnidia): a globose to flask-shaped asexual fruiting body with the interior lined with conidiogenous cells.

PYRIFORM: pear-shaped.

RACQUET HYPHA: a series of club-shaped cells in a single hypha.

RHIZOIDS: the rootlike hyphae occurring at nodes of stolons in some fungi. Example: *Rhizopus*.

SAPROBE: an organism that uses non-living organic matter for energy sources.

SCUTULUM (pl. scutulum): cup-shaped crust of hyphae and spores in favus of the skin.

SEPTATE: hyphae with cross-walls.

SEPTUM (pl. septa): a cross wall in a hypha.

SESSILE: attached directly to a hypha without a stalk (conidiophore).

SPIRAL HYPHA: coiled or corkscrew-like turns in a hypha.

SPORANGIOPHORE: a special hypha bearing a sporangium.

SPORANGIOSPORE: a spore borne within a sporangium.

SPORANGIUM: a sac or cell with the entire contents becoming converted into a number of asexual spores by cleavage.

SPORE: a small reproductive unit functioning like a "seed", as a result of asexual or sexual reproduction.

SPOROPHORE: a specialized hypha that develops spores.

STERIGMA (sterigmata): a small pointed hyphal branch or structure which supports a sporangium, a conidium, or basidiospore.

STOLON: a hypha from which rhizoids and sporangiophores are developed. Example: *Rhizopus*.

SYNONYM: another name considered acceptablee for a species or taxonomic group.

TELEOMORPH: the sexual or perfect state.

THALLUS: the vegetative growth or somatic phase of a fungus.

TINEA: ringworm or a skin disease occuring in different locations on the body due to a fungus. Example: Tinea pedis.

VERRUCOSE: surface with wartlike projections.

VESICLE: a swollen apex of a conidiophore or sporogenous cell having a bladder-like appearance. Example: *Aspergillus*.

VERTICILLATE: with branches arranged in verticils or whorls.

ZOOPHILIC: fungi that grow preferentially on animals.

ZOOSPORE: a motile asexual spore.

ZYGOSPORE: a thick-walled sexual spore formed by the fusion of two gametangia in the Zygomycetes. Example: *Rhizopus*.

INDEX

NOTE: *Page numbers followed by* t *refer to tables. Page numbers followed by* f *refer to figures.*

A

Abbott Quantum carbohydrate assimilation test kit, 156
Abscesses, specimen selection and preparation from, 28
Absidia spp., 192–193, 192f, 193f
  corymbifera
    laboratory examination of, 100t
    as zygomycosis cause, 189
Acetate agar, 38
Acicular, defined, 227
Acid-fast stain (Kinyoun's modification), 34–35
Acquired immune deficiency syndrome. *See* AIDS
Acremonium (Cephalosporium), 10, 10f, 179, 179t
  alabamensis, 179t
  conidiophores and conidia, 10f, 103f
  as eumycetic mycetoma cause, 102
  falciforme, 103, 103f, 179t
    as eumycetic mycetoma cause, 102
    laboratory examination of, 101t
  as hyalohyphomycosis cause, 179
  as keratomycosis cause, 202
  kiliense, 102, 103, 179t
  potroni, 179t
  recifei, 102, 103, 179t
  roseogriseum, 179t
  strictum, 179t
Acridinium ester-labeled DNA probes, 45–46
Acrogenous, defined, 227
Acropetal, defined, 227
ACTH, pityriasis versicolor and, 54
Actidione. *See* Cycloheximide
Actinobacillus ligieriesii, 101t
Actinomadura spp.
  as actinomycete, 207
  as actinomycotic mycetoma cause, 102, 214, 215
  culture medium for, 40
  madurae, 2, 102, 214, 215, 217f
    identification of, 101t, 216t, 217, 219
  pelletieri, 102, 215, 219
    identification of, 216t, 218
  physiologic characteristics of, 216t, 219
Actinomyces, 208–213, 208f, 211f
  See also Actinomycosis
  as actinomycete, 207
  bovis, 208, 209, 210–211, 212t, 213
  culture medium for, 43
  israelii, 208, 208f, 209f, 210f
    identification of, 100t, 209, 210, 212t, 213
    occurrence of, 208
  meyeri, 208, 211
  naeslundii, 208, 209, 211, 212t 213
  odontolyticus, 208, 211, 213
  viscosus, 208, 211, 212t, 213
Actinomycetes, 207–221
  culture media for, 31t, 41–42, 45
  infections caused by
    actinomycosis, 207–214
    dermatophilosis, 220–221
    nocardiosis, 214–220
  organisms listed, 207
  specimen types, 31t
Actinomycosis, 207–214, 208f
  See also Actinomyces spp.
  in animals, 207, 208
  etiologic agents, 208
  laboratory procedures, 100t, 208–211, 213
    animal inoculation, 213
    culture, 209
    direct examination, 209
    histopathology, 211, 213
    physiologic tests, 210, 212t
    serologic tests, 213
    specimen collection, 208
    specimen types and culture media, 31t
    stock culture maintenance, 48, 213
  occurrence of, 208

pulmonary, 208f
Actinomycotic mycetoma
  etiologic agents, 102, 214–215, 216t, 217, 218
  laboratory examination in, 101t
  physiologic characteristics of, 216t
Acuminate, 227
Addelloconidia, defined, 227
Adelaide Children's Hospital, teaching slides from, 225
Adiaconidium/Adiaconidia, defined, 227
Adiaspiromycosis, 198–199
  etiologic agents, 198
  hyalohyphomycosis and, 171
  laboratory procedures, 198
  occurrence of, 198
Adiasporosis. *See* Adiaspiromycosis
Aerobic, defined, 227
Aflatoxin, 177
African histoplasmosis, 145–146
AIDS
  aspergillosis and, 172
  nocardiosis and, 215
  opportunistic saprophytes and, 5
  Penicillium spp. and, 185
  torulopsosis and, 160
  yeast infections and, 149
Airborne fungi, laboratory exercise, 7
Ajellomyces spp.
  capsulatus, Histoplasma capsulatum and, 141, 144
  dermatitidis
    Blastomyces dermatitidis and, 129, 130
    classification example, 3
Aleurioconidium/aleurioconidia, defined, 227
Allergies, Alternaria spp. and, 17
Allescheria boydii. *See* Pseudallescheria boydii
Allescheriasis. *See* Pseudallescheriasis
Alopecia, in dermatophilosis, 220
Alphacel-yeast extract agar, 38–39
Alternaria, 17–18, 17f–18f, 118–119
  as airborne fungi, 7
  alternata, 118–119
  chief characteristics of, 116t
  conidia, 18f
  as phaeohyphomycosis cause, 118
  as poroconidia, 2
Aman's medium. *See* Lactophenol cotton blue
American Laboratory Supply, Inc., 224
American Registry of Pathology, 225
American Society of Clinical Pathologists, 225
American Society for Microbiology, 224
American Type Culture Collection, 223
Amium, as phaeohyphomycosis cause, 118
Ammonium nitrate, in Trichophyton agar, 44
Anaerobic, defined, 227
Analytab Products, Inc., 225
  API 20 C test kit from, 157
Anamorph, defined, 227
Animal inoculations
  actinomycosis and, 213
  Aspergillus spp., 174, 176
  Blastomyces dermatitidis, 131
  Candida spp., 157
  Coccidioides immitis, 138–139
  Cryptococcus neoformans, 164–165
  Dermatophilus congolensis and, 221
  Histoplasma capsulatum, 144
  Microsporum spp., 81
  mycetoma and, 105
  Nocardia spp. and, 218–219
  Paracoccidioides brasiliensis, 135
  Pseudallescheria boydii, 188
  Rhinosporidum seeberi, 115
  Rhizopus oryzae, 196
  Scedosporium apiospermum, 188
  Sporothrix schenckii, 99, 113
  zygomycosis and, 196
Animals
  actinomycosis in, 207, 208
  adiaspiromycosis in, 198
  aspergillosis in, 171, 172
  blastomycosis in, 129
  candidiasis in, 152
  coccidioidomycosis in, 137
  cryptococcosis in, 162
  dermatophilosis in, 220

Fusarium infection in, 181
  geotrichosis in, 200
  histoplasmosis in, 142
  keratomycosis in, 202
  lobomycosis in, 114
  Malassezia pachydermatis infection in, 54
  mycetoma in, 102
  paracoccidioidomycosis in, 133
  Penicillium marneffei infection in, 203
  piedra in, 52
  pseudallescheriasis in, 187
  pythiosis insidiosi in, 204, 205
  Rhizomucor pusillus in, 195
  ringworm in, 60t, 61f
    laboratory guidelines, 68, 69
  ringworm causes in, 60t, 61
    Trichophyton ajelloi, 92
    Trichophyton equinum, 87
    Trichophyton megninii, 89
    Trichophyton mentagrophytes, 86
    Trichophyton rubrum, 88
    Trichophyton schoenleinii, 90
    Trichophyton simii, 89
    Trichophyton tonsurans, 90
    Trichophyton verrucosum, 88
    Trichophyton violaceum, 91
  zygomycosis in, 190
Anxiopsis spp.
  fulvescens, 179t, 186
  stericoraria, 186
  sterocari, 179t
Annellides, 2
  defined, 227
Annelloconidium/Annelloconidia, 2
  defined, 226
Antheridium/Antheridia, defined, 227
Anthopsis, 119
  deltoidea, 117t, 119
  as phaeohyphomycosis cause, 117t, 118, 119
Anthropophilic, defined, 227
Antibacterial drugs, saprophytic fungi and, 5
Antibiotic production, Streptomyces spp. and, 24
Antibiotic treatment
  aspergillosis and, 171, 172
  candidiasis and, 151
  keratomycosis and, 202
  zygomycosis and, 190
Antibody, defined, 227
Antigen, defined, 227
Antigenemia tests, for aspergillosis, 177
Antineoplastic drugs, saprophytic fungi and, 5
API 20 C Yeast Identification System, 156, 164
Apiculus, defined, 227
Apophysis, defined, 227
Apophysomyces elegans, 193f
  as zygomycosis cause, 189, 193
Arachnia propionica, 211, 212t
  as actinomycosis cause, 208
Arnium leporinum, as phaeohyphomycosis cause, 117t
Arthritis
  Fusarium moniliforme and, 183t
  Pseudallescheria boydii and, 187
Arthroconidia (arthrospores), 1, 2, 70
  defined, 227
Arthroderma, 59, 66t–68t, 74
  appearance described, 74
  as Ascomycota, 2, 3, 66t
  benhamiae, 67t
    Trichophyton mentagrophytes and, 87
  borelii, 66t
  cajetani, 66t
    Microsporum cookei and, 77–78
  ciferrii, 68t
    Trichophyton georgiae and, 85, 92
  corniculatum, 66t
  flavescens, 67t
  fulvum, 66t
  gertleri, 68t
    Trichophyton vanbreuseghemii and, 85, 94
  gloriae, 68t
    Trichophyton gloriae and, 85
  grubyi, 66t
    Microsporum vanbreuseghemii and, 81
  gypseum, 66t

Microsporum gypseum and, 79
  incingulare, 68t
  incurvatum, 66t
    laboratory guidelines, 69
    Microsporum gypseum and, 79
  insingulare, Trichophyton terrestre and, 92
  lenticulare, 68t
    Trichophyton terrestre and, 92
Microsporum spp. and, 74, 76, 77–78, 79, 80, 81
  obstusa, Microsporum nanum and, 80
  obtusum, 66t
  otae, 66t
    Microsporum canis and, 76
  persicolor, 66t
    Microsporum persicolor and, 81
  quadrifidum, 68t
    Trichophyton terrestre and, 85
  racemosum, 66t
  simii, 67t
    Trichophyton simii and, 89
  soil-hair culture technique for, 69
  Trichophyton spp. and, 74, 80
  uncinatum, 67t
    Trichophyton ajelloi and, 85, 93
  vanbreuseghemii, 67t
    Trichophyton mentagrophytes and, 87
Arthrodermataceae, dermatophytes as, 59
Arthrographis kalrae, 179t, 186
Arthrospores. *See* Arthroconidia
Arthur H. Thomas Co., 224
Asci, 2, 3, 3f
  defined, 227
Ascocarp, defined, 227
Ascocarp production, by dermatophytes, 69
Ascomycetes, 3f
Ascomycota, 3, 23–24
  See also Hemiascomycetes (Ascomycota)
  dermatophytes as, 59
  as hyalohyphomycosis cause, 178
  as phaeohyphomycosis cause, 117t
  Plectomycetes, Chaetomium spp., 23–24, 24f
Ascospores, 2
  culture medium for, 42
  defined, 227
Ascus. *See* Asci
Aseptate (coenocytic) hyphae, 1
  defined, 227
Asexual reproduction, 1–2
  classification and, 3
  defined, 227
Asparagine broth, 39
Aspergillaceae, film on, 225
Aspergilloma, 171, 172
  ID test and, 177
Aspergillosis, 171f
  in animals, 171, 172
  candidiasis with, 176f
  described, 171
  etiologic agents, 171, 179t
  in eye, 171f, 176f
  hyalohyphomycosis and, 171, 178
  laboratory procedures, 100t, 172–177
    animal inoculation, 174, 176
    culture, 172–174, 175t–176t
    direct examination, 172
    histopathology, 174
    serologic tests, 177
    specimen collection, 172
    specimen types and culture medium, 31t
  in lung, 171, 172f
  occurrence of, 172
  as opportunistic infection, 127t
Aspergillus, 10–11, 11f
  as airborne fungi, 7
  amstelodami, 171, 176t, 179t
  candidus, 171, 176t, 179t
  carneus, 171, 179t
  clavatus, 176t, 179t
  conicus, 179t
  conidiophores, 11f, 173, 173f, 174f
  deflectus, 179t
  endotoxin production and, 177
  fischeri, 179t
  flavipes, 171, 176t, 179t
  flavus, 11, 175t, 176t
    aflatoxin and, 177

dermatomycoses and, 96
identification of, 173, 174f
as keratomycosis cause, 202
as opportunistic infection cause, 171, 179t
serologic test and, 177
fumigatus, 11, 172, 172f, 173, 173f, 175t, 176t
culture media for, 37
in eye, 171f
film on, 225
as keratomycosis cause, 202
laboratory examination of, 100t
as opportunistic infection cause, 171, 179t
serologic test and, 177
as keratomycosis cause, 202
laboratory identification of, 172–177, 175t, 176t
neveus, 171
nidulans, 103, 171, 176t
as eumycetic mycetoma cause, 102
as opportunistic infection cause, 179t
niger, 11, 173–174, 174f, 175t, 176t
as keratomycosis cause, 202
as opportunistic infection cause, 171, 179t
in otomycosis, 51f
serologic test and, 177
niveus, 179t
ochraceus, 171, 176t, 179t
as opportunistic infection cause, 127, 171, 179t
oryzae, 171, 176t, 179t
in otomycosis, 51, 52
parasiticus, 179t
phialides, 173
repens, 171, 179t
restrictus, 171, 176t, 179t
ruber, 179t
stock culture maintenance, 48
sydowi, 171, 176t, 179t
terreus, 11, 173, 174f, 175t, 176t
as opportunistic infection cause, 171, 179t
ustus, 171, 176t, 179t
versicolor, 171, 176t, 179t
Assimilation, defined, 227
Assimilation medium for carbohydrates, 39
Association Films, Inc., 224
Athlete's foot. *See* Tinea pedis
Atmospheric fungi, 5
Aureobasidium, 119
chief characteristics of, 116t
as phaeohyphomycosis cause, 118
Aureobasidium (Pullularia) pullulans, 18, 18f, 119
Exophiala werneckii and, 57
hyphae and conidia, 18f
Auxanographic technic, defined, 227
Axillary hairs, trichomycosis axillaris of, 56

B

BACTEC high-blood-volume fungal medium (HBV-FM), 158
BACTEC Plus 26 (BP26) media, 158
Bacteria
actinomycetes compared to, 207
actinomycosis and, 207
fungi compared to, 1
otomycosis and, 51
trichomycosis axillaris and, 56
Baker's yeast. *See Saccharomyces cerevisiae*
Basidia, 3, 3f
defined, 227
Basidiobolus haptosporus. See Basidiobolus ranarum
Basidiobolus ranarum, 195, 195f
histopathology, 196
laboratory procedures and, 190
zygomycosis and, 189, 190
Basidiomycetes, 3
Basidiomycosis, 199–200
etiologic agents, 199, 199f
hyalohyphomycosis and, 178
Basidiomycota, 3, 199
as hyalohyphomycosis cause, 178

Basidiospores, 3, 3f
defined, 227
Basidium. *See* Basidia
Baxter Microscan, 223, 225
serologic test kit by, 165
yeast identification system by, 148
Baxter Scientific Products Division, 224
Bayer Film Service, 224
BBL/Becton Dickinson Microbiology Systems, 223, 225
BBL Minitek System, 158, 164
Beard, ringworm of. *See* Tinea barbae
Beauveria, 179–180, 180f
alba, 179t
bassiana, 179t
as keratomycosis cause, 202
Becton Dickinson Diagnostic Instrument Systems, 158
Becton Dickinson Microbiology Systems, 223, 224, 225
Bifidobacterium dentium (B. eriksonii)
as actinomycosis cause, 208
identification of, 209, 210, 211, 212t, 213
BioMerieux, 223
Biomerieux Vitek System, 158
Biphasic vented blood culture bottles, 36
Bipolaris, 119, 119t, 120f, 121
australiensis, 118, 119, 121
as cerebral phaeohyphomycosis cause, 118
chief characteristics of, 116t, 119t
hawaiiensis, 118, 119, 120f, 121
as keratomycosis cause, 202
as paranasal sinus phaeohyphomycosis cause, 118, 119
as phaeohyphomycosis cause, 118
spicifera, 118, 119, 120f, 121
Black piedra, 52, 52–54, 53f
Piedraia hortai and, 27
Blastic, defined, 227
Blastic conidiogenesis, 1
Blastoconidia, 2
defined, 227
Blastomyces, as true pathogenic fungi, 127
Blastomyces brasiliensis. See Paracoccidioides brasiliensis
Blastomyces dermatitidis, 130f
Ajellomyces dermatitidis and, 129, 130
ascospores produced by, 2
classification example, 3
culture media for, 36, 38, 43
as dimorphic, 128t
DNA probes for, 45–46
exoantigen test for, 45
keratomycosis and, 202
laboratory procedures, 100t, 129–132
animal inoculation, 131
colonies, 129–130, 130f
culture, 129
direct examination, 129
DNA probe, 132
histopathologic studies, 130–131
nutritional requirements, 132
serology and immunology, 131
specimen collection, 129
Blastomycetes (Deuteromycota or Fungi Imperfecti), 22–23, 149
Rhodotorula spp., 22, 22f
Saccharomyces spp., 22–23, 23f
Blastomycosis, 128–133, 129f
in animals, 129
described, 128–129
etiologic agent, 128t, 129
European. *See* Cryptococcosis
film on, 224
keloid. *See* Lobo's disease
laboratory examination in, 100t
laboratory procedures for. *See*
Blastomyces dermatitidis
occurrence of, 129
South American. *See*
Paracoccidioidomycosis
as true pathogenic infection, 127t
Blastomycota (Heterobasidiomycetes), 149
Blastoschizomyces capitatus
Geotrichum candidum and, 200
opportunistic infections by, 169
Blood
Candida culture from, 153

culture media for, 29
serologic techniques, 45
specimen selection and preparation, 29
Bone marrow
Candida culture from, 153
Fusarium spp. and, 12, 183t
specimen selection and preparation, 28
Bone marrow transplants
aspergillosis and, 171, 172
Fusarium infection and, 12, 180
Botryodiplodia, keratomycosis and, 118, 202
Botryomycosis, laboratory examination in, 101t
Botrytis, 11, 11f
as airborne fungi, 7
conidiophore, 11f
as keratomycosis cause, 202
Brain abscess, *Pseudallescheria boydii* and, 187
Brain biopsy, *Drechslera biseptata* isolated from, 20
Brain-heart-infusion agar, 36
uses for, 30t–31t
Bromcresol purple, in fermentation medium, 41
Bud, defined, 227
Burns
Fusarium infection and, 12, 180, 183t
Phialenonium obovatum and, 186
zygomycosis and, 189
Bursitis, in hyalohyphomycosis, 10
Buschke's disease. *See* Cryptococcosis

C

Calcofluor white (CFW), laboratory procedures with, 32
Canavanine-glycine-bromthymol blue (CGB) agar, 39–40
Cancer, "opportunistic" saprophytes and, 5
Candida
See also Candidiasis
albicans, 151
as chlamydoconidia, 2
colony and microscopic morphology, 156
culture media for, 40, 41
diseases caused by, 61
fermentation/assimilation patterns, 155t
laboratory examination of, 71t, 100t, 153
skin scraping preparation, 28
specimen media and mounting procedure, 33
ubiquity of, 149
as blastoconidia, 2
as Blastomycetes, 149
brumpti. See Candida parapsilosis
culture media for, 37, 40, 41, 153
dermatomycoses and, 96
diseases caused by, 151
Exophiala werneckii and, 57
guilliermondii, 151
colony and microscopic morphology, 156
fermentation/assimilation patterns, 155t
Pichia guilliermondi and, 151
kefyr, 151
colony and microscopic morphology, 156
fermentation/assimilation patterns, 155t
Kluyveromyces fragilis and, 151
as keratomycosis cause, 202
krusei, 151
colony and microscopic morphology, 156
culture media for, 37, 153
fermentation/assimilation patterns, 155t
Pichia kudriavezii and, 151
laboratory identification of, 71t, 152–158, 153f, 154f, 155t, 157f
colony and microscopic morphology, 156–157
histopathology and, 157
significant numbers, 149
lusitaniae, 151–152
Clavispora lusitaniae and, 152

colony and microscopic morphology, 156
fermentation/assimilation patterns, 155t
obtusa. See Candida lusitaniae
opportunistic infection by, 127
parapsilosis 152
colony and microscopic morphology, 156
culture media for, 37, 153
fermentation/assimilation patterns, 155t
parapsilosis var. *obtusa. See Candida lusitaniae*
pseudotropicalis. See Candida kefyr
stellatoidea. See Candida albicans
tropicalis, 152
colony and microscopic morphology, 156–157
culture media for, 37, 153
fermentation/assimilation patterns, 155t
ubiquity of, 149
viswanathii, 152
colony and microscopic morphology, 157
fermentation/assimilation patterns, 155t
Candida endocarditis. *See* Candidiasis
Candida paronychia. *See* Candidiasis
Candidiasis, 151–160, 151f, 153f
in animals, 152
aspergillosis with, 176f
described, 151
etiologic agents, 151–152
film on, 224
laboratory examination in, 71t, 100t
laboratory procedures, 152–158
animal inoculations, 157
carbohydrate fermentation/assimilation tests, 154, 155t, 156
colonies, 153–154, 153f
culture, 153
culture media, 30t, 40, 41, 153
direct examination, 152
histopathology, 157
serologic studies, 157, 158
specimen collection and preparation, 28, 33, 152, 153
specimen types, 30t
occurrence of, 152
as opportunistic infection, 127t
Candidosis moniliasis. *See* Candidiasis
Cand-Tec serology kit, 157, 158
Carbohydrate fermentation/assimilation tests
for *Actinomyces* spp., 210, 212t
for *Candida* spp., 154, 155t, 156
for *Cryptococcus* spp., 164, 164t
media for, 39, 41, 154
in nocardiosis/actinomycotic mycetoma, 216t
Carolina Biological Supply Co., Inc., 223, 224
Casein medium, 40
Catalase test, for *Actinomyces* spp., 210
Catheter use, *Fusarium* infection and, 180
Cellophane tape-coverglass mounts, 5–6, 32
Cellufluor, laboratory procedures with, 32
Cellulitis, in hyalohyphomycosis, 10
Centers for Disease Control, as fungal culture source, 223
Central bureau Voor Schimelcultures, 224
Cephaliophora spp., as keratomycosis cause, 202
Cephalosporium spp. See *Acremonium (Cephalosporium)*
Ceratocystis stenoceras, Sporothrix schenckii and, 112
Cerebral phaeohyphomycosis, etiologic agents, 118
Cerebrospinal fluid
Candida culture from, 153
Schizophyllum commune in, 199
serologic techniques, 45
specimen selection and preparation, 28
Cerebrospinal fluid shunt, *Paecilomyces* spp. and, 14
CF test. *See* Complement fixation (CF) test
CFW. *See* Calcofluor white

B (canavanine-glycine-bromthymol blue)
agar, 39–40
aetoconidium spp., 186
aetomium, 23–24, 24f, 121
as airborne fungi, 7
cochliodes, 117t, 121
funicolum, 117t, 121
globosum, 117t, 118, 121
perithecium and ascospores, 24f
as phaeohyphomycosis cause, 117t, 118
askes-Tyndall medium, modified (L-Dopa
medium), 40–41
emical industry, Streptomyces spp. and, 24
icago disease. See Blastomycosis
lamydoconidia, 2, 70, 72f
in Candida albicans, 153–154, 154f
defined, 227
in Fusarium spp., 183, 184
lamydospore agar, 40
loramphenicol (Chloromycetin)
in brain heart infusion agar, 36
in Sabouraud agar, 37–38
risope Technology, 224
ristensen's test medium, urease test medium
and, 44
romoblastomycosis, 106–110, 106f, 107f
animal inoculation and, 109
in animals, 106
defined, 106
etiologic agents, 106
chief characteristics of, 109t–110t
as dimorphic, 128
laboratory procedures, 101t, 106–107
culture, 107
direct examination, 106–107
serologic tests, 109
specimen collection and preparation,
28
specimen type and culture medium,
30t
occurrence of, 106
sclerotic bodies, 107f
romomycosis. See Chromoblastomycosis
ronic diseases, Rhodotorula spp. and, 22
rysosporium parvum var. parvum. See
Emmonsia parva var. parva
rysosporium, 186
panorum, 186
E (counterimmunoelectrophoresis), 45
adorrhinum, keratomycosis and, 118, 202
adosporium, 18–19, 19f, 121
as airborne fungi, 7
animal inoculation with, 109
bantiana, 121
as blastoconidia, 2
carrionii
chief characteristics of, 109t
as chromoblastomycosis cause, 106
laboratory examination of, 109
chief characteristics of, 110t, 116t
cladosporioides, 121
conidiophore type, 107
culture medium for, 41
devriesii, 121
as keratomycosis cause, 202
laboratory examination of, 109
as phaeohyphomycosis cause, 118, 121
tinea nigra and, 61
trichoides, 121
animal inoculation with, 109
as cerebral phaeohyphomycosis
cause, 118
laboratory examination of, 100t, 101t
as paranasal sinus phaeohyphomycosis cause, 118
werneckii
Exophiala werneckii and, 57. See also
Exophiala werneckii
tinea nigra and, 64f
assification of fungi, 3
avate, defined, 227
avispora lusitanae, Candida lusitaniae and,
152
eistothecium (gymnothecium), 2, 3f
defined, 227
nical Laboratory Improvement Amendments
of 1988 (CLIA '88), 27
nical Sciences, Inc., yeast identification kit
by, 158

Coccidioides, as true pathogenic fungi, 127
Coccidioides immitis, 136, 137f, 138f
colonies, 137–138, 138f
as dimorphic, 128t
laboratory procedures, 101t, 137–140
animal inoculation, 138–139
culture, 137
culture medium, 38
direct examination, 137
DNA probes, 45–46, 139–140
exoantigen test, 45
histopathology, 138
safety concerns, 137, 138
serology, 139
specimen collection, 137
Coccidioidin (asparagine) broth, 39
Coccidioidomycosis (Coccidioidal granuloma;
Valley fever; San Joaquin fever), 136–141,
136f, 137f
in animals, 137
described, 136
etiologic agent, 136
laboratory examination in, 101t
occurrence of, 136–137
pulmonary, 136f
as true pathogenic infection, 127t
Coelomycetes, 23
Coenocytic (aseptate) hyphae, 1
defined, 227
Coils, microscopic view of, 72f
Cokeromyces recurvatus, 193f
as zygomycosis cause, 189, 193–194
Colab Laboratories, 224
Colletotrichum, keratomycosis and, 118, 202
Columella/columellae, defined, 227
Complement fixation (CF) test, 45
for coccidioidomycosis, 139
EIA and ID tests vs., 131
for histoplasmosis, 144, 145
for paracoccidioidomycosis, 135
Conidia, 1–2
defined, 1, 227
Conidiobolus coronatus, 196, 196f
histopathology, 196
laboratory procedures and, 190
zygomycosis and, 189, 190, 195
Conidiogenesis, thallic vs. blastic, 1
Conidiogenous (sporogenous) cells, 1
Conidiophores, 1
defined, 227
Coniothyrium fuckelii
as opportunistic infection cause, 186
as phaeohyphomycosis cause, 117t
Contaminant fungi, 5–24
Ascomycota, 23–24, 24f
Deuteromycota (Fungi Imperfecti), 10–23,
10f–23f
Blastomycetes, 22–23, 22f–23f
Coelomycetes, 23, 23f
Dematiaceae, 17–21, 17f–22f
Hyphomycetes, 10–17, 10f–17f
laboratory procedures with, 5–7
Schizomycota, 24, 24f
Zygomycetes (Phycomycetes), 8–9,
8f–10f
Coprinus
cinereus, 199
micaceous, 199
Coremium/coremia, defined, 228
Corneal infection. See Keratomycosis
Cornmeal agars, 40
Corticosteroids
aspergillosis and, 171, 172
Fusarium infection and, 180
keratomycosis and, 202
pityriasis versicolor and, 54
zygomycosis and, 190
Corynebacterium tenuis, trichomycosis axillaris
and, 56, 56f
Corynespora cassicola, as eumycetic mycetoma
cause, 102
Counterimmunoelectrophoresis (CIE), 45
for actinomycotic mycetoma, 219
for aspergillosis, 177
for candidiasis, 157
for nocardiosis, 219
Coverglass procedures, 5–6, 32
Cow, tinea on, 61f. See also Animals
Cryogenic storage, for stock cultures, 49

Cryptococcosis, 161–167, 161f, 162f
in animals, 162
in brain tissue, 162f
described, 161
etiologic agent, 162
laboratory procedures, 100t, 162–166
animal inoculation, 164–165
colonies, 163
culture, 162–163
direct examination, 162
DNA probes, 165
histopathology, 164
physiologic tests, 163–164, 164t
serologic tests, 165
specimen collection and preparation,
28, 162
specimen types and culture media,
31t
occurrence of, 162
as opportunistic infection, 127t
pulmonary, 161f
on skin, 162f
Cryptococcus
bacillispora. See Cryptococcus neoformans
var. gattii
bacillisporus. See Cryptococcus neoformans var. neoformans
neoformans, 162, 162f, 163f
basidiospores developed by, 3
culture media for, 37, 39, 40–41, 44
DNA probes for, 45–46
Filobasidiella spp. and, 3, 162, 163
laboratory identification of, 100t,
163–166
mounting procedure for, 33
physiologic tests for, 163–164, 164t
ubiquity of, 149
var. gattii, 39–40, 162, 163
var. neoformans, 162, 163
opportunistic infection by, 127
Crypto-LA test kit, 165
Crystal violet, in direct staining method, 33, 34
Culture collections
maintenance of, 48–49
sources for, 223
Culture media, 36–46
dermatophyte study guidelines, 68, 69
mounting procedures, 32–35
sources for, 223–224
Cunninghamella, 192, 192f
bertholletiae, 189, 192
elegans, 192
Cunninghamellaceae, characteristics of, 191t
Curtis-Matheson Scientific, 224
Curvularia, 19, 19f, 121–122, 122f
chief characteristics of, 116t
conidia and conidiophore, 19f
geniculata, 102, 103, 122
lunata, 102, 118, 122
opportunistic infections caused by, 121
eumycetic mycetoma, 102
keratomycosis, 118, 202
phaeohyphomycosis, 118, 121–122
pallescens, 122
senegalensis, 122
Cutaneous mycoses
See also Dermatophytoses
Cladosporium spp. and, 19
etiologic agents, 118
Fusarium moniliforme and, 180f, 183t
Pseudallescheria boydii and, 187
Rhizomucor pusillus and, 195
specimen collection and preparation, 28
specimen type and culture medium type,
30t, 59
Cycloheximide (Actidione)
in brain heart infusion agar, 36
in hair-bait technique, 41
in Sabouraud agar, 37–38
Cylindrocarpon
destructans, as eumycetic mycetoma
cause, 102
Fusarium spp. and, 181
as keratomycosis cause, 202
Cysteine blood agar, 40
Cytotoxin use, aspergillosis and, 172
Czapek's agar, 40

D

Dactylaria, 122
as cerebral phaeohyphomycosis cause,
118
chief characteristics of, 116t
gallopava, 118, 122, 122f
as phaeohyphomycosis cause, 118, 122
Debaryomyces
hansenii, as opportunistic infection cause,
169
hominis. See Cryptococcus neoformans
var. neoformans
Deep freeze storage, for stock culture, 48
Dematiaceae, 8
Dematiaceous, defined, 228
Dematiaceous hyphomycetes, 8, 17–21,
17f–22f
See also Deuteromycota (Fungi Imperfecti)
Alternaria spp., 17–18, 17f–18f
Aureobasidium (Pullularia) pullulans, 18,
18f
Cladosporium spp., 18–19, 19f
Curvularia spp., 19, 19f
Drechslera spp., 20, 20f
Epiococcum spp., 20, 20f
identification problems, 117
Nigrospora spp., 21, 21f
opportunistic infections and, 7–8
Ulocladiuim spp., 21, 21f–22f
Dermatomycosis, 96
defined, 59, 228
Dermatophilosis, 220–221
Dermatophilus congolensis, 220–221, 220f,
221f
Dermatophytes, 59
defined, 228
diseases caused by, 60t
films on, 225
imperfect and perfect states of, 66t–68t
laboratory identification of, 59, 68–73, 71t,
72f–73f
colony characteristics, 70, 71t
microscopic characteristics, 70, 72f,
73, 73f
by physiologic requirements, 70
specimen collection, 70
specimen examination, 70
Dermatophyte Test Medium, 36–37
uses of, 30, 30t
Dermatophytoses, 59–97
See also Cutaneous mycoses;
Dermatophytes
classification of, 59, 68
clinical types of, 59, 60t, 61f–65f. See also
specific types
defined, 228
tinea capitis, 60t, 61f–62f
Deuteromycota (Fungi Imperfecti), 3, 10–21
See also Dematiaceous hyphomycetes
Blastomycetes, 22–23
Coelomycetes, 23
dermatophytes, 59, 66t–68t
as hyalohyphomycosis cause, 178
opportunistic infections and, 7
otomycosis and, 52
Diabetes
candidiasis and, 151f
"opportunistic" saprophytes and, 5
zygomycosis and, 190
Dichotomous, defined, 228
Dictyoconidium/dictyoconidia, defined, 228
Difco Laboratories, Inc., 223
Dimorphic fungi, 1
defined, 228
specimen types and culture medium, 31t
systemic infections and, 128, 128t
Diploid, defined, 228
Diplosporium, as keratomycosis cause, 202
Direct examination of cultures, 32
Direct mount procedure, 5
Dissecting needles, use of, 29
Disseminated infection
Fusarium spp. and, 183t
nocardiosis, 214
Pseudallescheria boydii and, 187
Rhizomucor pusillus and, 195
DNA probes, 45–46
in blastomycosis, 132

in coccidioidomycosis, 139–140
in cryptococcosis, 165
in histoplasmosis, 145
in paracoccidioidomycosis, 135
sources for, 224
Dog, tinea on, 61f. *See also* Animals
Dolphins, lobomycosis in, 114. *See also* Animals
Drechslera, 20, 20f, 121
avenae, 120f
bisepata, 20, 118
chief characteristics of, 119, 119t
conidiophores and conidia, 20f
dictyoides, 120f
as poroconidia, 2
rostrata. See Exserohilum rostratum

E

Echinulate, defined, 228
Ectothrix, defined, 228
Eczema, epidemic. *See* Dermatophilosis
EIA. *See* Enzyme-linked immunosorbent assay (EIA)
Eiken Chemical Co., 223
serologic test kit by, 165
Emmonsia parva, 198
var. *crescens*, 198, 198f
var. *parva*, 198
Emmonsiella capsulata. See Histoplasma capsulatum
Emmon's modification, Sabouraud glucose agar, 38
Endocarditis
Actinomyces odontolyticus and, 208
Actinomycosis viscosus and, 208
Chrysosporium spp. and, 186
Coprinus cinereus and, 199
hyalohyphomycosis and, 10
Paecilomyces spp. and, 14
Penicillium spp. and, 185
Pseudallescheria boydii and, 187
Rhizomucor pusillus and, 195
Rhodotorula spp. and, 22
Thermomyces lanuginosus and, 186
Endomyces albicans. See Candida albicans
Endomyces guilliermondii. See Candida guilliermondii
Endomyces pseudotropicalis. See Candida kefyr
Endophthalmitis
Fusarium spp. and, 183t
Neurospora sitophila and, 186
Paecilomyces spp. and, 14
Pseudallescheria boydii and, 187
Endospore, defined, 228
Endothrix, defined, 228
Endotoxins, *Aspergillus* spp. and, 176–177
Enterothallic or enteroblastic conidia, 1–2
Entomophthorales, zygomycosis and, 189, 190, 195–196
Entomophthoramycosis, 189, 195
Enzyme-linked immunosorbent assay (EIA), 45
in blastomycosis, 131
in candidiasis, 157
in cryptococcosis, 165
test kits for, 165
in zygomycosis, 196
Epidermophyton, 82–84
as dermatophytes, 59, 66t
floccosum, 66t, 82–84, 83f, 84f
diseases caused by, 60t, 82
laboratory examination of, 70, 71t, 73, 75t, 83–84
macrocondia, 84f
stock culture maintenance, 48, 84
laboratory procedures, 83
stockdaleae, 82–83
Epilated hair, culture media for, 30t
Epiococcum, 20, 20f
Epizootic lymphangitis, *Histoplasma capsulatum* var. *farciminosum* and, 145–146
Equipment, for laboratory procedures, 27, 224
Escherichia coli, laboratory examination of, 101t
Eumycotic mycetoma
etiologic agents, 102
laboratory examination in, 101t
Eupenicillium, 3f
European blastomycosis. *See* Cryptococcosis

Exerophilum, keratomycosis and, 118
Exoantigen test, 45
for *Exophiala werneckii*, 57
Exophiala
chief characteristics of, 116t
dermatitidis, 122, 123f
animal inoculation with, 109
chief characteristics of, 109t
as phaeohyphomycosis cause, 118
jeanselmei, 103–104, 122–123, 123f
chief characteristics of, 109t
as eumycetic mycetoma cause, 102
laboratory examination of, 71t, 103–104
keratomycosis and, 118, 202
laboratory examination of, 71t
moniliae, 123
as phaeohyphomycosis cause, 118, 122
spinifera, 123
chief characteristics of, 109t
laboratory examination of, 71t, 100t, 101t, 123
werneckii
Cladosporium werneckii and, 57. *See also Cladosporium werneckii*
specimen selection and preparation, 27
tinea nigra and, 27, 57, 61, 118
Exserohilum, 119, 121, 123–124
chief characteristics of, 116t, 119t
as keratomycosis cause, 202
longirostratum, 123, 124
mcginnisii, 118, 120f, 123, 124
as phaeohyphomycosis cause, 118
rostratum, 118, 120f, 123–124, 124f
Exudate specimens
mailing procedures, 29
selection and preparation, 28
Eye infections
aspergillosis, 171f, 172, 176f
Cladosporium spp. and, 19
keratomycosis, 201–202, 202f
pythiosis insidiosi, 205, 205f

F

Facial granuloma, *Fusarium* spp. and, 12
Favic chandeliers, 70, 72f, 91f
defined, 228
Favus in animals (tinea favosa), 60t
Female urogenital tract, *Candida albicans* in, 149
Fermentation industry, *Streptomyces* spp. and, 24
Fermentation medium for carbohydrates, 41
Filobasidiella, 3f
as Basidiomycota, 3, 199
culture medium for, 43, 44–45
Cryptococcus spp. and, 3, 44–45, 162, 163
as Heterobasidiomycetes (Blastomycota), 149
neoformans
culture medium for, 44–45
var. *bacillispora*, 162, 163
var. *neoformans*, 162, 163
Fisher Scientific Co., 224
Fission, defined, 228
Floccose, defined, 228
Flow Laboratories, Inc., 158, 223
Fluorescence, defined, 228
Fluorescent antibody test. See Indirect fluorescent antibody test
Fluorescent brightener, laboratory procedures with, 32
Fonsecaea, 124
chief characteristics of, 116t
compacta, 108, 108f, 124
animal inoculation with, 109
chief characteristics of, 109t
as chromoblastomycosis cause, 106
laboratory examination of, 108
pedrosoi, 107–108, 107f, 124
animal inoculation with, 109
as cerebral phaeohyphomycosis cause, 118
chief characteristics of, 109t
as chromoblastomycosis cause, 106
laboratory examination of, 101t

Foodborne infections
aspergillosis, 171, 172
geotrichosis, 200
hyalohyphomycosis, 179
Foot
fungus infections of, film on, 224
mycetoma on, 99, 102f
ringworm on. *See* Tinea pedis
Foot rot, strawberry. *See* Dermatophilosis
Fragmentation, defined, 228
Freezing stock cultures, 48
Fruiting body, defined, 228
Fungal cultures
sources for, 223
stock culture maintenance, 48–49
Fungemia
blood specimen collection and preparation, 29
commercial media for detecting, 158
Fusarium spp. and, 12, 183t
in hyalohyphomycosis, 10
Malassezia furfur and, 54
Penicillium spp. and, 185
Rhodotorula spp. and, 22
Saccharomyces spp. and, 23
Fungicides, laboratory use of, 32
Fungi Imperfecti. *See* Deuteromycota
Fungus ball
See also Aspergilloma
Pseudallescheria boydii and, 187, 189
Trichoderma spp. and, 16, 186
Fungus ear. *See* Otomycosis
Fusarium, 12, 12f, 180–184
in animals, 181
chlamydosporum, 180
conidia, 112f
Cylindrocarpon spp. and, 181
dimerum, 180
diseases caused by, 127, 180, 183t, 202
eumycetic mycetoma, 102
keratomycosis, 202
laboratory procedures, 181–183
culture, 181
specimen collection, 181
moniliforme, 104, 180f, 181, 181f, 182f
chlamydoconidia, and, 183
dermatomycoses and, 96
as eumycetic mycetoma cause, 102
nivale, 180
occurrence of, 180
oxysporum, 180, 181, 181f, 182f
chlamydoconidia and, 183
proliferatum, 180
roseum, 180
simifectum, 180
solani, 104, 180, 182–183, 183f
chlamydoconidia and, 183
as eumycetic mycetoma cause, 102
as keratomycosis cause, 202
laboratory examination of, 100t
verticillioides, 180
Fuseau, defined, 228
Fusiform, defined, 228

G

Gastric mucin, in animal inoculation, 47
Gastric zygomycosis, *Mucor* spp. and, 9
Gastrointestinal tract, *Candida albicans* in, 149
Gelatin liquefaction test
for *Actinomyces* spp., 210
for *Nocardia* spp., 218
for *Streptomyces* spp., 218
Gelatin medium, 41
Gen-Probe
in blastomycosis, 132
in coccidioidomycosis, 139–140
in cryptococcosis, 165
in histoplasmosis, 145
Gen-Probe, Inc., 224
Geophilic, defined, 228
Geotrichosis, 200–201
described, 200
etiologic agent, 200
laboratory procedures, 200
occurrence of, 200
specimen types and culture medium, 31t
Geotrichum, 12, 13f, 200–201, 200f, 201f
arthroconidia, 2, 13f, 200, 201f

candidum, 200–201
Blastoschizomyces capitatus and, 2
fermentation/assimilation patterns, 155t
Trichosporon beigelii and, 200
ubiquity of, 149
as keratomycosis cause, 202
nutritional requirements of, 201
sputum collection and preparation, 28
ubiquity of, 200
Germ tubes
for *Candida* identification, 153, 154, 154f
defined, 228
production of, 41
Gibberella, as keratomycosis cause, 202
Gibberella fujikuroi. See Fusarium moniliform
Gibco/BRL, Inc., 224
Gibson Laboratories, Inc., 223
Giemsa solution, direct staining method, 33, 3
Gilchrist's disease. *See* Blastomycosis
Glabrous, defined, 228
Glaucoma, keratomycosis and, 202
Gliocladium, 13, 13f
conidiophores and conidia, 13f–14f
as keratomycosis cause, 202
Glomerella, as keratomycosis cause, 202
Gomori methenamine-silver nitrate staining, uses for, 35
Grain, aflatoxin in, 177
Gram's method (Hucker modification), staining methods, 34
Granulomatous lesions
in dermatophytoses, 59
facial, *Fusarium* spp. and, 12, 180
in mycetoma, 99
paracoccidioidal. *See* Paracoccidioidomycosis
Greer Laboratories, Inc.
aspergillosis test kit by, 177
serologic test kit available from, 45
Gridley staining, uses for, 35
Groin, ringworm of. *See* Tinea cruris
Guinea pigs, inoculation methods, 47. *See also* Animals
Gym itch. *See* Tinea cruris
Gymnothecia production
defined, 228
laboratory guidelines, 69
Gymnothecium (cleistothecium), 2, 3f

H

Hair
culture media for, 30t
organisms attacking, 66t, 67t
specimen collection and preparation, 28, 68, 69, 70
Hair-bait technique, 41
Hamsters, inoculation methods, 47. *See also* Animals
Hands
blastomycosis on, 129f
mycetoma on, 99
tinea nigra on, 56–57
Hansenula
anomala, opportunistic infections by, 169
as Hemiascomycetes (Ascomycota), 149
Hans Media, inc., 223
Haploid, defined, 228
Haplomycosis. *See* Adiaspiromycosis
HBV-FM (BACTEC high-blood-volume fungal medium), 158
Helminthosporium, 119, 121
Drechslera spp. and, 20
Hemiascomycetes (Ascomycota), 149. *See als* Ascomycota
Hendersonula
as phaeohyphomycosis cause, 118
toruloidea
dermatomycoses and, 96
as phaeohyphomycosis cause, 117t
Scytalidium hyalinum and, 125
Heterobasidiomycetes (Blastomycota), 149
Heterothallic, defined, 228
Hilum, defined, 228
Histidine solution, for Trichophyton agar, 44
Histoplasma, as true pathogenic fungi, 127
Histoplasma capsulatum, 141f, 142f, 143f
Ajellomyces capsulatus and, 141, 144

culture media for, 36, 38, 40
as dimorphic, 128t
laboratory procedures, 100t, 142–145
  animal inoculation, 144
  cultures, 143
  direct examination, 142
  DNA probes, 45–46, 145
  histopathology, 144
  nutritional requirements, 145
  serologic tests, 45, 144–145
  specimen collection and preparation, 28, 142
  specimen types and culture media, 31t
  staining methods, 35
Sepedonium spp. and, 16, 143
var. *capsulatum*, 141, 142, 145
var. *duboisii*, 141, 142, 145
  culture medium for, 38–39
  laboratory examination of, 100t
var. *farciminosum*, 141, 142, 145–146
var. *histoplasmum*, 146
  yeast cells, 142f, 143f
Histoplasmin, skin test for, 144–145
Histoplasmin (asparagine) broth, 39
Histoplasmosis, 141–145
  African, 145–146
  in animals, 142
  described, 141
  etiologic agent, 141, 141f
  film on, 224
  laboratory examination in, 100t
  occurrence of, 141–142
  pulmonary, 141f
  as true pathogenic infection, 127t
Hollister-Stier Laboratories
  aspergillosis test kit by, 177
  serologic test kit by, 45
Holothallic or holoblastic conidia, 1
Homothallic, defined, 228
Hormodendrum. See Cladosporium
Hormonema dematioides, as phaeohyphomycosis cause, 117t
Hot weather ear. See Otomycosis
Hucker crystal violet, in direct staining method, 33, 34
Hyaline, defined, 228
Hyaline hyphomycetes. See Hyphomycetes, hyaline
Hyalohyphomycosis, 10, 178–180
  etiologic agents, 178, 179, 179t
  laboratory procedures, 100t, 178–179
    cultures, 178, 179
    specimen collection, 178
    specimen types and culture medium, 31t
  occurrence of, 178
  as opportunistic infection, 127, 171
Hyphae, 1
  defined, 228
  racquet, 70, 72f
  septate, 1
Hyphomycetes
  dematiaceous, 8, 17–21, 17f–22f
    Alternaria spp., 17–18, 17f–18f
    Aureobasidium (Pullularia) pullulans, 18, 18f
    Cladosporium spp., 18–19, 19f
    Curvularia spp., 19, 19f
    Drechslera spp., 20, 20f
    Epiococcum spp., 20, 20f
    Nigrospora spp., 21, 21f
    opportunistic infections and, 7–8
    Ulocladium spp., 21, 21f–22f
  hyaline (Moniliaceae), 8, 10–17, 10f–17f
    Acremonium (Cephalosporium) spp., 10, 10f
    Anixiopsis (Ahanoascus) spp., 186
    Arthrographis kalrae (Oidiodendron kalrai), 186
    Aspergillus spp., 10–11, 11f
    Botrytis spp., 11, 11f
    Chaetoconidium spp., 186
    Chrysosporium spp., 186
    Coniothyrium fuckelii, 186
    Fusarium spp., 12, 12f
    Geotrichum spp., 12, 13f
    Gliocladium spp., 13, 13f–14f

hyalohyphomycosis and, 171, 178, 179t
Microascus spp., 186
Myriodontium keratinophilum, 186
Neurospora sitophila, 186
Paecilomyces spp., 14, 14f
Penicillium spp., 14, 15f
Phialenonium obovatum, 186
Scopulariopsis spp., 15, 15f–16f
Scytalidium hyalinum, 186
Sepedonium spp., 16, 16f
Thermomyces lanuginosus, 186
Trichoderma spp., 16, 16f–17f
Trichoderma viride, 186
Verticillium spp., 17, 17f
Hyphomycosis destruens. See Pythiosis insidiosi
Hyplohyphomyosis, culture media for, 37
Hypomycetes, imperfect or anamorph states, 66t–68t

I

ID test. See Immunodiffusion test
IFA test. See Indirect fluorescent antibody test
Immune system disorders
  aspergillosis and, 172
  blood specimen collection and preparation, 29
  culture medium for, 38
  Fusarium infection and, 180
  nocardiosis and, 214
  opportunistic infections and
    See also specific types
    mycelial fungal infections, 171
    systemic infections, 127
    yeast infections, 149
  Paecilomyces spp. and, 14
  phaeohyphomycosis and, 118
  saprophytic fungi and, 5
  zygomycosis and, 189
Immunodiffusion (ID) test, 45.
  for actinomycotic mycetoma, 219
  for aspergillosis, 177
  for blastomycosis, 131
  for candidiasis, 157
  for coccidioidomycosis, 139
  fungal reagent sources, 131
  for histoplasmosis, 145
  for nocardiosis, 219
  for paracoccioidomycosis, 135
  for pythiosis insidiosi, 206
  for zygomycosis, 196
Immuno-Mycologics, Inc., 223
  serologic test kits by, 45
    for aspergillosis, 177
    for blastomycosis, 131
    for cryptococcosis, 165
Immunsuppressive drugs
  Chaetoconidium spp. and, 186
  Curvularia spp. and, 19
  opportunistic yeast infections and, 149
  saprophytic fungi and, 5
  Trichosporon infection and, 167–168
  zygomycosis and, 189
Immy test kit, 165
"Imperfect fungi." See Deuteromycota (Fungi Imperfecti)
Imperfect state, defined, 228
Indirect fluorescent antibody (IFA) test
  for Actinomyces spp., 213
  for Cryptococcus neoformans, 165
Ink, laboratory procedures with, 32, 33
Inositol solution, for Trichophyton agar, 44
Insects, Beauveria spp. in, 179
Institut für den Wissenschaftlichen Film, 225
International Biological Laboratories, Crypto-LA test kit by, 165
Intestinal tract, geotrichosis in, 200
Intravenous (IV) infusions, contaminated, Trichoderma spp. and, 16
In vitro antifungal susceptibility tests, 46
Isolator (IS) Centrifugation-Lysis Blood Culture System, 158

J

Jamaica, dermatomycoses in, 96
Jaw, lumpy. See Actinomycosis

Jock itch. See Tinea cruris
Joint aspirates, Candida culture from, 153

K

Kaminskis Teaching Slides on Medical Mycology, 225
Keloid blastomycosis. See Lobomycosis
Keratinomyces ajelloi. See Trichophyton
Keratinomycosis
  Beauveria spp. and, 179
  Fusarium spp. and, 12
  hyalohyphomycosis and, 178
  Penicillium spp. and, 185
Keratinophilic, defined, 228
Keratomycosis (mycotic keratitis), 201–203, 202f
  described, 201–202
  etiologic agents, 118, 202
  Fusarium spp. and, 180
  laboratory procedures, 202–203
  occurrence of, 202
Kerion, Microsporum distortum and, 74
Kidney
  candidasis in, 157f
  nocardiosis in, 214
Kinyoun's stain, procedures, 34–35
Kluyveromyces
  fragilis, Candida kefyr and, 151
  marsianus, as opportunistic infection cause, 169
KOH. See Potassium hydroxide

L

Laboratory exercises, soilborne and airborne fungi, 7
Laboratory procedures, 5–7, 27–49
  See also specific disorders; specific fungi
  animal inoculations, 47–48, 69
  cultivation of fungi, 29–35, 30t–31t
    examination of cultures, 32
    mounting media, stains, and staining methods, 32–35
    culture media, 36–46
  DNA probes, 45–46
  equipment needs, 27
  equipment sources, 224
  handling cautions, 29, 32
  in vitro antifungal susceptibility tests, 46
  mailing of specimens, 29
  regulations and, 27
  serologic techniques, 45
  specimen selection and preparation, 27–29
  stock culture maintenance, 48–49
  visual aids sources, 224–225
Lacrimal canaliculitis, 208
Lactophenol cotton blue (Aman's medium), laboratory procedures with, 33
Lanose, defined, 228
Lasiodiplodia, keratomycosis and, 118, 202
Latex agglutination (LA) test, 45
  for candidiasis, 157
  for cryptococcosis, 165
  for histoplasmosis, 145
Latex particle agglutination (LPA) test, for coccidioidomycosis, 139
L-Dopa medium (Modified Chaskes-Tyndall medium), 40–41
Lecythophora
  hoffmannii, 117t
  mutabilis, 117t
  as phaeohyphomycosis cause, 117t, 118
Legal regulations, laboratory procedures and, 27
Leptosphaeria
  senegalensis
    as eumycetic mycetoma cause, 102
    laboratory examination of, 104
  tompkinsii
    as eumycetic mycetoma cause, 102
    laboratory examination of, 104
Leptothrix (trichomycosis axillaris), 56, 56f
Leucosporidium, as Heterobasidiomycetes (Blastomycota), 149
Leukemia
  aspergillosis and, 171, 172
  Coniothyrium fuckelii and, 186

Penicillium spp. and, 185
Scopulariopsis spp. and, 185
zygomycosis and, 190
Litmus milk medium, 41–42
Liver
  Histoplasma capsulatum in, 142
  nocardiosis in, 214
  Penicillium marneffei in, 203
Liver spots. See Pityriasis versicolor
Loboa laboii, laboratory examination of, 101t
Lobomycosis (Lobo's disease; keloidal blasto-
  mycosis), 99, 114
  described, 114
  laboratory procedures, 28, 101t, 114
  occurrence of, 114
Loeffler methylene blue, in direct staining method, 33
LPA test. See Latex particle agglutination test
Lumpy jaw. See Actinomycosis
Lumpy wool. See Dermatophilosis
Lung lesions
  See also terms beginning with Pulmonary
  Actinomadura spp. and, 214
  Actinomyces israelii and, 208f
  Aspergillus and, 171, 172f
  Beauveria spp. and, 179
  Curvularia spp. and, 19
  Emmonsia parva and, 198
  Geotrichum candidum and, 200
  Nocardia spp. and, 214, 214f, 218f
  Penicillium marneffei and, 203
  Pseudallescheria boydii and, 187, 188
  Rhizomucor pusillus and, 195
  Streptomyces spp. and, 214
Lymph node infections, Penicillium marneffei and, 203
Lyophilization of stock cultures, 48

M

M.A. Bioproducts, serologic test kits by, 45
  for aspergillosis, 177
Macroconidia, 1, 70, 72f, 73, 73f
  defined, 228
Macrophoma, as keratomycosis cause, 202
Madura foot. See Mycetoma
Madurella
  grisea, 104
    as eumycetic mycetoma cause, 102
    laboratory examination of, 101t, 104
  mycetomatis, 104
    as eumycetic mycetoma cause, 102
    laboratory examination of, 104
Maduromycosis. See Mycetoma
Mailing of specimens, 29
Malassezia furfur, 55f
  laboratory procedures, 71t, 167
    culture, 55
    direct examination, 54–55
    mounting procedures, 33, 55
    specimen collection and preparation, 27, 54
  pityriasis versicolor and, 27, 54, 61, 64f
  as systemic infection cause, 167
Malassezia pachydermatis, 54
  laboratory procedures, 55, 167
  as systemic infection cause, 167
Malnutrition, zygomycosis and, 190
Matheson Scientific, 224
Media, 36–46
  dermatophyte study guidelines, 68, 69
  mounting procedures, 32–35
  sources for, 223–224
Meningitis
  Pseudallescheria boydii and, 187
  Rhodotorula spp. and, 22
Meridian Diagnostics, Inc., serologic test kits by, 45, 223
  for aspergillosis, 177
  for cryptococcosis, 165
Merosporangia, defined, 228
Metabolic acidosis, zygomycosis and, 189, 190
Methylene blue, in direct staining method, 33
Mice, inoculation methods, 47–48. See also Animals
Michigan State University Instructional Media Center, teaching slides from, 225
Microascus, 186
  cinereus, 186

desmosporus, 186
Microbiological Associates, 223
Micrococcus, otomycosis and, 51
Microconidia, 1, 70, 72f, 73
  defined, 228
Microdrop Yeast Identification System, 157
Micromonospora, 207
Microscan Division. See Baxter Microscan
Microscan Yeast, 158
Microsporosis nigra. See Tinea nigra
Microsporum, 73–74, 75t, 76–82
  See also Dermatophytes
  amazonicum, 66t
  Arthroderma spp. and, 74, 76, 77–78, 79,
    80, 81
  ascospores produced by, 2, 59
  audouinii, 66t, 74f, 76f
    as chlamydoconidia, 2
    culture medium for, 43
    diseases caused by, 60t
    laboratory examination of, 71t, 74,
      75t, 76
    stock culture maintenance, 48
    tinea capitis and, 61f, 73
    tinea corporis and, 63f
    Wood's lamp and, 73
  boullardii, 66t
  canis, 76, 76f
    Arthroderma otae and, 76
    culture medium for, 43
    diseases caused by, 60t, 76
    films on, 225
    laboratory examination of, 71t, 75t, 76
    laboratory guidelines, 68, 69
    tinea capitis and, 61f, 62f, 73–74
    tinea corporis and, 63f, 73–74
    Wood's lamp and, 73, 73f
  canis var *canis,* animal ringworm and, 60t
  canis var. *distortum,* 66t, 77, 77f
    animal ringworm and, 60t
  cookei, 66t, 74, 75t, 77–78, 77f
    animal ringworm and, 60t
    Arthroderma cajetani and, 77–78
    laboratory guidelines, 69
  as dermatophytes, 59
    in imperfect or anamorph state, 66t
  diseases caused by, 60t. *See also specific*
    species
  distortum
    tinea capitis and, 74
    Wood's lamp and, 73
  ferrugineum, 66t, 78, 78f
    diseases caused by, 60, 74
    nutritional tests for, 87t
    Wood's lamp and, 73
  fulvum (gypseum), 66t, 73, 75t, 79–80
    Arthroderma fulvum and, 80
  gallinae, 66t, 75t, 78–79, 78f
    favus in animals and, 60t, 78
    nutritional tests for, 85, 87t
  gypseum, 59, 66t, 73, 74, 79, 79f
    Arthroderma gypseum and, 79
    Arthroderma incurvatum and, 79
    diseases caused by, 60t, 79
    film on, 225
    hair specimens and, 28
    laboratory examination of, 71t, 75t
    laboratory guidelines, 69
    Scopulariopsis spp. and, 15
    tinea manuum and, 63f
  hair and skin attacked by, 66t
  kerion and, 74
  laboratory identification of, 70, 71t, 73, 74,
    75t
  laboratory procedures, 74. *See also specif-*
    ic species
  nanum, 66t, 73, 74, 75t, 80, 80f
    animal ringworm and, 60t
    Arthroderma obtusa and, 80
  persicolor, 66t, 75t, 80–81
    animal ringworm and, 60t
    Arthroderma persicolor and, 81
  praecox, 66t
  racemosum, 66t
  scalp ringworm and, hair specimen collec-
    tion, 28
  soil-hair culture technique for, 68–69
  vanbreuseghemii, 75t
  vanbreuseghemii, 66t, 74, 81, 81f

animal ringworm and, 60t
  Arthroderma grubyi and, 81
  Trichophyton ajelloi compared to, 81
Mineral oil, maintaining stock cultures in, 48
Mississippi Valley disease. *See* Histoplasmosis
Molds, defined, 1
Moniliaceae. *See* Hyphomycetes, hyaline
Moniliasis, candidosis. *See* Candidiasis
Monilia spp.
  as airborne fungi, 7
  albicans. See Candida albicans
  candida. See Candida tropicalis
  krusei. See Candida krusei
  mortifera. See Candida kefyr
  parakrusei. See Candida parapsilosis
  parapsilosis. See Candida parapsilosis
  pseudotropicalis. See Candida kefyr
Monosporiosis. *See* Pseudallescheriasis
Monosporium apiospermum. See Scedosporium
  apiospermum
Mortierellaceae, characteristics of, 191t
Mortierella, 194f
  as zygomycosis cause, 194
Mouth
  actinomycosis in, 208
  candidiasis in, 151, 151f
  geotrichosis in, 200
Mucocutaneous scrapings, culture medium for,
  30t
Mucor, 8–9, 9f, 190f, 194–195, 194f
  as airborne fungi, 7
  circinelloides, 189, 194
  circinelloides f. *circinelloides,* 194
  circinelloides f. *lusitanicus,* 194
  hiemalis, 195
  indicus, 100t, 195
  in otomycosis, 51, 52
  pusillus, 194f
  ramosissimus, 189, 194–195
  rhizopodiformis. See Rhizopus microsporus
    var. rhizopodiformis
  rouxii. See Mucor indicus
  sporangiophores, 9f
  as Zygomycota, 2, 3
Mucoraceae, characteristics of, 191t
Mucorales, characteristics of, 191t
Mucormycosis. See Zygomycosis
Muriform, defined, 228
Mushroom poisoning, Basidiomycota and, 3
Mycelia, defined, 1, 228
Mycelial fungi, opportunistic infections by,
  171–206
  See also specific infections and etiologic
    agents
  Acremonium infection, 179
  adiaspiromycosis, 198–199
  aspergillosis, 171–178
  basidiomycosis, 199–200
  Beauveria infection, 179–180
  Fusarium infection, 180–184
  geotrichosis, 200–201
  hyalohyphomycosis, 171, 178–180
  Paecilomyces infection, 184
  Penicillium infection, 184–185
    penicilliosis/penicilliosis marneffei,
      203–204
  pseudallescheriasis, 187–189
  pythiosis insidiosi, 204–206
  Scopulariopsis infection, 185–186
  zygomycosis, 189–198
Mycelia sterilia, defined, 228
Mycelium, defined, 1, 228
Mycetoma (maduromycosis), 99, 102–106
  Acremonium (Cephalosporium) spp. as
    cause of, 10
  actinomycotic
    etiologic agents, 102, 214–215
    laboratory examination in, 101t
  in animals, 102
  defined, 99, 102
  etiologic agents, 102, 103–105, 180, 187
  eumycetic
    etiologic agents, 102
    laboratory examination in, 101t
  laboratory procedures, 100t–101t,
    102–103
    culture, 103
    direct examination, 102–103

specimen collection and preparation,
  28, 102
  specimen type and culture media, 30t
  occurrence of, 102
  Pseudallescheria boydii and, 187
Mycetoma pedis, 99, 102f
Mycobacteriaceae, actinomycetes and, 207
Mycobacterium, Actinomycetaceae and, 207
Mycobiotic Agar, 37
Mycogel Labs, Inc., 223
Myco-Immune LA test kit, 165
Mycosel Agar, 37
Mycoses. *See* Cutaneous mycoses;
  Subcutaneous mycoses; Superficial
  mycoses; Systemic mycoses
Mycosis fungoides, on skin, *Malassezia pachy-*
  dermatis and, 54
Mycotic keratomycosis. *See* Keratomycosis
Mycotorula dimorpha; M. trimorpha. See
  Candida tropicalis
Myocentrospora
  acerina, as phaeohyphomycosis cause,
    117t
  as phaeohyphomycosis cause, 118
Myringomycosis. *See* Otomycosis
Myriodontium keratinophilum, 186
Myrothecium, as keratomycosis cause, 202

N

Nail infections
  See also Onychomycosis
  Cladosporium spp. and, 19
  organisms causing, 66t
  ringworm. *See* Tinea unguium
  Scopulariopsis spp. and, 15, 185
  Scytalidium hyalinum and, 186
Nail scrapings
  culture medium for, 30t
  specimen collection and preparation, 28
  for dermatophytes, 70
Nannizzia. See Arthroderma spp.
Neonates, *Malassezia pachydermatis* infection
  in, 54
Neotestudina rosatii, 102, 104
Nephritis, in hyalohyphomycosis, 10
Neurospora sitophila, 186
Nichrome wire needle, use of, 29
Nicotinic acid solution, for Trichophyton agar, 44
Niger (thistle) seed agar (Staib's Medium), 37
Nigrospora, 21, 21f
  conidia and conidiophores, 21f
  sphaerica, as phaeohyphomycosis cause,
    117t, 125
Nitrate assimilation test
  for *Cryptococcus* spp., 164, 164t
  medium for, 42
Nitrate reduction test, for *Actinomyces* spp.,
  210
Nocardia
  acid-fast stain method for, 34–35
  as actinomycete, 207
  animal inoculation and, 218–219
  asteroides, 215, 215f, 216t, 217f, 218f
    as actinomycotic mycetoma cause,
      102, 214, 215
    culture media for, 37, 42
    laboratory identification of, 100t, 215,
      216t
    as nocardiosis cause, 214
    occurrence of, 215
    stain appearance of, 34
  brasiliensis, 217f
    as actinomycotic mycetoma cause,
      102, 214, 215
    laboratory identification of, 34, 101t,
      216t, 217
    as nocardiosis cause, 214
    occurrence of, 215
  caviae, 216t, 217
  culture media for, 37, 40
  histopathology tests for, 218
  physiologic characteristics of, 216t
  serologic tests for, 219
  special tests for, 219
  sputum collection and preparation, 28
Nocardiosis, 214–220
  described, 214
  etiologic agents, 214–215

laboratory procedures, 31t, 100t, 215
  occurrence of, 215
  pulmonary, 214f
  Nodular bodies, 70, 72f
    defined, 228
Nolan-Scott Biological Laboratories, serologic
  test kit available from, 45
Nonseptate, defined, 228
Nose, ulcerated lesion on, *Nigrospora* spp. and
  21

O

Oatmeal tomato-paste agar, 42
  for dermatophyte study, 69
Oidiodendron
  cerealis, 117t, 125
  kalrai. See Arthrographis kalrae
  as phaeohyphomycosis cause, 117t, 118,
    125
Oidium
  albicans. See Candida albicans
  tropicalis. See Candida tropicalis
Onychomycosis
  See also Nail infections; *Tinea unguium*
  Candida, 151f. *See also* Candididiasis
  Fusarium spp. and, 180
  Microascus spp. and, 186
  Schizophyllum commune and, 199
  specimen examination, 71t
Opportunistic fungus infections, 127t
  See also specific infections and etiologic
    agents
  contaminant fungi and, 5
  culture medium for, 38
  mycelial fungi, 171–206
    Acremonium infection, 179
    adiaspiromycosis, 198–199
    aspergillosis, 171–178
    basidiomycosis, 199–200
    Beauveria infection, 179–180
    Fusarium infection, 180–184
    geotrichosis, 200–201
    hyalohyphomycosis, 171, 178–180
    miscellaneous hyaline hyphomycetes
      186
    Paecilomyces infection, 184
    penicilliosis/penicilliosis marneffei,
      203–204
    Penicillium infection, 184–185,
      203–204
    pseudallescheriasis, 187–189
    pythiosis insidiosi, 204–206
    Scopulariopsis infection, 185–186
    zygomycosis, 189–198
  nocardiosis, 214
  yeasts, 149–170
    See also specific types
    Blastoschizomyces capitatus, 169
    Hansenula anomala, 169
    Malassezia infection, 167
    protothecosis, 168–169
    Rhodotorula infection, 168
    Saccharomyces infection, 168
    Sarcinosporon inkin, 169
    trichosporonosis, 167–168
Oral thrush, 151, 151f. *See also* Candidiasis
Organ transplants
  See also Renal transplants
  Acremonium spp. and, 179
  aspergillosis and, 171, 172
  Fusarium infection and, 12, 180
  "opportunistic" saprophytes and, 5
OSHA regulations, for clinical laboratories, 27
Osteomyelitis
  Chrysosporium spp. and, 186
  Fusarium spp. and, 183t
  Pseudallescheria boydii and, 187
Otomycosis (external otitis), 51–52
  specimen types and culture medium, 31t

P

Paecilomyces, 14, 14f, 184
  conidiophores and conidia, 14, 14f
  javanicus, 184
  as keratomycosis cause, 202
  laboratory procedures, 100t, 184
  lilacinus, 100t, 184

marquandii, 184
varioti, 184
viridis, 184
racoccidioides, as true pathogenic fungi, 127
racoccidioides brasiliensis, 133, 134f, 135f
　as dimorphic, 128t
　laboratory procedures, 45, 100t, 134–135
racoccidioidomycosis, 133–135, 134f
　in animals, 133
　described, 133
　etiologic agent, 133
　laboratory examination in, 100t
　occurrence of, 133–134
　specimen types and culture media, 31t
　as true pathogenic infection, 127t
raffin bait technique, 41
ranasal sinus, phaeohyphomycosis of, 118
thogenic fungus infections, 127t
anuts, aflatoxin on, 177
ctinate bodies, 70, 72f
　defined, 228
nicillin, in hair-bait technique, 41
nicilliosis, 203
　Penicilliosis marneffei, 203f
nicillium, 14, 15f, 184–185
　as airborne fungi, 7
　bertai, 185
　bicolor, 185
　chrysogenum, 185
　citrinum, 185
　commune, 185
　conidiophores andd conidia, 15f
　crustaceum, 185
　decumbens, 185
　expansum, 185
　glaucum, 185
　Gliocladium spp. vs., 13
　as keratomycosis cause, 202
　laboratory procedures, 185
　　stock culture maintenance, 48
　marneffei, 14, 100t, 184, 203–204, 204t
　　occurrence of, 184, 203
　　in otomycosis, 51, 52
　　as phialoconidia, 2
　　septate hyphae in, 1
　　spinulosum, 185
rfect state, defined, 228
rianal candidiasis, 151f
riconia, as keratomycosis cause, 202
ridium, 2
riodic acid-Schiff stain, laboratory proce-
　dures with, 33–34, 35
rioral lesions, *Phoma* spp. and, 23
rithecia, defined, 228
ritoneum, *Candida* culture from, 153
ritonitis
　Fusarium moniliforme and, 183t
　in hyaluphomycosis, 171
　Rhodotorula spp. and, 22
　Saccharomyces spp. and, 23
　Trichoderma spp. and, 16
　Trichoderma viride and, 186
tri dish culture, 5
　disadvantages of, 30
　hair-bait technique, 41
triellidiosis. *See* Pseudallescheriasis
etriellidium boydii. *See* Pseudallescheria
　boydii
zer Diagnostics Division, 224
aeltrichoconis, as keratomycosis cause, 202
haeoannellomyces, 124
　chief characteristics of, 116t
　elegans. *See* Exophiala jeanselmei
　werneckii. *See* Exophiala werneckii
aeococcomyces, 124
　chief characteristics of, 116t
haeohyphomycosis, 99, 116–126
　Cladosporium spp. and, 19
　culture media for, 30t, 37
　dematiaceous hyphomycetes and, 7–8,
　116
　etiologic agents, 116t–117t
　clinical groupings of, 118
　laboratory procedures, 100t, 117–118
　　culture, 118
　　direct examination, 117–118
　　specimen collection and preparation,
　　28, 117
　　specimen examination, 71t

specimen type, 30t
Ulocladium spp. and, 21
Pharynx, candidiasis in, 151f
Phialdemmonium obovatum
　as hyalohyphomycosis cause, 186
　as opportunistic pathogen, 186
　as phaeohyphomycosis cause, 117t
Phialides (sterigmata), 2
　Aspergillus, 173
　defined, 228
Phialoconidia, 2
　defined, 228
Phialophora, 124–125
　aquaspersa, chief characteristics of, 109t
　bubakii, 124
　chief characteristics of, 117t
　compacta. See Fonsecaea compacta
　conidia type, 107–108
　dermatitidis. See Exophiala dermatitidis
　jeanselmei. See Exophiala jeanselmei
　keratomycosis and, 118, 202
　parasitica, 124, 125f
　pedrosi. See Fonsecaea pedrosoi
　as phaeohyphomycosis cause, 118, 124
　as phialoconidia, 2
　repens, 124
　richardsiae, 124–125, 125f
　　chief characteristics of, 109t
　verrucosa, 108, 108f, 124, 125
　　chief characteristics of, 109t
　　as chromoblastomycosis cause, 106,
　　125
　　laboratory examination of, 100t, 101t,
　　108
Phoma, 23, 23f
　as airborne fungi, 7
　eupyrena, 117t, 125
　hibernica, 117t, 125
　keratomycosis and, 118
　minutella, 117t, 125
　as phaeohyphomycosis cause, 117t, 118,
　125
　pycnidium and conidia, 23f
Phycomycetes. *See* Zygomycetes
Phycomycosis. *See* Zygomycosis
Phyllosticta, onychomycosis and, 118
Pichia
　farinosa, as opportunistic infection cause,
　169
　guilliermondi, Candida guilliermondii and,
　151
　as Hemiascomycetes (Ascomycota), 149
　kudriavezii, Candida krusei and, 151
Piedra, 52–54, 53f
　specimen collection and preparation, 27,
　53
　specimen examination, 71t
　specimen type and culture medium, 30t
Piedra, black, 52, 53f
　Piedraia hortai and, 27, 52, 118
　specimen examination, 71t
Piedraia hortai, 53f
　black piedra and, 27, 52, 118
　culture results, 53
　laboratory examination, 53, 71t
　specimen selection and preparation, 27
Piedraia quintanilhae, primate piedra and, 52
Piedra, white, 52, 53f
　specimen examination, 71t
　Trichosporon beigelii and, 27
Pityriasis nigra. See Tinea nigra
Pityriasis versicolor, 54–56
　Malassezia furfur and, 27, 54, 61, 64f
　specimen examination, 71t
　specimen type, 30t
Pityrosporum orbiculare. See Malassezia furfur
Plant diseases, *Verticillium* spp. and, 17
Plastic tape, direct staining on, 33
Plectomycetes
　Chaetomium spp., 23–24, 24f
　perfect or telemorph states, 66t–68t
Pleomorphism, defined, 229
Pleospora, as keratomycosis cause, 202
Pneumonitis, *Pseudallescheria boydii* and, 187
Polycytella hominis, as eumycetic mycetoma
　cause, 102
Polysciences, Inc., 224
Poroconidia, 2

Potassium hydroxide (KOH), laboratory proce-
　dures with, 32, 33
Potato dextrose agar, 42
Pour plate-disk media, for yeast identification,
　39
Prosthetic heart valves
　Paecilomyces spp. and, 14
　Penicillium spp. and, 185
　Saccharomyces spp. and, 23
　Thermomyces lanuginosus and, 186
Proteus
　otomycosis and, 51
　vulgaris, laboratory examination of, 101t
Prototheca spp.
　opportunistic infection by, 168–169
　wicherhamii, 169
　zopfi, 169
Prototheocosis (hyaline algae), 168–169
Pseudallescheria
　as keratomycosis cause, 202
　opportunistic infection by, 127
Pseudallescheria boydii, 104–105, 105f
　conidia, 105f
　culture media for, 37
　diseases caused by, 187
　as eumycetic mycetoma cause, 102
　laboratory examination of, 100t, 101t,
　104–105
　Scedosporium apiospermum and, 125
　Scedosporium prolificans and, 187
Pseudallescheriasis, 187–189, 188f
　in animals, 187
　etiologic agents, 187
　hyalohyphomycosis and, 171, 178
　laboratory procedures, 187–188
　occurrence of, 187
Pseudochaetosphaeronema larense, as
　eumycetic mycetoma cause, 102
Pseudohyphae, defined, 1, 229
Pseudomonas
　aeruginosa, laboratory examination of,
　101t
　otomycosis and, 51
Psoriasis, *Malassezia pachydermatis* and, 54
Pubic hairs, trichomycosis axillaris of, 56
Pullularia, as keratomycosis cause, 202
Pullularia pullulans. See Aureobasidium
　(Pullularia) pullulans
Pulmonary blastomycosis, 129f
Pulmonary coccidioidomycosis, 136f
Pulmonary cryptococcosis, 161, 161f
Pulmonary fungus ball, *Trichoderma* spp. and,
　16, 186
Pulmonary histoplasmosis, 141f
Pulmonary lesions. *See* Lung lesions
Pustular lesions
　Candida culture from, 153
　Phoma spp. and, 23
　specimen selection and preparation, 28
Pycnidia, defined, 228
Pyrenochaeta
　onychomycosis and, 118
　romeroi, as eumycetic mycetoma cause,
　102
Pyriform, defined, 229
Pythiosis insidiosi, 204–206, 205f
　described, 204–205
　etiologic agent, 205, 205f
　laboratory procedures, 205–206
　occurrence of, 205
Pythium
　destruens. See Pythium insidiosum
　gracile. See Pythium insidiosum
　insidiosum, 205, 206
　　eye infection caused by, 205f
　　from bone biopsy, 206f
　　as keratomycosis cause, 202

R

Rabbits, inoculation methods, 47
Racquet hyphae, 70, 72f
　defined, 229
Radioimmunoassay (RIA), 45
　for aspergillosis, 177
Ramco Laboratories, Inc., 158, 223
Ramichloridium
　as phaeohyphomycosis cause, 117t, 118
　schulzeri, 117t

Refrigerating stock cultures, 48
Regulations, laboratory procedures and, 27
REMEL, 224, 225
Renal transplants
　See also Organ transplants
　Chaetoconidium spp. and, 186
　Phoma spp. and, 23
Reproduction of fungi, 1–3
　asexual, 1–2
　classification and, 3
　sexual, 2–3
Rhinocerebral zygomycosis, *Mucor* spp. and, 9
Rhinocladiella, 125
　aquaspersa
　　chief characteristics of, 109t
　　as chromoblastomycosis cause, 106
　　chief characteristics of, 117t
　　conidia type, 107
Rhinofacial zygomycosis, Entomophthorales
　and, 195
Rhinosporidiosis, 99, 114–115, 115f
　animal inoculation and, 115
　defined, 114
　etiologic agent, 114
　laboratory procedures, 101t, 115
　　specimen collection and preparation,
　　28, 115
　　specimen type, 30t
　occurrence of, 114–115
Rhinosporidium seeberi, 114
　laboratory procedures, 28, 101t, 115
Rhizoctonia, keratomycosis and, 118, 202
Rhizoids, defined, 229
Rhizomucor pusillus, 195
　laboratory examination of, 100t
　as zygomycosis cause, 189
Rhizopus, 8, 8f, 191–192, 191f
　as airborne fungi, 7
　arrhizus, 189
　aseptate hyhphae in, 1
　microsporus, as zygomycosis cause, 189,
　191
　microsporus var. oligosporum, 189
　microsporus var. rhizopodiformis, 189, 191
　oryzae, 8, 191
　　animal inoculation with, 196
　　laboratory examination of, 100t
　　sporangial production by, 1
　　as zygomycosis cause, 189
　　in otomycosis, 51, 52
　　sphorangiophores, 8f
　　as Zygomycota, 2, 3
Rhodotorula, 22, 22f
　as blastoconidia, 2
　budding cells, 22f
　Cryptococcus spp. vs., 163, 165
　culture medium for, 44
　mucilaginosa. See Rhodotorula rubra
　rubra, opportunistic infection by, 168
RIA. See Radioimmunoassay
Rice grain medium, 43
Riddell slide culture, 6–7, 32
Ringworm, 59, 60t, 61f–65f
　See also terms beginning with Tinea
　in animals
　　laboratory guidelines, 68, 69
　　organisms causing, 60t, 61f
　Microsporum spp. and, 28, 73
Room temperature, maintaining stock cultures
　at, 48
Rothia dentocariosa, 211

S

Sabhi, Inc., 224
Sabouraud-brain-heart-infusion (Sabhi) agar, 38
Sabouraud glucose agar
　Emmons' modification of, 38
　uses for, 30, 30t–31t, 38
　with cycloheximide and chloramphenicol,
　37–38
Saccharomyces, 22–23, 23f
　asci formed by, 2
　budding cells, 23f
　cerevisiae (baker's or brewer's yeast), 22,
　23f, 96
　　fermentation/assimilation patterns,
　　155t
　　opportunistic infection by, 168

as Hemiascomycetes (Ascomycota), 149
krusei. See Candida krusei
neoformans. See Cryptococcus neoformans var. *neoformans*
Rhodotorula spp. and, 22
as systemic infection cause, 168
Safety considerations in laboratory, 29, 32
with *Coccidioides immitis*, 137, 138
Saksenaea vasiformis, 192f
as zygomycosis cause, 189, 192
Sakseneacae, characteristics of, 191t
Saprobe, defined, 229
Saprophytic fungi, 7–24
dermatophytes, imperfect and perfect states, 67t–68t
opportunistic infections and, 5
Sarcinomyces phareomuriformis, as phaeohyphomycosis cause, 117t
Sarcinosporon inkin, opportunistic infections by, 169
Sargent-Welch Co., 224
Scalp ringworm. *See* Tinea capitis
Scedosporiosis. *See* Pseudallescheriasis
Scedosporium, 125, 187
apiospermum, 125, 187, 188
chief characteristics of, 117t
prolificans, 188, 188f
Pseudallescheria boydii and, 187
Schiff reagent, laboratory procedures with, 33–34
Schizomycota, 24, 24f, 207
Schizophyllum commune, 199, 199f
Scientific Products, 224
Scopulariopsis, 15, 15f–16f, 185–186
acremonium, 185
as annelloconidia, 2
brevicaulis, 185
dermatomycoses and, 96
laboratory examination of, 71t
brumptii, 185
condiophores and conidia, 15f–16f
fusca, 185
as keratomycosis cause, 202
koningii, 185
laboratory examination of, 71t, 185
occurrence of, 185
Scutulum, defined, 229
Scytalidium, 125, 186
chief characteristics of, 117t
cutaneous dematiaceous infections and, 118
hyalinum, 125, 186
dermatomycoses and, 96
as hyalohyphomycosis cause, 186
lignicola, 125
as phaeohyphomycosis cause, 118, 125, 186
Sepedonium, 16, 16f
conidia, 16f
Septa, defined, 229
Septate hyphae, 1
defined, 229
Septic arthritis, *Fusarium* spp. and, 183t
Septicemia
blood specimen collection and preparation, 29
from contaminated IV infusions, *Trichoderma* spp. and, 16
Septum, defined, 229
Serodirect Eiken Cryptococcus test kit, 165
Serologic techniques, 45. *See also specific fungi; specific tests*
Serologic test kits, sources for, 223
Serum, for germ tubes, 41
Sessile, defined, 229
Sexual reproduction, 2–3
classification and, 3
Silkworms, *Beauveria* spp. in, 179
Sinus infections
actinomycosis, 207
nocardiosis, 214
specimen selection and preparation, 28
Sinusitis
Myriodontium keratinophilum and, 186
paranasal, *Curvularia* spp. and, 19
Pseudallescheria boydii and, 187
Skin infections
Anixiopsis spp. and, 186
candidiasis, 151, 151f

Cladosporium spp. and, 19
dermatophilosis, 220–221
Fusarium oxysporum and, 183t
geotrichosis, 200
Mucor spp. and, 9
organisms causing, 60–61, 66t. *See also specific types of organisms*
Penicillium marneffei and, 203
Scytalidium hyalinum and, 186
Skin scrapings
culture media for, 30t
direct staining methods with, 33–34
specimen collection and preparation, 28, 33, 70
Skin testing
for coccidioidomycosis, 139
for histoplasmosis, 144–145
for paracoccidioidomycosis, 135
Slide culture techniques, 6–7, 6f, 32
Smith's systemic fungal medium, 38
Software program, 225
Soil extract agar, 43
Soil fungi, 5
Acremonium spp., 179
Anixiopsis spp., 186
Beauveria spp., 179
Blastomyces dermatitidis, 129
culture media for, 41
dermatomycoses and, 96
Exophiala werneckii, 57
Histoplasma capsulatum, 142
as hyalohyphomycosis cause, 171
isolation of with mice, 47–48
laboratory exercise, 7
laboratory guidelines, 68–69
mycetoma and, 102
Paracoccidioides brasiliensis, 134
as phaeohyphomycosis cause, 117, 118
Pseudallescheria boydii, 187
zygomytosis and, 189–190
Soil-hair culture technique, for dermatophyte study, 68–69
South Central Association for Clinical Microbiology, teaching slides from, 225
Specimen handling. *See* Laboratory procedures
Sphaeropsis, as keratomycosis cause, 202
Spiral coils or cords, 70, 72f
Spiral hypha, defined, 229
Sporangiophores, 8f
in asexual reproduction, 1
defined, 229
Sporangiospores, 9f
in asexual reproduction, 1
defined, 229
Sporangium
in asexual reproduction, 1
defined, 229
Spores, defined, 229
Sporobolomyces, as opportunistic infection cause, 169
Sporogenous (conidiogenous) cells, 1
Sporophores, defined, 229
Sporothrix schenckii, 111f, 112f
as dimorphic, 128
laboratory identification of, 100t, 111–113
Sporotrichosis, 99, 110–114, 111f, 112f
defined, 110–111
etiologic agent, 111, 128
laboratory procedures, 100t, 111–113
animal inoculation, 99, 113
culture, 111–112
histopathologic studies, 112
serologic studies, 112–113
special nutritional requirements, 112
specimen collection and preparation, 28, 111
specimen type and culture medium, 30t
occurrence of, 111
Sputum
Candida culture from, 153
Geotrichum in, 200, 200f
specimen mailing procedures, 29
specimen selection and preparation, 28
Staib's Medium. *See* Niger (thistle) seed agar
Staphylococcus
aureus, laboratory examination of, 101t
otomycosis and, 51, 52

Starch hydrolysis test
for *Actinomyces* spp., 210
medium for, 43
Starvation, zygomycosis and, 189
Stemphyllium, Alternaria spp. and, 17
Stenella araguata, tinea nigra and, 118
Sterigmata. *See* Phialides
Sterile distilled water, maintaining stock cultures in, 48
Steroids. *See* Corticosteroids
Stock culture maintenance, 48–49
Stolon, defined, 229
Strawberry foot rot. *See* Dermatophilosis
Streptococcus
otomycosis and, 51
pyogenes, laboratory examination of, 101t
Streptomyces, 24, 24f
as actinomycete, 207
as actinomycotic mycetoma cause, 102, 214, 215
as airborne fungi, 7
hyphae, conidiophores, and conidia, 24f
laboratory identification of, 216t, 218
paraguayensis, 215
somaliensis, 102, 214, 215, 216t, 218
Streptomycin, in hair-bait technique, 41
Streptotrichosis. *See* Dermatophilosis
Subcutaneous granuloma, *Fusarium* spp. and, 183t
Subcutaneous granulomata, *Pseudallescheria boydii* and, 187
Subcutaneous mycoses, 99–126
See also specific infections
chromoblastomycosis, 106–110
etiologic agents, 100t, 101t
laboratory procedures, 99, 100t–101t
specimen selection and preparation, 28
specimen type and culture medium, 30t
lobomycosis, 114
mycetoma, 99, 102–106
phaeohyphomycosis, 116–25
rhinosporidiosis, 114–115
Scopulariopsis spp. and, 15
sporotrichosis, 110–114
Sucrose-yeast extract agar, 43
Sugar assimilation tests. *See* Carbohydrate fermentation/assimilation tests
Superficial mycoses, 51–57
See also specific infections
etiologic agents of, 118
films on, 224
otomycosis, 51–52
piedra, 52–54
pityriasis versicolor, 54–56
specimen collection and preparation, 27
specimen type and culture medium, 30t
tinea nigra, 56–57
trichomycosis axillaris, 56
Swamp cancer. *See* Pythiosis insidiosi
Syncephalastraceae, characteristics of, 191t
Syncephalastrum, 9, 9f, 195, 195f
merosporangia, 8f, 9f, 195f
racemosum, 189, 195
Synonym, defined, 229
Systemic mycoses, 127–147
See also specific etiologic agents; specific infections
blastomycosis, 128–133, 129f
dimorphic fungi and, 128, 128t
etiologic agents
opportunistic fungi, 127
phaeohyphomycosis, 118
true pathogens, 127
film on, 224
opportunistic fungus infections, 127t
phaeohyphomycosis, etiologic agents, 118
specimen selection and preparation, 28–29
specimen type and culture medium, 30t–31t
true pathogenic fungus infections, 127t, 128

as phaeohyphomycosis cause, 117t, 118
stilbospora, 117t
TA test. *See* Tube agglutination (TA) test
Teaching aids, 224–225
Teleomorph, defined, 229
Terminal illness, *Rhodotorula* spp. and, 22
Test tube culture, 5
cultivation procedures, 29–35, 30t–31t
Tetraploa
arilstata, as phaeohyphomycosis cause, 117t
keratomycosis and, 118, 202
Thalassemia, pythiosis insidiosi and, 204–20
Thallic conidiogenesis, 1
Thallus, defined, 229
Thermomyces lanuginosus, 186
Thiamine solution, for Trichophyton agar, 44
Thioglycollate medium, 43
Thistle seed agar. *See* Niger (thistle) seed aga
Thomas, Arthur H. Co., 224
Thrush, 151, 151f. *See also* Candidiasis
Thyroid abscess, *Pseudallescheria boydii* and 187
Tinea, defined, 229
Tinea barbae (ringworm of the beard)
organisms causing, 60t, 64f, 73
Tinea capitis, 59, 60t, 61f–62f
hair specimen procedure, 28, 70
Microsporum spp. and, 28, 62f, 73, 73f
organisms causing, 60t, 62f. *See also specific organisms*
specimen examination, 71t
specimen type and culture media, 30t
Trichophyton spp. and, 62f
Tinea corporis (ringworm of the body), 65f
organisms causing, 60t, 63f, 73–74
specimen examination, 71t
specimen type and culture media, 30t
Tinea cruris (jock itch, gym itch, ringworm of the groin), 60t, 65f
organisms causing, 60t, 61
Tinea favosa, 60t
Tinea imbricata, *Trichophyton concentricum* and, 60t, 63f
Tinea manuum, organisms causing, 61, 63f, 6
Tinea nigra, 56–57
Cladosporium werneckii and, 64f
Exophiala werneckii and, 27, 57
laboratory procedures, 30t, 57
organisms causing, 61, 64f
specimen type and culture medium, 30t
Tinea nodosa. *See* Piedra
Tinea pedis (athlete's foot, ringworm of the feet), 59, 60t, 65f
organisms causing, 60t, 61
Tinea unguium (onychomycosis, ringworm of the nail), 60t, 65f
organisms causing, 60t, 61
specimen examination, 71t
specimen type and culture medium, 30t
Tinea versicolor. *See* Pityriasis versicolor
Tissue biopsy
Candida culture from, 153
specimen selection and preparation, 29
Tissue sections, direct staining methods with 34
Torula
histolytica. See Cryptococcus neoforman var. *neoformans*
neoformans. See Cryptococcus neoformans var. *neoformans*
Torulopsis
as Blastomycetes, 149
glabrata, 160–161, 160f
fermentation/assimilation patterns, 155t
laboratory examination of, 100t
ubiquity of, 149
haemulonii, 160, 161
Torulopsosis, 160–161
etiologic agents, 160
laboratory procedures, 100t, 160–161
Toruloisis. *See* Cryptococcosis
TP test. *See* Tube precipitin (TP) test
Trauma
Fusarium infection and, 12, 180
keratomycosis and, 200–201
zygomycosis and, 189
Triarch, Inc., 223

T

Taeniolella
dematiaceous dermatomycosis and, 118

ichoderma, 16, 16f–17f
  as airborne fungi, 7
  conidiophores and conidia, 16f–17f
  viride, 186
ichomycosis axillaris (trichomycosis nodosa),
  56, 56f
chophyton, 84–94
  See also Dermatophytes
  ajelloi, 59, 67t, 84, 92–93, 92f
    Arthroderma uncinatum and, 85, 93
    laboratory guidelines, 69
    Microsporum vanbreuseghemii com-
      pared to, 81
    as soilborne, 85, 92
  Arthroderma spp. and, 74, 85, 87, 89, 92,
    93, 94
  characteristics of, 84
  concentricum, 67t, 85, 91, 91f
    nutritional tests for, 87t
    tinea imbricata and, 60t, 63f, 91
  as dermatophytes, 59
  diseases caused by, 60t
    ecothrix-type hair infections, 84–85
    endothrix-type hair infections, 85
  etiologic agents, 84–85
  ferrugineum. See Microsporum ferrug-
    ineum
  flavescens, 67t
  gallinae. See Microsporum gallinae
  georgiae, 68t, 91–92
    Arthroderma ciferrii and, 85, 92
    as soilborne, 85, 91
  gloriae, 68t, 84, 93
    Arthroderma gloriae and, 85
    as soilborne, 85, 93
  gourvillii, 67t, 93, 93f
    endothrix-type hair infection by, 85
  hair, skin, and nails attacked by, 66t–67t
  as imperfect or anamorph states, 66t–68t
  as keratomycosis cause, 202
  laboratory procedures, 70, 71t, 72f, 73,
    73f, 75t, 84, 85
    culture media, 38, 40, 42, 43–44
    hair specimens, 28
    nutritional tests, 85
    soil-hair culture technique, 68–69
    stock culture maintenance, 48
  longifusum, 84
  megninii, 67t, 75t, 89, 89f
    diseases caused by, 60t, 89
    ecothrix-type hair infection by, 84
    nutritional tests for, 85, 87t
  mentagrophytes, 59, 67t, 85–87, 86f
    animal infections by, 86
    Arthroderma benhamiae and, 87
    Arthroderma vanbreuseghemii and, 87
    culture media for, 40, 42, 44
    diseases caused by, 60t, 85–86
    ecothrix-type hair infection by, 84
    laboratory examination of, 71t, 75t, 86
    microconidia, 72f, 86f
    Microsporum persicolor and, 80
    nutritional tests for, 85, 87t
    tinea barbae and, 64f
    tinea capitis and, 62f
    tinea manuum and, 64f
    T. rubrum vs., 86, 88
    var. *erinacei,* 86, 86f
    var. *interdigitale,* 86
    var. *quinckeanum,* 86
  rubrum, 67t, 88, 88f
    animal infections by, 88
    culture media for, 40, 42, 44
    diseases caused by, 60t, 61, 88
    ecothrix-type hair infection by, 84
    laboratory examination of, 71t, 75t, 86
    macroconidia, 73f, 88f
    nutritional tests for, 87t
    tinea corporis and, 63t
    tinea manuum and, 64f
    T. mentagrophytes vs., 86, 88
  schoenleinii, 67t, 90–91, 90f
    endothrix-type hair infection by, 85

laboratory examination of, 71t, 75t,
    85, 90–91, 91f
  nutritional tests for, 85, 87t
  tinea capitis and, 62f
  tinea unguium and, 60t
  simii, 67t, 89–90
    Arthroderma simii and, 89
    endothrix-type hair infection by, 85
    favus in animals and, 60t
  soudanense, 67t, 85, 93, 93f
  terrestre, 59, 68t, 92, 92f
    Arthroderma insingulare and, 92
    Arthroderma lenticularum and, 92
    Arthroderma quadrifidum and, 85, 92
    conidia, 73f, 92f
    laboratory guidelines, 69
    as soilborne, 85, 92
  tonsurans, 67t, 90, 90f
    diseases caused by, 90
    endothrix-type hair infection by, 85
    laboratory examination of, 71t, 75t, 90
    microconidia, 73f, 90f
    nutritional tests for, 85, 87t
    tinea capitis and, 62f
    tinea corporis and, 63f
    tinea unguium and, 60t
  vanbreuseghemii, 68t, 94
    Arthroderma gertleri and, 85, 94
    as soilborne, 85, 94
  verrucosum, 67t, 75t, 88–89, 89f
    animal infections by, 88
    diseases caused by, 60t, 61, 88
    ecothrix-type hair infection by, 84–85
    laboratory examination of, 85, 88–89
    nutritional tests for, 85, 87t
  violaceum, 67t, 90f, 91, 91f
    diseases caused by, 60t, 91
    endothrix-type hair infection by, 85,
      90f
    laboratory examination of, 75t, 85, 91
    nutritional tests for, 87t
    tinea capitis and, 62f
  yaoundei, 67t, 85, 93–94
Trichophyton agars, 43–44
Trichosporon
  beigelii, 53f
    biochemical test results, 54
    culture media for, 37
    fermentation/assimilation patterns,
      155t
    Geotrichum candidum and, 200
    laboratory examination of, 53, 71t
    specimen collection and preparation,
      27
    as systemic infection cause, 167–168
    white piedra and, 27, 52
  capitatum, 96
  cutaneum. See Trichosporon beigelii
  inkin. See Sarcinosporon inkin
  pullulans, *Cryptococcus* spp. vs., 163
  ubiquity of, 149
Trichosporonosis, 167–168
Tritirachium, as keratomycosis cause, 202
Trypan blue, laboratory procedures with, 33
Tube agglutination (TA) test, 45
  for cryptococcosis, 165
Tube precipitin (TP) test, for coccidioidomyco-
  sis, 139
Tuberculosis, aspergillosis and, 172
Turtox, 223, 224
Tyrosine agar, 45

U

Ulcerated lesions, *Nigrospora* spp. and, 21
Ulocladiuim, 21, 21f–22f
  chartarum, 117t
  conidiophore and conidia, 22f
  as phaeohyphomycosis cause, 117t, 118
Uni-Yeast-Tek System, 158, 164, 225
Urea medium, 44
Urease test, for *Cryptococcus* spp., 163, 164t
Urease test medium, 44
Urinary tract disorders
  Fusarium spp. and, 183t
  Penicillium spp. and, 185
Urine
  Candida culture from, 153
  medically significant yeasts in, 149

specimen mailing procedures, 29
Urogenital tract (female), *Candida albicans* in,
  149
Ustilago spp.
  basidiomycosis and, 199
  as keratomycosis cause, 202

V

V-8 juice agar, 44–45
Vagina
  candidiasis in, 151, 151f
  geotrichosis in, 200
  Vaginal scrapings, culture medium for, 30t
Vegetation, decaying, fungi in, 5
Ventriculitis, *Rhodotorula* spp. and, 22
Verrucose, defined, 229
Verticillate, defined, 229
Verticillium, 17, 17f
  conidiophores, 17f
Vesicle, defined, 229
Vinyl plastic tape, direct staining on, 33
Visual aids, sources for, 224–225
Vitek Systems, 156, 225
Volutella, as keratomycosis cause, 202
Vulvovaginitis, mycotic. *See* Candidiasis

W

Wampole Laboratories, 158, 223
Wangiella, 125
  chief characteristics of, 117t
  dermatitidis. See Exophiala dermatitidis
Warlock Productions, software program for, 225
Weitzman's culture medium, for dermatophyte
  studdy, 69
White piedra, 52, 53f
  specimen examination, 71t
  Trichosporon beigelii and, 27

X

Xanthine agar, 45
Xylohypha bantiana (synonym), chief character-
  istics. *See Cladosporium trichoides*
Xylohypha emmonsii (synonym). *See*
  Cladosporium bantianum.

Y

Yeast extract phosphate medium, 38
Yeasts; Yeastlike fungi
  See also specific species; specific types
  baker's. *See Saccharomyces cerevisiae*
  Blastomycetes (Deuteromycota or Fungi
    Imperfecti), 149
  culture media for, 30t–31t, 42
  defined, 1
  identification of, 149, 150t
    media and kits for, 225
  in normal environment, 149
  opportunistic infections by, 149–170
    Blastoschizomyces capitatus, 169
    candidiasis, 151–160
    cryptococcosis, 161–167
    Hansenula anomala, 169
    incidence of, 149
    Malassezia infections, 167
    protothecosis, 168–169
    Rhodotorula infections, 168
    Saccharomyces infections, 168
    Sarcinosporon inkin, 169
    torulopsosis, 160–161
    trichosporonosis, 167–168
  Rhodotorula spp., 22, 22f
  sexual reproduction and types of, 149
  specimen types, 30t–31t
  stock culture maintenance, 48

Z

Zoophilic, defined, 229
Zoospore, defined, 229
Zygomycetes (Phycomycetes), 8–9, 8f–10f. *See*
  also specific species
Zygomycosis (mucormycosis), 189–198, 190f
  in animals, 190
  classification, 190–191
  described, 189

etiologic agents, 189
laboratory procedures, 100t, 190–196
  animal inoculation, 196
  culture, 190
  direct examination, 190
  histopathology, 196
  serologic tests, 196
  specimen collection, 190
  specimen types and culture medium,
    31t
Mucor spp. and, 9
occurrence of, 189Sauvignon 190
as opportunistic infection, 127t
Rhizopus spp. and, 8
Zygomycota, 3
Zygospores, 2, 2f, 3
  defined, 229